Curandero Conversations

El Niño Fidencio, Shamanism and
Healing Traditions of the Borderlands

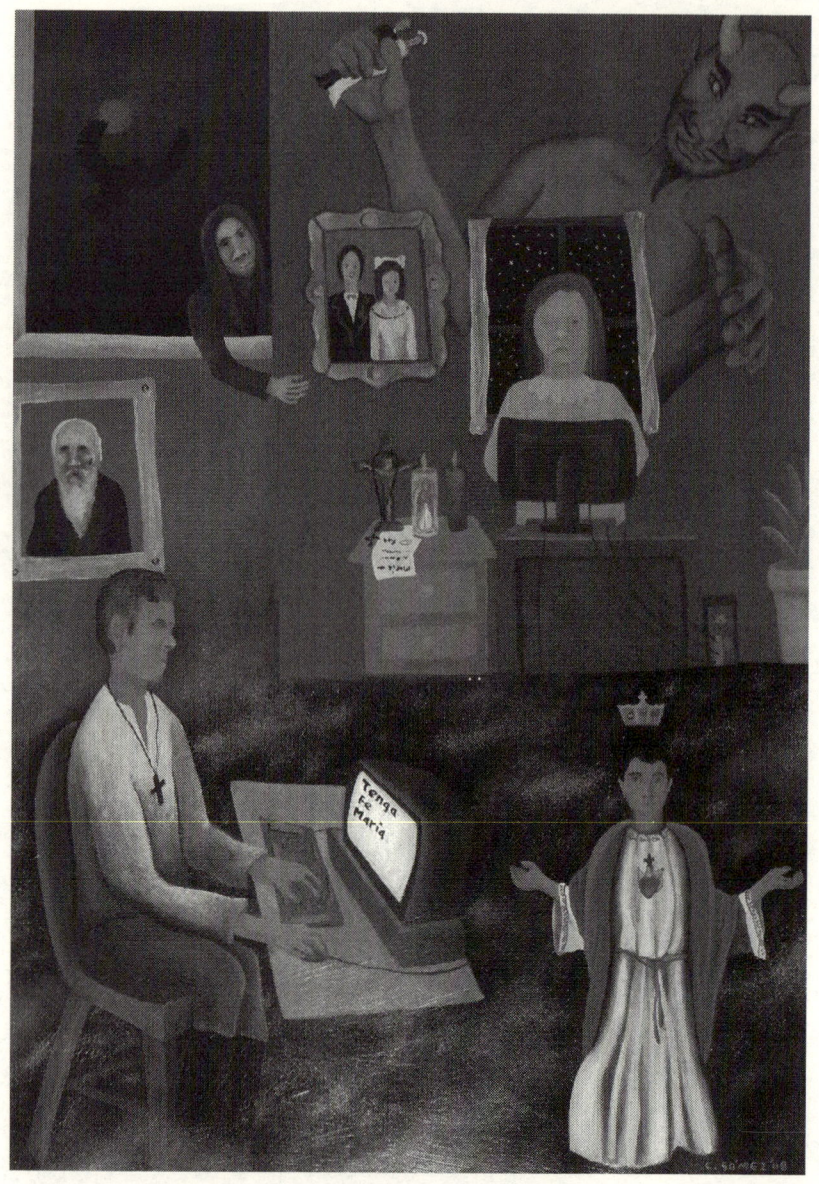

"*Tenga Fe María*" - "Have Faith Maria"
Artist Carlos G. Gómez

Curandero Conversations

El Niño Fidencio, Shamanism and Healing Traditions of the Borderlands

Antonio Zavaleta

and

Alberto Salinas Jr.

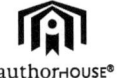

The University of Texas at Brownsville
And Texas Southmost College

AuthorHouse™
1663 Liberty Drive
Bloomington, IN 47403
www.authorhouse.com
Phone: 1-800-839-8640

©2009 Antonio Zavaleta and Alberto Salinas Jr. All rights reserved.

No part of this book may be reproduced, stored in a retrieval system, or transmitted by any means without the written permission of the author.

First published by AuthorHouse 8/26/2009

ISBN: 978-1-4490-0087-5 (e)
ISBN: 978-1-4490-0088-2 (sc)
ISBN: 978-1-4490-0089-9 (hc)

Library of Congress Control Number: 2009906889

Includes bibliographical references and index
1. Curandero-Curanderismo
2. El Niño Fidencio-Shamanism
3. U.S.-Mexico Border Health
4. Folk Medicine and Healing Traditions
5. Cultural Competencies in Latino Health Care
6. Border Herbal

Printed in the United States of America
Bloomington, Indiana

This book is printed on acid-free paper.

Artist and Cover Art

The cover art for *Curandero Conversations* is by artist Carlos G. Gómez. Born in Mexico City, Carlos found his first artistic expression in the Tex–Mex culture of the Rio Grande Valley in Brownsville where he was raised. "Brightly colored buildings and the surreal atmosphere of the Mexican border towns gave me the first appreciation of color, line, and the generalization that my chosen images would have to be bold and realistic," explains Gómez. Currently, he is a professor of fine art at The University of Texas at Brownsville and Texas Southmost College where he teaches a wide range of classes in painting and drawing.

The cover art by Carlos G. Gómez is an original painting commissioned for *Curandero Conversations,* entitled, *Tenga Fe María,* (Oil on Printers Vellum, 24" x 18," 2008). This marvelous painting depicts, in traditional ex-voto style, the story of a life's struggle in art. María, the petitioner, sits at her computer corresponding with the *curandero* via the Internet. Protected by her home altar and patron saints, she is attacked by a witch at the window who has sent the devil to destroy her marriage. Presumably, the witch has been hired by María's husband's lover. The *curandero* is surrounded by his patron folk saints Don Pedrito Jaramillo and El Niño Fidencio as he works. He responds to her e-mail, consoling her via the Internet, to have faith, and all will be resolved.

Dedication

This book is dedicated to all the *curanderos* and *curanderas* whose names will never be known, but who have dedicated their lives for the benefit of their communities and to those people who share their personal stories in this book and to all who will read, learn and benefit from their collective cultural knowledge.

José Fidencio Síntora Constantino
El Niño Fidencio
Mexico's greatest *curandero*
November 13, 1898 – October 19, 1938

An Important Message For Our Readers

Curandero Conversations: El Niño Fidencio, Shamanism and Healing Traditions of the Borderlands, is not intended to serve as medical advice and is only for informational and educational purposes. Do not use the plants, remedies, practices or information from the resource links described in this book for medical purposes. Please immediately contact a health-care professional about any condition that requires a diagnosis or medical attention. The numerous resource links referenced in this book are provided as an example of additional information which exist on the Internet but their content is not endorsed by the authors nor the publishers and this disclaimer applies to all material referenced on those websites. Always consult a medical doctor first before considering or using any complementary or alternative health care material. The authors and The University of Texas at Brownsville and Texas Southmost College and Authorhouse disclaim any liability arising directly or indirectly from the use of any of the plants or remedies or practices listed in this book.

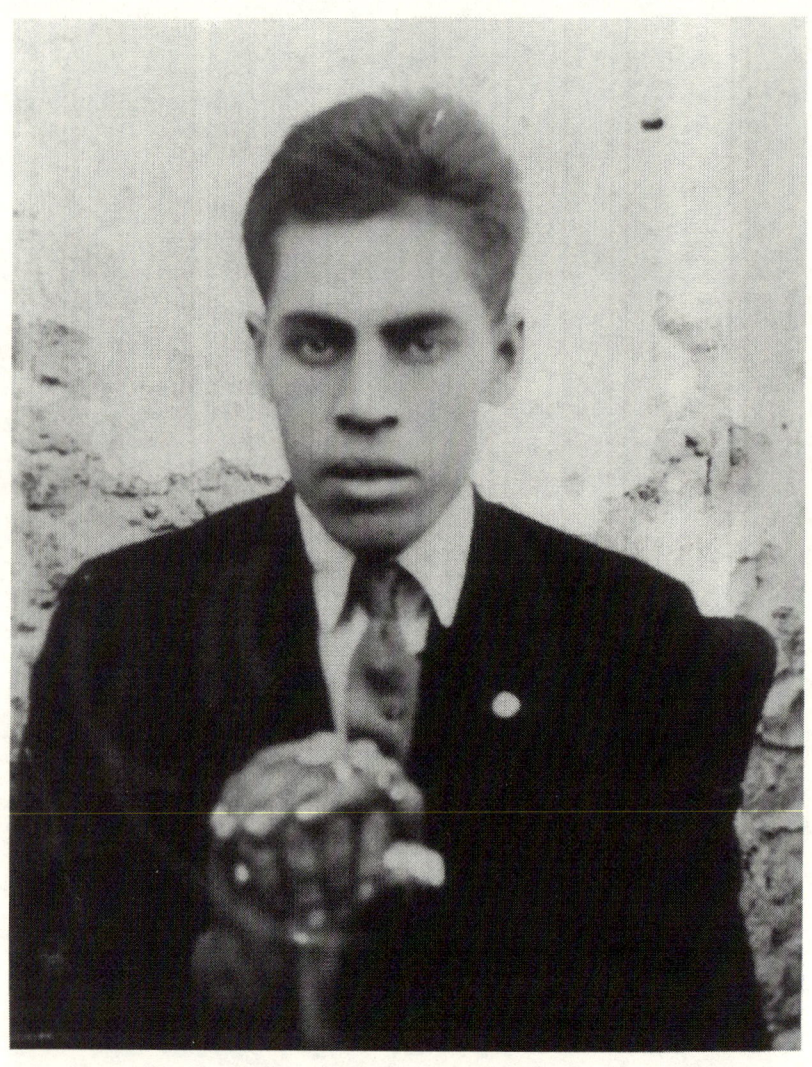

This is a photograph of El Niño Fidencio dressed as the people's lawyer and taken in Espinazo, Nuevo León, México around 1928. (Photo from Zavaleta collection)

Acknowledgments

The authors acknowledge the support of Dr. Juliet V. García, President, and Dr. José G. Martín, Provost Emeritus, of The University of Texas at Brownsville and Texas Southmost College for their unfailing support of the preservation of U.S.-Mexico border history and culture.

We thank our families who have supported and encouraged us throughout the time we have worked on this book, especially our wives, Lydia Posas-Salinas and Gabriela Sosa-Zavaleta and son Michael Anthony Zavaleta.

The gift of time cannot ever be fully repaid. We acknowledge the leadership of the Fidencista movement for 25 years of support and especially those who have gone before us: †Ciprianita "Panita" Zapata de Robles and †Manuel Robles. We especially thank María Tamayo, †Josefa Contreras and †Don Perfecto Rodríguez for their faith and support over a 40-year journey in the study of *curanderismo*.

We thank all of the faithful followers of the Fidencista movement we have encountered over the last 25 years. For their kind thoughts about our book we thank: Dr. Philip Kendall; Michael Van Wagenen; Oscar Casares; Bill Minutaglio; Dr. Joseph Spielberg and Dr. Miguel Alemán. We acknowledge and thank all of those who labored on the production of this book including: Ms. Yolanda Zamarripa, research analyst; Ms. Jamie Sams, author; Jefferson Cortinas-Walker, text editor (English/Spanish); Sra. Carmelita Ramos, translation expert; Ms. Rachel E. Barrera, doctoral student; †José M. Duarte, loyal friend and photographer; Carlos Gómez, artist; Ms. Camilla Montoya, design consultant; Dr. Suzanne Simon, anthropologist; Ms. Jacqueline Cooke, research assistant; Martha P. Espinoza, administrative assistant; Milton C. Rodríguez, technical assistant; Juan Miguel González, photographer. A special acknowledgement is given to anthropology professors Robert M. Malina and †Don Américo Paredes, and to all my professors at the University of Texas at Austin, Department of Anthropology.

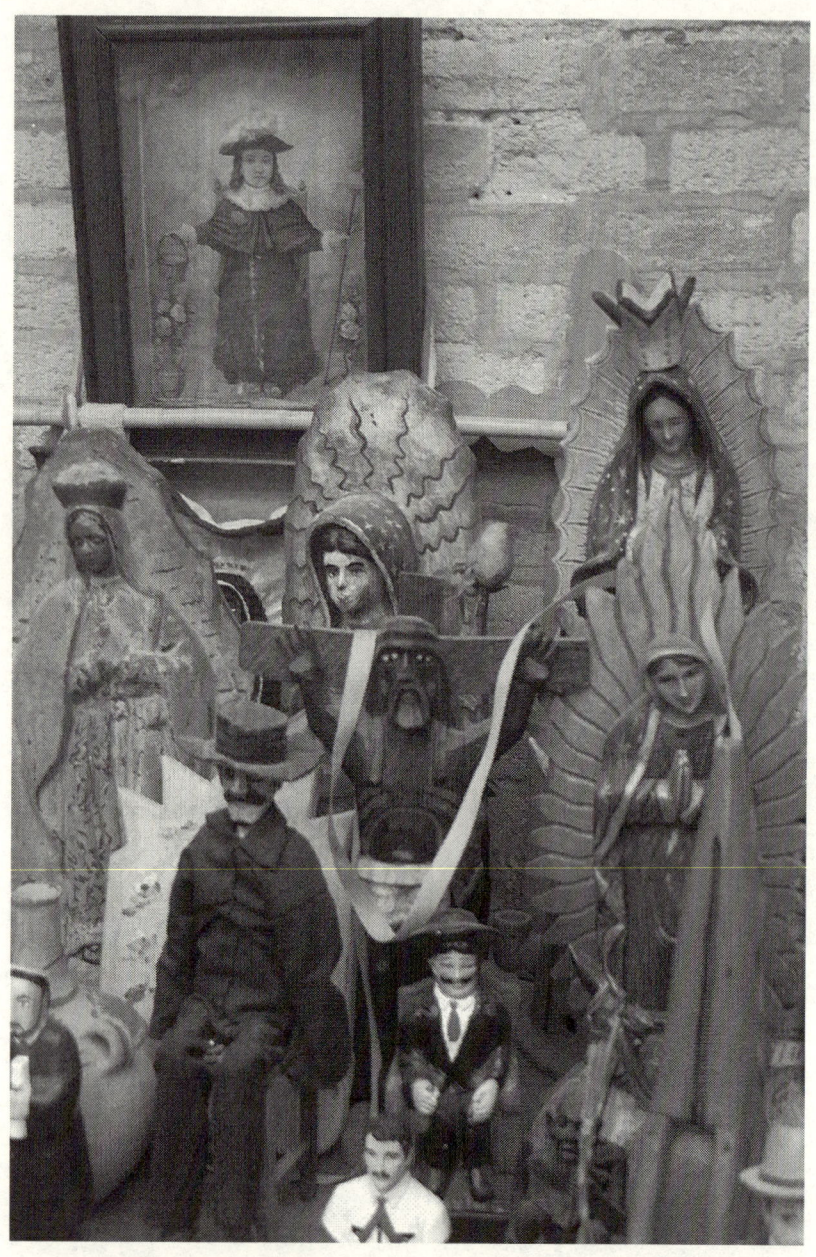

A typical home altar displaying patron saints and offerings.
(Photo by Zavaleta)

Table of Contents

Artist and Cover Art v

Dedication vi

An Important Message For Our Readers vii

Acknowledgments ix

Introduction by Jamie Sams xix

Part 1. A Testimonial 1

Part 2. Healing the Spirit: Life as a Spiritual Journey 11

1. The Life of El Niño Fidencio   *Vida del Niño Fidencio* 12
2. Niño's Spiritual Helpers   *Guardias* 15
3. Bracero Campfire Tale   *Cuentos de mi Abuelito* 18
4. Niño Fidencio's Blessing   *Una Bendición* 20
5. Searching for El Niño Fidencio   *Buscando al Niño* 22
6. Answered Prayer   *Oración Contestada* 23
7. Native Americans   *Indios Americanos* 25
8. We Believe in El Niño Fidencio   *Creemos en el Niño Fidencio* 26
9. Healing Mission   *Misión de Curación* 28
10. El Niño on the Internet   *La Red Espiritual* 30
11. El Niño's Helpers   *Sus Ayudantes* 31
12. Waiting for a Blessing   *Esperando su Bendición* 33

Part 3. Curanderismo: The Healing Arts and Sciences 37

13. The Specialists   *Los Especialistas* 37
14. The Folk Pharmacy   *Hierbería-Botánica* 43
15. Spirits and Folk Saints   *Santos Populares* 47
16. Liturgical Holy Days   *El Santoral* 48
17. The Folk Psychiatrist   *Cura Mentes* 52
18. Home Remedies   *Remedios Caseros* 54

19.	Faith and Folk-healers	*Don de Curar*...................56
20.	Mistrust of Curanderos	*Desconfianza*.....................57
21.	Fake Curanderos	*Charlatánes*......................59
22.	Santería	*Creencias Afro-Caribeñas* 60
23.	Card Reader	*La Baraja Española* 62
24.	Incantations and Rituals	*Encantos y Rituales*............. 64
25.	Amulets and Talismans	*El Libro del Rey Salomón*.........66
26.	Dancing with the Devil	*Bailando con el Diablo* 67
27.	The Pastorela and Posada	*Fiestas Navideñas* 70
28.	Ex-Votos	*Milagros Pintados*..................72
29.	The Home Altar	*El Altar Familiar*...................74
30.	Promise and Pilgrimage	*Promesa y Peregrinación* 76

Part 4. Curanderismo: Healing the Body's Aches and Pains 81

31.	Colds and Flu	*La Gripa y Resfriados* 81
32.	Fallen Fontanel	*Mollera Caída*......................84
33.	The Midwife	*La Partera*.........................85
34.	Stomachaches	*Empacho, Cólico, y Latido* 87
35.	Back Problem Poultice	*El Parche Guadalupano*............90
36.	Earache Funnel	*El Cucurucho* 91
37.	Caring for Father	*Cuidando Papá*.....................93
38.	Grandmother's Rheumatism	*Las Reumas*........................95
39.	Please Help My Little Son	*Ayuda mi Pequeño* 97
40.	Like Other Children	*Como otros Niños* 98
41.	Angry Little Boy	*Enmuinado y Encorajinado*.....100
42.	Pray for Us	*Reza por Nosotros* 101
43.	Very Sick Little Girl	*La Enfermita*...................... 102
44.	Pregnancy and Birth	*Encinta y Dar a Luz*............... 103
45.	The Family is Sick	*Estamos Enfermos*................106
46.	Herbal Remedies	*La Herbolaria* 109
47.	Hot Cold Wet Dry	*Teoría Humoral* 110
48.	Old Fashioned Grandmother	*Abuelita Anticuada* 112
49.	Advice on my Condition	*Pide Consejos*...................... 114
50.	My Dad has Cancer	*Canceroso*........................ 115
51.	When There is No Cure	*Desahuciado*...................... 117
52.	Diabetes is Eating Me	*Me está Comiendo* 119

53.	My Baby is Sick	*Bebé Enfermito* 120
54.	Body Rash and Itching	*La Comezón y Ronchas* 122
55.	Bare Feet	*La Frialdad* 123
56.	Medicinal Plants	*Plantas Medicinales* 125
57.	Candles Helped Us	*Las Velas Sirvieron* 126

Part 5. Curanderismo: Healing the Frailties of the Mind 129

58.	Bogus Healers	*El Engaño Cuesta* 129
59.	Lost the Will to Live	*Quiere Morir* 130
60.	Fright Sickness	*El Susto* 132
61.	Envy and Jealousy	*Envidia y Celos* 134
62.	Strong Dream Man	*El Soñador* 136
63.	Pray for My Soldier	*Oracion por mi Soldado* 138
64.	A Run of Bad Luck	*La Mala Suerte* 139
65.	The Prodigal Son	*El Hijo Pródigo* 140
66.	Family Issues	*Problemas Familiares* 142
67.	Nervous Breakdown	*Ataque de Nervios* 143
68.	Death of a Loved One	*Un Pesar* 145
69.	Life is a Nightmare	*Mi Pesadilla* 146
70.	Baby Cries in the Womb	*Llanto del Bebé* 147
71.	Frightened before Birth	*Asustado en el Vientre* 148
72.	Candle Doesn't Smoke	*No hay Maldad* 150
73.	Bad Air	*Mal de Aire* 151
74.	Evil Eye	*Mal de Ojo* 153
75.	Baby Scared in Sleep	*Sueño Asustado* 154
76.	We are Suffering	*El Sufrimiento* 156
77.	Abused Grandchild	*Nieto Violado* 158
78.	Moonbeams Hurt my Baby	*Eclipse de Luna* 159
79.	Dew Harms Baby	*El Sereno* 161
80.	Lost Valuables	*Ayúdame San Antonio* 162
81.	Clean Grandmother's House	*El Despojo* 162
82.	Our Family Curse	*Maldición* 164
83.	Help Sell My Home	*Ayúdame San José* 166
84.	Cleansing and Sweeping	*Limpia y Barridas* 167
85.	Healing Psalms	*Los Salmos Sanan* 168

Part 6. Healing the Heart: Cheating Husbands and the Other Woman 171

86. My Husband Left Me	*La Abandonada*	171
87. Destroyed Marriage	*Brujería Destruye*	173
88. Arguing Grandparents	*Abuelos Peleoneros*	176
89. He Doesn't Love Me	*Ya no me Quiere*	177
90. It's Definitely Over	*Hasta aquí*	178
91. Drunk and Using	*Vicioso*	179
92. Nobody Understands	*Nadie me Entiende*	181
93. Mending Fences	*Metiendo la Paz*	183
94. He Doesn't Help Us	*No nos Ayuda*	184
95. Daughter's Baby's Father	*Enredado*	186
96. Doesn't Know His Son	*Desobligado*	188
97. Life's Trouble	*Dilemas*	189
98. Life is Terrible	*Errores*	191
99. Someone for Me	*Alguien para Mi*	192
100. The Other Woman	*La Otra*	194
101. Guy Problems	*El Tonto*	195
102. Vanquish the Other	*Librame*	196
103. The Divorce	*El Divorcio*	197
104. My Rival	*Mi Rival*	199
105. Bring Him Back	*Ven a Mi*	201
106. My Husband's Affair	*El Engaño*	201
107. Mother Accused Father	*El Acusado*	202
108. The Other Man	*Desamárrame*	204
109. Let Him Go	*Déjalo Ir*	205
110. Couple Problems	*Entre Dos*	206
111. Candle Magic	*La Vela Magica*	208
112. Spiteful Stepfather	*Malicioso*	210
113. Remove this Woman	*Quítamela*	212
114. Manipulative Women	*Controladora*	213
115. Differences of Opinion	*Punto De Vista*	214

Part 7. Healing the Workplace: The Treacherous World Beyond the Home 217

116. Bad People	Gente Mala	217
117. Change My Luck	Estoy Salada	218
118. She Needs Her Job	Necesita su Trabajo	220
119. Gossipy Workmates	Chismes	221
120. Teacher Needs a Job	Abre Camino	223
121. She Burned Me	Me Quemó	224
122. The Bureaucracy	Enredado en la Política	226
123. Success	Éxito	228
124. Father's Credit	El Buen Nombre	229
125. A Spiritual Test	Una Prueba Espiritual	230
126. I Need Work	Necesito Trabajar	232
127. Lonely	La Soledad	232
128. Need Guidance	Oriéntenme	234
129. Anguish	La Angustia	236
130. Homeless	Sin Techo	237
131. Bad Luck	Mala Suerte	238

Part 8. Healing Injustice: In and Out of Jail 241

132. Dark Secret	Secreto Obscuro	241
133. Arrested for Drugs	Drogadicta	244
134. Hard Time	Encarcelado	245
135. Winning in Court	Justo Juez	247
136. Drugs Kill	Drogas Destruyen	248
137. The Big Law Firm	Ganando la Causa	249
138. Going Crazy	Volviéndome Loca	250
139. Molesting Stepfather	Abusada	252
140. Plea Agreement	Un Acuerdo	253
141. Can't be Good	Malo Maloso	254
142. Temptation	Tentación	255
143. Pray for Father	Orar Por mi Padre	256
144. Going to Court	Corriendo Corte	257
145. No More Jail	Nunca Más	259

Part 9. Healing the Evil Around Us: Witches, Spirits & Demon Possession 263

146. Witchcraft Signs	*Reconoce las Señales*	263
147. Mother is Calling Me	*Me está Llamando*	265
148. The She Devil	*La Diabla*	266
149. Exorcism	*El Exorcismo*	267
150. Smoking Out Bad Spirits	*El Sahumerio*	270
151. Owls and Omens	*Lechuzas y Agüeros*	272
152. Scared of the Unseen	*El Miedoso*	273
153. Toad Spell	*El Sapo Tonto*	274
154. The Mind Reader	*El Clarividente*	276
155. Dark Shadow	*Una Sombra Negra*	277
156. Spirit Door	*La Ouija*	278
157. Working Me	*Trabajándome*	280
158. Witchcraft Dolls	*Muñecos*	281
159. I'm Cursed	*Maldición*	282
160. The Witch	*La Bruja*	283
161. Home Spirits	*Espíritus Malignos*	284
162. Darkness	*Las Tinieblas*	286
163. Exorcising Demons	*Sacando Demonios*	287
164. Freed of Demons	*Liberado*	290
165. Tormented	*El Diablo*	292
166. Grandma is a Witch	*La Hechicera*	293
167. Guardian Angel	*Angel Guardián*	295
168. Evil Spirits	*Veo lo Malo*	296
169. Bewitched	*Embrujamiento*	297
170. Afraid of Witchcraft	*Espantado*	299
171. The Conjure	*Conjuro*	300
172. I'm Surrounded	*Perseguido*	301
173. Cursed	*Me Maldijo*	302
174. The Hex	*El Hechizo*	303
175. Pins and Needles	*Alfileres*	305
176. Crazy Toddler	*El Loquito*	307
177. Protecting Ours	*Lo Nuestro*	309
178. Fixing the Game	*Conjurando el Futbol*	310
179. Holy Death	*La Santisima Muerte*	312

Part 10. Giving Thanks: Prayers Answered and Miracles Received 317

180. Personal Pilgrimage	*Peregrinación* 317
181. Grant Us a Miracle	*Un Milagro* 319
182. Good Medicine	*La Buena Medicina* 320
183. Our Luck Changed	*La Buena Suerte* 323
184. Praying	*Orando* 324
185. Grant Me Strength	*Fortaléceme* 326
186. Spiritual Assistance	*Ayuda Espiritual* 327
187. Niño is Love	*Niño es Amor* 328
188. Promoted	*Promovida* 330
189. Good to Us	*Nos Trata Bien* 331
190. Garden of Healing	*Jardín de Curación* 333

Appendix I.   **Cultural Competency** 343

Appendix II.   **Important Internet Resource Links** 367

Appendix III. **A Border Herbal** 381

References 417

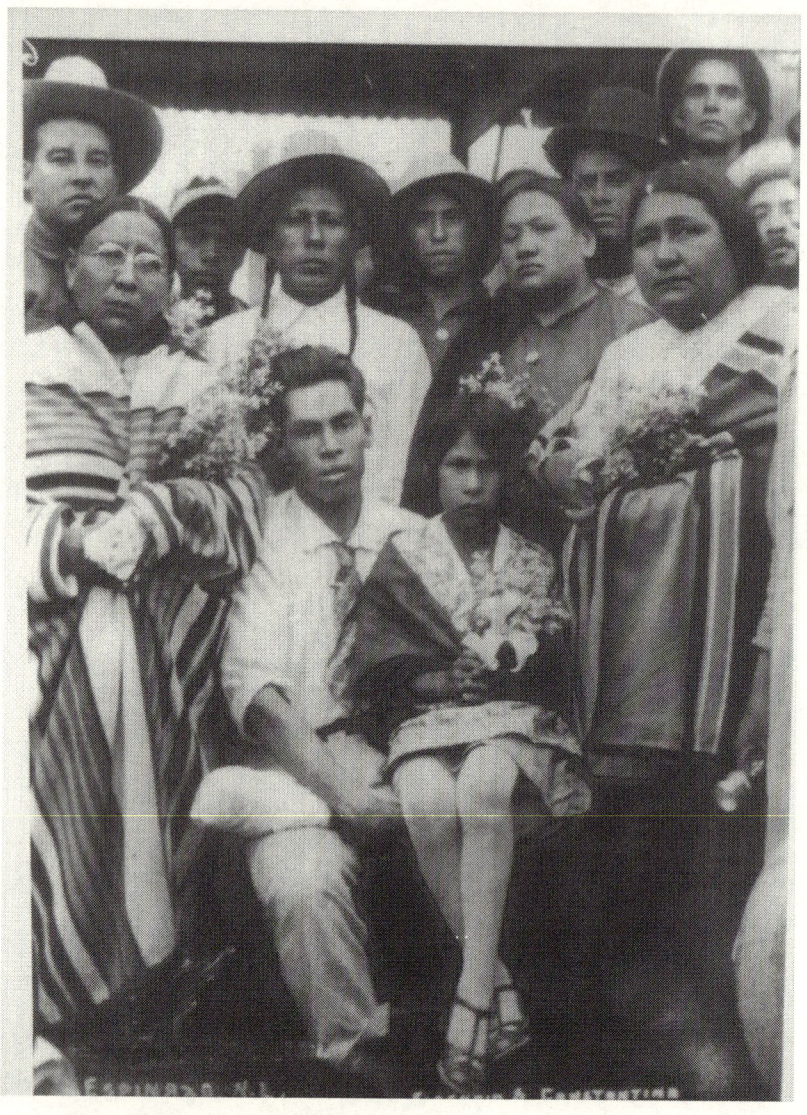

In the late 1920's at the height of his fame, El Niño Fidencio was visited by a delegation of Southwestern Native Americans who recognized him as a great shaman.
(Photo from Zavaleta collection)

Introduction
by Jamie Sams

I am honored to introduce Dr. Antonio *"Tony"* Zavaleta and Alberto Salinas Jr. to the readers of *Curandero Conversations*, a book of great importance to all those seeking understanding in these times of uncertainty. I am grateful that these two men have included the essential female-healing viewpoints of Latina academic, Rachel Edith Barrera, who wrote a personal testimonial, and my own Native American healing traditions. In the Cherokee way, we honor the male and female balance in the Circle of Life, creating wholeness. These two gifted men have chosen to honor that same sense of wholeness within their literary co-creation.

There is a special fellowship between people who have embraced the rich healing heritages of the American Southwest border region and Mexico. These spiritual practices may often include ancient Toltec, Mayan, Aztec, and Hispanic cures and remedies passed from one gifted family member to another for centuries. Many of these sacred healing traditions would be lost forever if not recorded for posterity and for the benefit of future generations.

In 1973, I met Tony Zavaleta, who was then a dedicated anthropology graduate student at the University of Texas at Austin. I had just returned from living in Mexico, studying with my *curandero* and Native American healing teachers. For over 30 years, we have shared many intersecting paths in life that have shown me his desire for authentic knowledge, his high personal integrity, as well as his devotion to helping Latinos who have lost parts of their cultural heritages and their personal sense of identity. Dr. Zavaleta's years of personal investigation into cultural knowledge and healing practices have put him in touch with credible shaman and healers from many races, faiths, and traditions. His explorations have allowed him to respect all those seeking healing from their own lineages, as well as the traditions of other cultures.

Alberto Salinas Jr. is an honored Latino elder, a living treasure of a healer, who has devoted his life to the service of others over many decades. His tireless efforts have helped hundreds of Latinos and non-Latinos throughout the years. The rich heritage that he embodies expands every time it is used to help another person and when they pass that cure or wisdom to the next generation.

The questions asked of the healer or *curandero*, Alberto Salinas Jr., apply to the physical, psychological, and spiritual well-being of those seeking consultation. These requests also include advice and help in how to face life's many challenges. This set of abilities would normally confound medical practitioners and academics who are only trained in general medicine and the specialized fields they chose in medical school. An authentic *curandero* must often times be a shaman, a diagnostician, a psychologist, a seer, a healer, an herbalist, as well as an interpreter of dreams. Not every *curandero* possesses all of these gifts; just as many human beings are gifted mathematicians while others excel in art, cooking or engineering.

Dr. Zavaleta's commentaries enlighten areas of Mr. Salinas' answers that may not be readily understood by a first-time seeker looking into *curanderismo*. Tony Zavaleta's academic, anthropological, personal, and experiential healing viewpoints allow readers to better understand and to apply the wisdom offered by Salinas.

These two extraordinary men have come together to offer traditional cures; interpretations of clarity, and to show others how healing practices can apply to every situation. This book applies to human beings from all walks of life and embraces any person seeking the enrichment of healing. Naturopathic doctors, medical doctors, alternative and complementary medical professionals would do well to take note of this book since it embodies the very essence of compassion that most of us find missing from the health care systems of today.

For years pharmaceutical companies have tried to duplicate simple plant remedies to sell to the public at astronomical prices when those very remedies cannot be chemically copied since they come from Mother Earth's natural pharmacy. For example, few people know that aspirin comes from willow bark. We may take a pill to get rid of a headache but if we contract chronic illnesses we may wonder why they keep re-occurring. *Curandero Conversations* reminds us on every page that faith and prayer are the mystical, healing ingredients and preventative medicine that many people have forgotten to use on a daily basis.

It is my personal hope that more books will be written that are bridging the differences between races, forging sturdy links of understanding and mending the broken or missing pieces of diverse healing heritages. Together, all traditions of healing are teaching humanity that there are alternatives to losing your sense of self or your hope for a better life. These authors demonstrate how to reclaim your internal healing heritage and how to find the courage to approach life head on.

As ancient scribes chronicled the new discoveries and ancient wisdom known in their own times, so these two men have reclaimed lost wisdom and placed it in written form for humankind. Like the scribes and pathfinders who walked before them to make our world a better place, Zavaleta and Salinas are blazing trails that can lead each individual to his or her next step of becoming the best human being they can be.

My reply is, "BRAVO! Well done!"

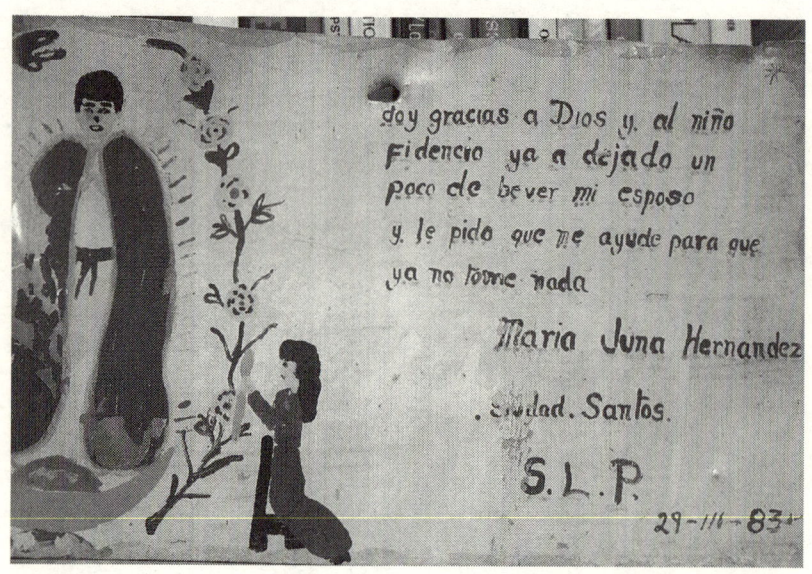

An authentic ex-voto is dedicated to El Niño Fidencio from Espinazo, Nuevo León. (Photo by Zavaleta).

PART ONE
A Testimonial

"I came to the realization that the lack of cultural knowledge is like soul loss initiated by the void of our ancestral and family legacies."

—Rachel Edith Barrera, doctoral candidate

Learning to Walk Between Worlds: A Latina's Spiritual Journey

by Rachel Edith Barrera

The Spanish word for healer is *curandero/a*, and comes from the verb *curar* meaning to heal. Healing is the defining part of the word *curandera*. A *curandera* is a female healer and a *curandero* is a male healer. In Latino culture there are those who are born with a special gift called *el don*. This gift of healing can manifest itself in a variety of different ways: *parteras* (midwives), *hierberas* (herbalists), *hueseras* (bonesetters), *sobadoras* (massage specialists), *materias* (spirit mediums) and other types of healers who are as unique as the people they help. The gift can manifest in both men and women at any point in their lives; from the moment they are born to the time they become grandparents. The gift can also be passed on from generation to generation like it has with mine.

The mystical world of *curanderos/as* has been a part of my family for generations. I was born with a special awareness. From my earliest recollection, family, friends and strangers noticed this difference. Some described it as a *luz,* or light, while others told me I had the gift of healing. Since I was a child, information about and experiences with *curanderismo* have come to me through a variety of ways, transforming my life into a unique and wonderful apprenticeship in healing and shamanism.

My mother's stories were an early chapter in my apprenticeship. Stories like the time a young girl was possessed in my mother's village or the time my grandmother saw a black cat visit her grandfather, who was a known *brujo*, warlock, in the community. He lived until my mother was 10 and was easily over a century old. My great-grandfather was also a *curandero* in the same community. My mother's experiences within the context of her *curandera* heritage taught her many things, some practical and others esoteric, which she passed on to me. Through these stories, I learned the healing beliefs and practices of my mother's family. I learned the practical application of this knowledge. As a child I eavesdropped on my mother's consulting sessions, as she gave advice to those who came to her for help. I can still smell the herbs she used in her *barridas*, or ritual sweepings of the body. I learned the art of passing a fertile hen's egg over the body as a cure for *mal de ojo*, evil eye. I learned the many rituals one must know by heart including those that offered protection against enemies and those which broke *trabajos*, works of witchcraft. I learned how to identify and prepare medicinal plants for healing. My childhood was filled with wonder and magic. But that soon changed.

During my teenage years my mother became part of an evangelical sect and stopped healing in the ways she learned from her family. Her new church saw her "old ways" as evil, and, little by little, my mother "forgot" the healing ways of our ancestors. However, I did not forget. My mother could not erase what I had learned. My memories resonate with a vital part of my being and define who I am today. Against my mother's wishes, I continued to learn the ways of my ancestors. Luckily, and unintentionally, early in my childhood I learned to interact within the non-ordinary reality, a unique world where shamans and *curanderos/as* interact. When my mother no longer shared her knowledge, I continued to be taught and to learn through dreams and visitations from my ancestors and by one very special teacher. My mother will never cease being a healer. My mother's *don*, or her gift of healing and intuition, has not abandoned her. She continues to apply her medicinal plant knowledge, and her other more esoteric practices continue to evolve. Prayer is now my mother's tool of choice to heal and interact with God. Just as my mother's gift evolved over the years, so did my apprenticeship.

The next part of my apprenticeship began during my undergraduate work at The University of Texas at Brownsville and Texas Southmost College, where I crossed paths with Dr. Antonio Zavaleta. I visited his office one day and we began a conversation and a collaboration that has spanned two decades. It was then that I began my deconstruction and re-interpretation of *curanderismo* through an academic lens. I learned of the syncretic nature of the healing traditions I had been taught—the mixture of the Old World and New World ways. I've read the different histories that created many of the practices seen today in *curanderismo*. I also worked alongside *materias*, or trance mediums, of El Niño Fidencio, Mexico's most important folk saint. I learned their traditions, rituals and beliefs. I documented the practices via multi-media techniques; including digital photography, field research, participant observation, and I translated these experiences into the *El Niño Fidencio Curanderismo Research Project's* initial website. Through these projects, I found myself researching spirit channeling, possession and the ethno-pharmacology related to traditional medicinal plant uses. I delved ever deeper into the knowledge base established by my heritage. I learned the significance of spirits, saints and angels within different contexts, and learned more of the vast richness and resources that *curanderos/as* use in their healing repertoire. I learned how votive candles are used, about oils, amulets and talismans, and countless other items used by folk practitioners. I visited the crowded and mysterious Mercado Sonora, Sonora Market, known as the Witches' Market, in the heart of Mexico City, and walked alongside countless healers, witches and shamans. I learned to recognize the material resources used by the darker arts, *brujería*, witchcraft, as well as those of the light.

I have also witnessed how *curanderismo* is constantly evolving such as *curanderos/as*, who now use concepts like *chakras*, understand the positive use of meditation, and blend traditions from around the world. Because of the knowledge gathered through my unique learning opportunities, I formed two conclusions. One conclusion, based on my collaborations with the *El Niño Fidencio Curanderismo Research Project*, is the lack of knowledge and understanding that the newly trained generations of health care providers possess regarding cultural healing beliefs and practices of the Latino/a community. This failure to incorporate traditional knowledge into the health care delivery system affects the availability of medical treatment options. The other is based on my personal experiences and reflections: some of my generation and younger Latino/as, especially those of Mexican descent are losing vital parts of their diverse cultural heritage. This includes folk beliefs, family traditions and their native Spanish and/or their indigenous language. Some are intentionally no longer being taught their family histories and language. This is especially true of the art of healing and spirituality. I may have the rituals and beliefs that were passed down from my mother's family, but I don't know the specific indigenous group my mother's great grandparents came from because it was shameful to acknowledge *Indio*, or Indian, blood. This is just one of many examples of how indigenous languages can be lost to future generations.

I have continuously encountered and conversed with other young Latinos/as from diverse communities and backgrounds throughout the United States. Through my interactions, I learned that many Latinos/as were not familiar with their family cultural heritage or those related to the wider Latino/a culture and history. This was especially true of healing and spirituality. I was intrigued and discovered that many were unaware of the practices and beliefs related to *curanderismo*. Realizing their lack of knowledge, I was shocked to learn that some even feared this part of their heritage and legacy.

I am a first generation Mexican American, but I see first, second, and third generation counterparts who have not been raised with the knowledge of the histories of their cultural and healing traditions. For different reasons, their parents did not teach them Spanish. I found that some Latinos/as, especially those of Mexican descent who lacked this knowledge, seemed lost, adrift, and hungry for opportunities to learn to speak Spanish. They were also interested in learning more about the esoteric cultural traditions related to their Latino/a culture. Once they began their own journeys of discovery, some soon found a rich and colorful family history of stories and traditions.

I have met many who would make amazing *curanderos/as*. They can sense their ancestors calling to them, but they do not know how to listen. I came to the realization that the lack of cultural knowledge is like soul loss initiated by the void of our ancestral and family legacies. Important traditions were not passed on to the next generation. This loss of heritage has become like a kind of *susto*, or fright sickness, a folk illness, typically initiated through some trauma, in which the soul or parts of the soul are separated from the body. The person who suffers from soul loss is not complete until all of the parts of the soul are returned to the body. By healing the soul, the body is subsequently healed. The reuniting of the lost parts of the soul with the body requires the skills of a knowledgeable cultural practitioner. This specialist performs a healing ritual to make the body whole again. The cultural soul loss I speak of has to do with the loss of the spiritual-healing heritage as well as other traditions which have been stripped from the ancestral consciousness of the soul because it no longer is being passed on to new generations. If it is not taught to future generations, the void caused by the loss is eventually filled with something else.

For those like me, who had the good fortune of learning our family's spiritual traditions and beliefs, we should not take for granted that other Latinos/as were exposed to similar ideas and practices and taught their own stories. I have found that many Latinos/as lack this kind of knowledge and at the same time, they long for it, sensing its absence. Often, they are eager to explore every aspect of their cultural heritage. I also found that non-Latinos/as are curious about *curanderismo* and welcome knowledge that can enrich their lives.

In my understanding, *curanderismo* deals with the essence of the person, the spirit, and the soul, that constitutes the life fire, along with the body and mind which makes *curanderismo* a healing modality taking into consideration every component of a human being. *Curanderismo* is not simply about diagnosing a condition or an illness; it's about treating an entire community through the individual treatment of each member, one by one. *Curanderismo* is about healing the most integral parts of our being: family and community. In doing so, that which makes us whole is healed: the connection between mind, body and spirit/soul. This connection, which functions through time and space, is where healing truly begins. I realize this connection can also serve as a metaphor for individuals and members of the family within the Latino/a culture, in which the spirit/soul can be represented through the community. *Curanderos/as* are entrusted to carry the soul and the spiritual essence of their respective communities. As we lose these gifted individuals who carry and protect our cultural and spiritual knowledge, we lose the heart and soul of our communities.

One way to keep the community heart alive is to document, share and pass on our rich cultural heritage. We must learn to treasure each individual's unique interpretation and life experience because each adds their essence to the ancestral soul as it passes to the next generation. The *curanderismo* of my mother is different from her mother's, which is different from my own. Each generation brings to bear its own thoughts, ideas, and beliefs resulting in a re-enculturation of beliefs. Because of the Latino/a community's ability to acculturate and adapt, we have continued to evolve our cultural beliefs and practices at the dawn of the 21st century. This is evident when Latinos/as use *curanderismo* to complement modern medicine. However, this may not be the case if it is not being passed on. New generations must ensure the rapidly evolving traditions of healing in the Latino/a community from disappearing all together.

Humankind needs new ways of learning, sharing and healing. Four hundred years ago, the Badianus Manuscript documented the use of medicinal plants by the Aztecs. This manuscript marked one of the earliest known attempts at recording the healing practices in Mexico. This manuscript was unknown to scholars until the early 20th century when it was discovered in the Vatican library. In 1940, a facsimile was published, making the knowledge of Aztec medicine widely available.

Nearly half a millennium after the initial creation of the Aztec herbal, healing knowledge can be recorded and shared in a way that the Aztecs may never have imagined: the Internet. Latinos/as who may not have access to a *curandero/a* in their community, can now utilize the Internet to access informational resources on *curanderismo*. And as this book will illustrate, access to a consultation with a *curandero* via e-mail is now possible. Through this medium, all generations are able to document, share and spread the knowledge of *curanderismo*. Latino/a esoteric knowledge and traditions are made accessible not only to those who wish to rediscover their own cultural heritage, but to non-Latinos/as as well. If the current generation is not proactive, it will not take long for our cultural knowledge base to eventually vanish. It took almost 500 years for a miniscule portion of the Aztec knowledge base to reappear in mainstream consciousness. We cannot afford to wait another 500 years for the current knowledge base of *curanderismo* to be explicitly incorporated with its cultural and historical context alongside other different modern healing modalities. It is possible that this critically important, yet mostly overlooked knowledge holds the key to understanding the health care delivery needs of the largest minority population in the United States. We also need to realize that within Latinos/as there exist many cultural and regional sub-groups from all over the world, including, but not limited to, Cuban, Puerto Rican, Guatemalan, Columbian and their children which may represent a plethora of mixed cultural heritages, healing beliefs and practices. These differences influence *curanderismo* because the healing modalities and the use of material resources of *curanderismo* differ by culture and region.

Currently, I am a doctoral candidate at the University of Texas at Austin. The alternative-healing community of Austin, Texas has offered me additional ways to expand my knowledge of healing modalities through the study of meditation, neo-shamanism, Native American and New Age healing techniques. However useful, these will never replace the *curanderismo* I learned from my family as the foundation of my spiritual-healing ancestral knowledge. I have found that modern medicine can sometimes be at odds with the healing ways I have been taught. The current Latino/a generation can help bridge both worlds while simultaneously teaching one another about healing and cultural beliefs. We must connect these worlds so that all can share, learn, and understand how to best heal and prevent further soul loss, or cultural *susto*. Through spiritual journeys of self-discovery, we will find that we share more than we know or can ever understand. We will find that we are all part of one family, of which everyone and everything that lives on Mother Earth is a member.

One way to connect these worlds is through the book you are about to read. This book also reflects another adaptive evolutionary step in *curanderismo*— consulting via e-mail in addition to face-to-face. These pages present a unique insight into the lives, cultural beliefs and practices of the Latino/a community expressed through their voices. Voices of people like you because illness and disease do not discriminate. The 190 e-mail exchanges in this book represent many of the current illnesses, worries, thoughts and concerns for which Latinos/as seek assistance from *curanderos/as*. By bringing these voices to you, we hope to bring a missing perspective in understanding our population. The dialogues are from actual individuals longing for physical and spiritual wholeness in their lives by which e-mail assisted in the process. We illustrate the healer's perspective through the native voice and life's work of *curandero* Alberto Salinas Jr. The commentaries of anthropologist Dr. Antonio N. Zavaleta elaborate the implications of *curanderismo* for health care providers who deliver treatment to the Latino/a community.

Of all that I have learned, the most important is that *el don*, the gift, is bestowed upon a *curandero/a* for the purpose of healing any and all who seek it.

One day, perhaps this day, the seeker may be you.

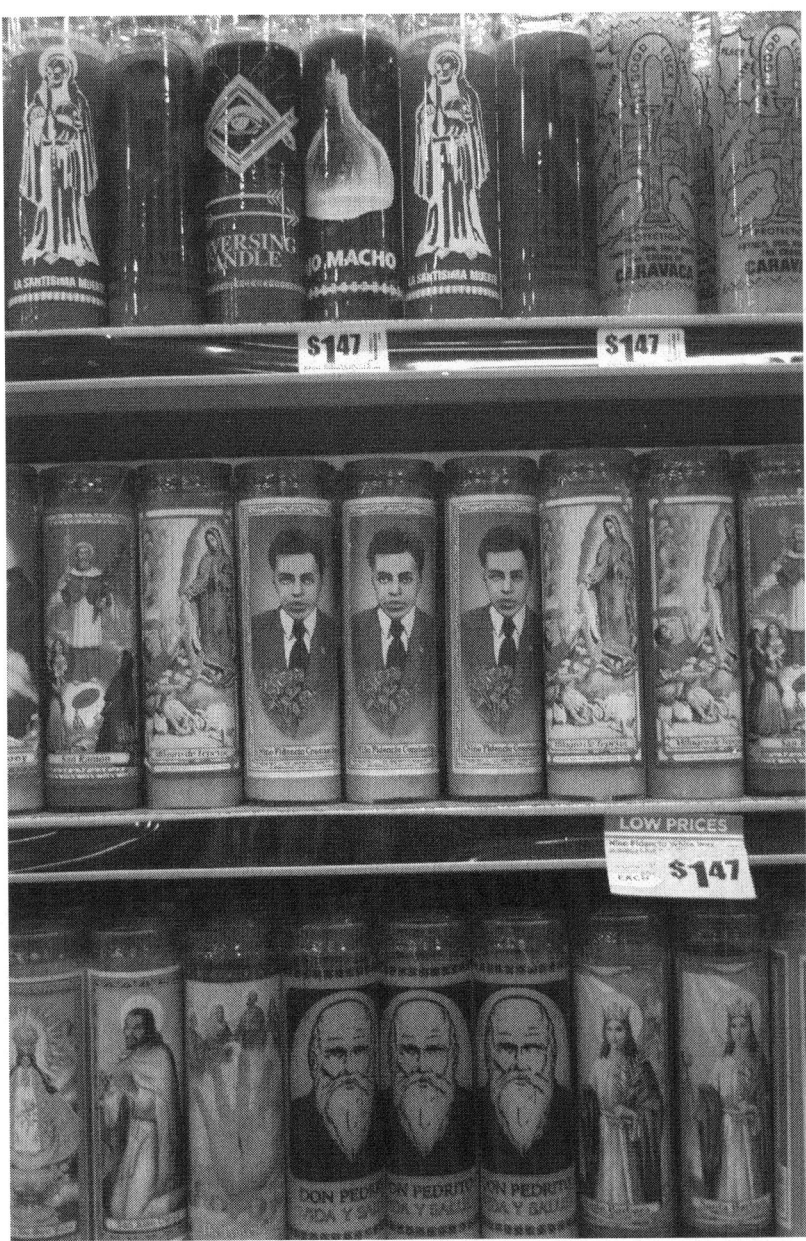

Display of votive candles to El Niño Fidencio, Pedrito Jaramillo, the Virgen de Guadalupe and others. Typical display found along the U.S. Mexico border in retail stores. (Photo by Zavaleta)

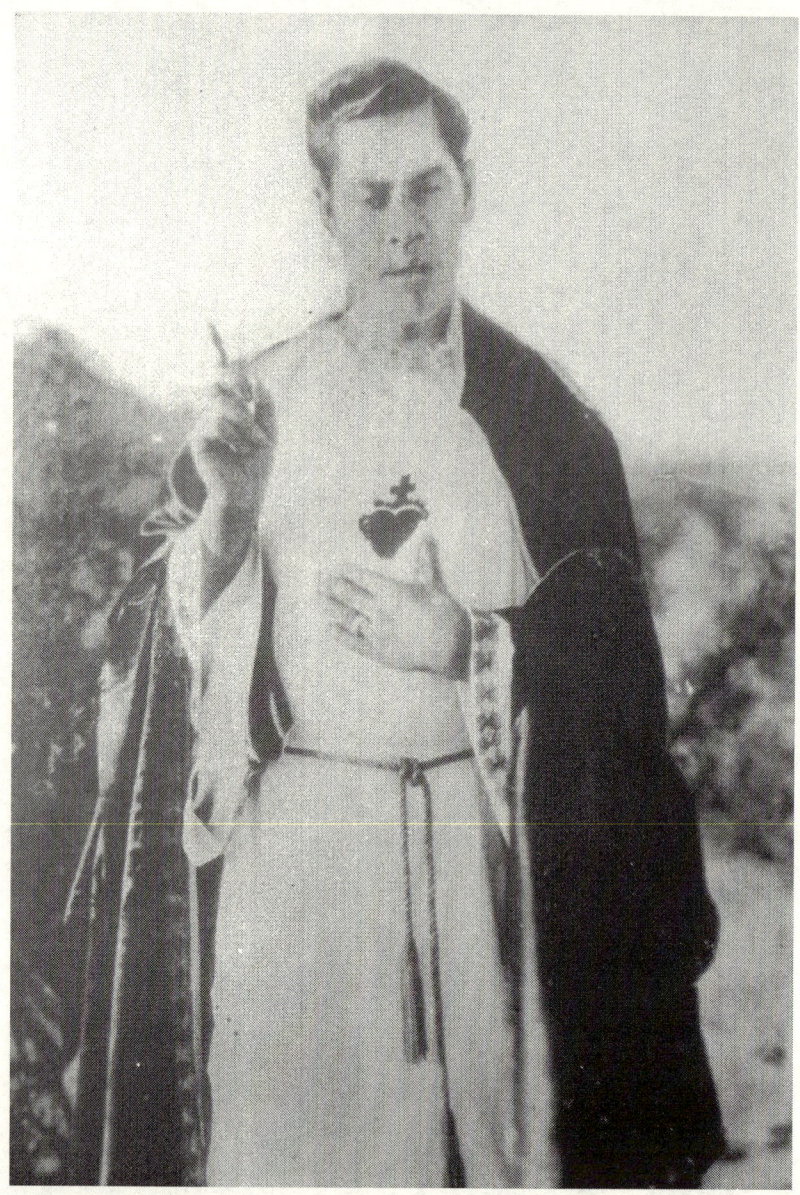

The Niño Fidencio was often represented as the Sacred Heart of Jesus and the Virgen of Guadalupe. (Photo from Zavaleta collection)

PART TWO

Healing the Spirit: Life as a Spiritual Journey

"Those who suffer have the grace of God. By suffering, health is reached, and it is necessary that this should be so, because those who desire to be well are strengthened by our sorrow and pain."

—*El Niño Fidencio, 1928*

(From Anita Brenner's "Idols Behind Altars" 1929, p.21)

The 190 stories and petitions you are about to read have been selected from more than 7,000 available. They are from people all across the United States and Mexico, just like you, and are for the most part published as they were received by the *curandero*. The stories in this book were chosen to represent the broad spectrum of the human condition and to reveal to you the vast diversity of the topic of *curanderismo*. The *curandero's* responses have, likewise, been changed very little. Together the petition and the response represent an accurate glimpse into the mostly unknown *curandero*-client dynamic. Commentaries are offered to explain material and/or to offer additional information for the reader.

Antonio Zavaleta and Alberto Salinas Jr.

1. THE LIFE OF THE NIÑO FIDENCIO — *VIDA DEL NIÑO FIDENCIO*

José Fidencio Síntora Constantino, known as El Niño Fidencio, was born in the Valley of Caves, or Valle de las Cuevas near Iramuco, Guanajuato, México on November 13, 1898. He was baptized on November 16, 1898. His father was Socorro Constantino and his mother was María Transito Síntora. Legend says that they had 25 children: 23 boys and two girls.

Most people believe that Fidencio began healing in Espinazo, Nuevo León, Mexico but that is not true. At the age of eight he performed his first cure, when he set his mother's broken arm. He used small sticks and a local root called *sacasil,* or the cactus cereus, to set the bone. She is said to have recovered promptly.

In 1921, Fidencio accompanied his childhood friend, Enrique López de la Fuente north to Nuevo León. Fidencio worked as a kitchen and house boy at the Loma Sola Ranch, which today is the abandoned Socorro Ranch.

At the Socorro Ranch his healing activities and his many cures were kept hidden from Enrique. Enrique did not approve of Fidencio working as a healer. When Enrique and Fidencio arrived in Espinazo he continued to heal albeit without Enrique's approval.

Although Fidencio called Enrique *papá,* father and considered him his stepfather, their relationship was always difficult at best.

For awhile, Fidencio lived in the home of Herculana de Rosales and it was there that he began to heal openly. One of his patients was Teodoro von Wernich, owner of the hacienda, or large estate, at Espinazo. Teodoro had an open sore, called a fistula, on his leg that refused to heal. After Fidencio treated him, the wound healed completely.

Teodoro was so impressed with Fidencio's remarkable ability that he published the story of his healing in the Mexico City newspapers. This is how Fidencio became a public figure in Mexico.

After the article was published, many people ventured from the interior of Mexico to the north seeking Fidencio's cures. It was only then that Enrique began to accept Fidencio's talent and allowed Fidencio to heal full-time. By that time, the people affectionately called him "El Niño" Fidencio because of his humble and childlike nature.

El Niño's pinnacle healing years were between 1927 and 1929, when the greatest number of people came to see him. Espinazo's population swelled to 50 thousand semi-permanent residents in 1928. Mexican president General Plutarco Elías Calles came aboard his train, Olivo, the olive, to see him. When the train arrived at Espinazo station Fidencio greeted President Calles. They are said to have spoken in private for six hours. It is not known if the president himself had an illness or if it was his daughter who was ill. We do know that something miraculous happened during that consultation that caused the president great joy and gratitude. Since Espinazo had no natural source of water, President Calles ordered a pipeline be built from a nearby mountain spring at La Gavia, to Espinazo, a distance of about five miles. To this day, that pipeline is the only source of water Espinazo has.

Although Fidencio never charged for his cures, thousands of gifts were left for him in Espinazo. He distributed all of the gifts and money he received to the needy or sometimes used the money to pay for the operation of his hospital facility. He never put aside any money for himself.

A wealthy family from Torreón, Coahuila, México purchased medical equipment and a surgical table for Fidencio, but he never used them, preferring to work outside and on the ground.

He is said to have healed lepers, persons with tuberculosis and the insane, simply by looking at them. He delivered babies and treated all manner of ailments.

There were 30 beds in his maternity clinic and they were always full. He liked to do his healing touching the earth and usually on the exact spot each time.

He would heal with water that had been left out overnight and which had gold and jewels placed in it and believed to enhance its powers. He would make special soaps and salves or *pomadas*, with cow lard, and he used an assortment of fruits such as bananas, lemons, tomatoes and apples.

Fidencio was very humble in his appearance and in his actions. He respected everyone and he was truly childlike. He rejected money and material things which were offered him in great amounts. He would never allow the practice of witchcraft, or *brujería*. He always stated that he healed in the name of God.

Fidencio would punish unruly persons by locking them inside a pen with his mountain lion. The lion did not harm them because it did not have teeth or claws. But it sure did scare them! Misbehaving children were also punished this way.

He had several trusted male and female followers who were his principal helpers, or *guardias*. They served as assistants when he was curing and throughout his operations. They prepared meals for many who attended. There were also designated helpers for the mentally ill.

Fidencio predicted his death months ahead of time; always stating that he would have to leave. He said that after his death, there would appear many who would claim to be him. So he reminded everyone that there was only one Fidencio and to be aware of charlatans. He died on October 19, 1938. (This story was translated from Spanish and has been circulated around Espinazo, Nuevo León for many years. It is attributed to the Nino's brother Joaquín but there is no way to know if that is true. The story itself is believed to be accurate).

COMMENTARY:

In the 1960s, Mexican American folklorist and anthropologist, Américo Paredes published "Folk Medicine and Intercultural Jest," examining the unique relationship that exists between doctors and curanderos/as viewed through the genre of jest. In order to honor Don Américo, I offer this brief exchange collected by Dr. Paredes in Brownsville, Texas in 1962.

"Somebody falls ill and is taken to a doctor, but the doctor can do nothing for him. The patient gets worse and worse. There may be a consultation attended by several doctors—"a meeting of the doctors," as the casos (folklore

cases) put it—but the men of science cannot find the cause of the disease or recommend a cure. Or perhaps they say the patient is beyond hope of recovery. Again, they may recommend a painful and costly operation requiring a long stay at the hospital. Then someone suggests going to Don Pedrito or El Niño Fidencio (altered by the authors) or some other curandero. The patient's relatives are skeptical at first, but they finally agree. The whole group journeys to the curandero, who receives them kindly but chides the doubters about their skepticism, which he has learned about by miraculous means even before they arrive. Then he asks a standard question, seemingly unnecessary for his diagnosis but very important to the structured arrangement of the narrative: 'And what do the doctors say?'"

"The curandero is told what the doctors say, and he smiles indulgently at their childish ignorance. Then he prescribes some deceptively simple remedy: An herb perhaps, drinking three swallows of water under special circumstances three times a day, washing at a certain well or spring or the like. The patient recovers completely. There may be a sequel in which the former patient goes and confronts the doctors. They are surprised, even incredulous. The doctors visit the old curandero, seeking to find out the secret of the cure. The old man tells them nothing, or he answers in words such as "God cured him, not I." The doctors leave, chastened and still mystified." (Paredes, 1993, p.52)

Many of the true stories you are about to read depict ordinary people whose encounters with the health care delivery system are no different today than they were decades ago. Thank you, Don Américo for being my professor, and for being the planter of seeds, El Sembrador. I am one of your seeds.

2. NIÑO'S SPIRITUAL HELPERS — *GUARDIAS*

My family is from the mountains of Nuevo León, México where El Niño Fidencio was a constant guest at the homes of my aunts, uncles and cousins. I was raised on the stories of his life and the multitude of blessings he brought to every member of our family.

During his years of helping others, El Niño became a surgeon, cutting out tumors, stitching up cuts from the many typical accidents of ranch life and hard work. He was an herbalist, a trusted *curandero*, healer, and a *partero*, or midwife. El Niño delivered my aunt's two children, a girl and a boy. When he began going into spiritual trances, that same aunt became his first *guardia*, or spiritual guardian who holds the protective space for the medium while he or she is out of body. She only performed this role for a year but she was his first *guardia*. Due to his travels and her small children at home, she was not able to leave her village and follow him on his many journeys through the rugged mountains to other villages.

Fidencio blessed our family and all of our generations to come before I was born. My mother was among the family members that he blessed. El Niño also gave my mother a prophecy that one of her female children would be born with the gift of clairvoyance. I was that child. When I was 13, I had a vision of Our Lady of Lourdes while I was praying. I told Our Lady that if I was blessed with a husband and a female child, I would name that child Lourdes. I was given that blessing and I have fulfilled my spiritual promise to Our Lady of Lourdes. That vision began another cycle in my life where I became aware of the gift from God that I believe came from El Niño's blessing the wombs of the older generation of women in my family.

In the seven and a half decades of my life, I have been a psychically-gifted Spanish tarot card reader. I have realized that the cards are just like a tiny road map that guides my vision of what those seeking advice need to know. There are many readers who are talented with reading the Spanish tarot cards, but most do not see deeply into the non-material world because they tell clients that things could go one way or another. That is simply life, you can turn left or right. Those types of readers are not directed by the spirit to see a person's past, present, and future and cannot usually reveal details of the person's personal life because the client is a stranger. I feel that my gift from God was begun before my birth and that El Niño's blessing on my family members has manifested in many ways.

Although I am semiretired, I see a new surge of people that want readings. Unfortunately, most of them simply go to any reader available. I believe that it is important for people to know the difference between fakers, readers who are just beginning the use Spanish tarot, readers who have good hearts but no real talent and those who are authentic. My question to you is: How do you teach these lessons to people who are living in the chaos and desperation of this new century?

CURANDERO'S RESPONSE:

Your family's connection to El Niño Fidencio is a rare treasure to those of us who did not witnesses his life nor the daily activities and interactions of his healing practices. His blessing your family's lineage is a story that should be passed down to every generation since it will always continue to carry his love and protection.

You ask about teaching others to look for authentic spiritual gifts and how not to be taken for an expensive ride. The discernment is always with the seeker. The person, who is searching, must do his/her homework just as he must seek out authentic healers. It is always proper to get many recommendations from people you trust and to see how you feel with the person before allowing them access to your personal life. By that I mean answering too many questions put to you by any spiritual advisor or Spanish tarot reader. The reader is supposed to be supplying the information to you, and not the person seeking advice providing the information to the reader. On a first reading, being as silent as possible will tell any seeker whether the reader really has the gift or not.

It is also good to remember that if you go to the same reader many times and develop a close relationship with that person, it causes the reader a lot of hard work to separate what they know about you from the messages that the spirit is trying to send you. There is not enough compensation in the world for harming the health of an authentic spiritual advisor by making constant demands or being needy.

COMMENTARY:

El Niño Fidencio's very first spiritual helpers or guardias were people he confided in, and had complete confidence and trust in. They were common people who lived as he did, humbly and in the desert. Their story has rarely, if ever, been told. The deep commitment and affection they had for El Niño were handed down through family lore for several generations and several of the most special of them have continued his spiritual work. This is the story of such a family. (This wonderful true story was submitted on behalf of the family in the story by Jamie Sams.)

3. BRACERO CAMPFIRE TALE — *CUENTOS DE MI ABUELITO*

My grandfather says that he first heard about the Niño Fidencio when he was a boy in the 1950s. He told me that he picked cotton on his grandmother's ranch and that the migrant farm workers called *braceros* would tell stories around the campfire at night. Do you know anything about this that you could share with me? I am taking an anthropology class at my local community college and I have chosen to write my semester paper about El Niño Fidencio. I know that you also had some of the same experiences that my grandfather had. Could you explain to me how the *braceros* and other Mexicans spread the tale of El Niño Fidencio into the United States?

CURANDERO'S RESPONSE:

You are correct. I had many of the same experiences your grandfather had when I was growing up about the same time. In the 1940s and 1950s the legend of El Niño Fidencio was in its formative stage and the stories of his miraculous cures were being carried northward from Mexico to the border with the United States and then into the American Southwest and Midwest. His name was carried by Mexican migrant farm workers called *braceros* as they migrated northward through the cotton fields, and from citrus orchards to garden patches. Many of the original storytelling *braceros*, being rural farm hands or *campesinos,* had actually been present at Espinazo during the peak years of the Niño Fidencio phenomenon in 1928-1929. Many had witnessed firsthand the Niño's healing, and had personal accounts to tell.

After a long day in the cotton fields it was not practical to walk the miles back to the farmhouse. I was a 12-year-old son of agricultural workers and I learned about Mexico's most famous folk healer around a *bracero* campfire just as many others my age did. That is exactly how the legends of the Niño were passed on from generation to generation in those days.

I made my bed on the ground around the campfires like all of the others. I was just another wide-eyed *bracero* kid, picking cotton under the hot Texas-Mexican sun hoping for September to come, crying out to

Barbas de Oro, to send the cooling winds indicating that it was time to go back to the comfort of the schoolhouse.

Over the years, I have recounted this story many times, whenever I am asked how I first learned about Fidencio.

The women in the field-camp made *tortillas* by hand and cooked up pots of delicious concoctions. There was always plenty of rice, beans and *tortillas.* We worked and sweated all day and ate and slept together in the field-camp at night. I marveled about how respectful the children were as they waited patiently to be fed. Our fathers, who had toiled all day under the July sun of the *canícula,* the dog days of summer, were always fed first, followed by the children, and always dutiful, the women would serve themselves last. As they did then, and so today, the women sacrificed themselves to support their hard-working families.

The campfire crackled and reflected ethereal flames on the bronzed faces of the workers, as each evening, one by one, someone would tell a tale, only to be bested by the next story. And so it went until the last tale was told or everyone had fallen asleep.

I learned about the dog days of summer, about saints and devils and heard stories about witches and forest elves called *duendes,* which were said to be all around us. It was then that I first heard about the mysterious miracle-working, man-child of the desert they called El Niño Fidencio. For reasons I do not understand, the stories about miracles and healing were always my favorite.

From the 1970s to this day, El Niño Fidencio has always been present in my life. For 25 years I have served and learned from his movement and his devoted followers. I think you have picked a wonderful topic to study and I will do everything I can to assist you with sources and explanations.

COMMENTARY:

I am often asked how I became interested in anthropology and in curanderismo. The curandero's story also reflects my personal recollection of childhood memories during the Bracero Era on the United States-Mexico border. It was in the cotton fields of northern Mexico and south Texas where many of my generation first heard about the Niño Fidencio, and his magic has followed us throughout our lives. This book is simply the most recent manifestation of Fidencio in our lives. My spiritual path as a Roman Catholic, my personal sojourn, and memories will endure for my lifetime but this little book will help them endure beyond our lifetimes. This is just the most recent installment. (This story was submitted by Dr. Tony Zavaleta.)

4. NIÑO FIDENCIO'S BLESSING — *SU BENDICIÓN*

Dear Niño Fidencio: I thank you for all the blessings, happiness, enlightenment, understanding, love and peace you have brought into my heart, my family, and my life. I thank you for the fellowship you bring to those of us who truly believe and follow you throughout life here on earth. I thank you for being my spiritual guide, my spiritual doctor, my spiritual lawyer and my protector in the course of my life's journey. I can ask for no more than strength, valor and the spirit of love to continue serving our Lord in heaven as you have instructed me. Please make me disciplined and worthy of the honor and privilege of serving the Lord.

CURANDERO'S RESPONSE:

May the spirit of El Niño Fidencio be always with you. I remember you and wish you the best in life. You have asked for guidance, help, and for something that would help you to understand the mystery of Fidencio. I remind you of what you already know in your heart and what is so simple. You think that you have forgotten, but you have not. Open your heart. You have experienced faith. You have known hope. And you prayed over it. You know what it was to have a longing and an unrequited spiritual need. There is something nagging at you that you cannot seem to put your finger on, something missing in your life. The feeling of not knowing puzzles you. You know intuitively that you are not getting the whole picture but you do not realize why God is keeping you on hold and has not answered your prayers.

You know something is wrong; you just cannot seem to grasp what it is. Allow me to help you understand. You have talked to God. God has talked to you. At some point in your lifetime, you met God and then you forgot Him. You went on about in your life not having realized how important it had been for you to believe in Him and how important you were to Him. He came to you in Spirit when you needed Him the most. Later in life, you needed God's help once again. You had faith, you had hope, you prayed and prayed and He did not seem to answer you. Your failure of realization caused you to question your faith. All you had left was hope with desperation and unknowing. You thought that God had not answered you. You felt that God would not meet with you. Your nights were filled with anguish, doubt and confusion. I believe God has not left your side. You just have to realize there is nothing more important in your life than He is. There is nothing more important than God. Once you have accepted God back into your life again, do not let Him go and He shall not abandon you and you shall want not. Your soul will be fully blessed.

In your life there shall be understanding, patience, fulfillment, knowledge, wisdom, answers, righteousness, fellowship, faith, hope, anointment and the blessing of the Spirit.

Many of Niño's teachings are in his greetings. One of his favorite greetings was *luz, entendimiento, amor y paz*, light, understanding, love and peace. Many of Niño's followers see him as their personal guide through life's journey. That is, their personal intermediary with God. Others see Niño as their spiritual doctor for all ailments, conditions or problems. Others see Niño as their lawyer who intercedes for them when in need for the troubles life may bring. Fidencio is also seen as a guardian angel and a protector by many who have faith in him.

COMMENTARY:

Curanderismo in the 21st century is an eclectic collection of beliefs, practices and traditions; including but not limited to belief in the Niño Fidencio. Fidencismo is a branch of curanderismo which channels the spirit of Fidencio. Only the spiritist branches of curanderismo channel spirits while the majority of curanderos/as heal on the physical level with the use of prayer and material items such as medicinal plants.

There is no single way or more correct practice of curanderismo than any other. Curanderos and curanderas are self-styled practitioners. They remind us of our familial and cultural traditions, regional or national variations, personal abilities and available healing materials and methods. Since the curandero, who is the focus of this work, is a materia or spirit trance medium of El Niño Fidencio, our journey begins there. In the tradition of curanderismo, the ability to channel spirits is considered to be a gift from God. The gifts of healing are discussed in 1 Corinthians 12:9 *"to another faith by the same Spirit, to another, gifts of healing by that one Spirit."*

5. SEARCHING FOR EL NIÑO FIDENCIO — *BUSCANDO AL NIÑO*

Since I was a child, I have been a great believer in El Niño Fidencio. I am compelled to speak with him again someday. I just don't know where to find him. El Niño predicted the birth of both my sons. I long to speak to him again can you help me find him?

CURANDERO'S RESPONSE:

Many people who met Niño Fidencio when he was living and had a personal encounter with him, would attest to his divine healing powers. They too continue believing in El Niño Fidencio throughout their lifetime. After Niño passed away, they carried their faith with them and would speak with the spirit of Niño through a *cajón/cajita*, or spirit box, the spirit channelers of the Niño Fidencio. During his life, Fidencio left his following with the understanding that his healing mission on earth would continue in the spirit after his death.

In every Latino community there are people who channel spirits and some who work specifically with the spirit of El Niño Fidencio. If for some reason you are unable to find or visit one of his *materias*, just call out his holy name Fidencio Síntora Constantino three straight times into a clear glass of water. Say a prayer and make your petition to his holy spirit and he will come to you in your dreams, in a vision or some other way. He will reveal himself to you through a sign or in a newspaper. If you really need him, look for him in your heart. You don't have to go any further than your heart for him to answer your prayers.

COMMENTARY:

Many followers of the Niño Fidencio have been so since childhood, having grown up in families with deep faith in Catholicism and in the Niño Fidencio. The Niño Fidencio always told his followers, "call out my name three times and I will be there in the spirit to attend to you in your hour of need." Spirit mediums that channel the spirit of El Niño Fidencio are found in every major Latino community in the United States. The Niño Fidencio movement is growing rapidly and is larger today than ever before. This is partially due to the socioeconomic marginality of many Latinos. Since Latinos have difficulty accessing health care they turn to time-tested cultural and alternative delivery systems. These systems are often neighborhood-based and very effective.

6. ANSWERED PRAYER — *ORACIÓN CONTESTADA*

I pray to El Niño Fidencio to help me not feel so bad. An hour after I pray, I feel a great relief come into my body and my sadness goes away. I pray to El Niño because only he can do the impossible for me and my family. We don't have any money. We asked El Niño to help us scrape together a little money and, as always, he answers my prayers and now I am going to be able to travel to visit my mother.

CURANDERO'S RESPONSE:

I share in your relief and happiness to hear that El Niño Fidencio has answered your prayers. Please give my regards to your mother and your friends at home. Please pray the prayer I sent you. Recite the prayer once a day for nine straight days making your petitions to the Lord God. I pray that you shall be rewarded very soon.

Check the *hierbería* or herb store for basil, rosemary, peppermint and boil them in water adding cinnamon sticks, coffee grounds and sugar. Bathe with this water for three straight days. I have listed a common prayer to the Niño Fidencio below. The Lord will answer your prayers through the intercession of the Niño Fidencio. Pray to Saint Bernadette, April 16 to save you from poverty and say the following prayer to El Niño Fidencio:

OH, POWERFUL SPIRIT OF FIDENCIO

Oh, powerful spirit of Fidencio, fill my heart full of contentment because you, with the power that God has given you will soften my suffering. I don't know how to respond to the love you have for those who ask for your protection.

Oh, miraculous Niño Fidencio, my language is very simple. I lack the words to express to you my gratitude and my love, but you that are so kind can see everything and know everything. You can see into my heart and see how much I love you. Look at me kneeling before you as an act of humility. I come to offer you repentance for all my faults with all my heart and to do all the good possible to my fellow man.

I confide in you and I await you, divine Niño. I offer you my heart as a sanctuary and my good works that I promise to do from here on, in your honor, for your spiritual progress. Give me your holy blessing and watch over me. Fill my heart full of fervor for your spiritual progress, I offer these three Our Fathers, may it be made so. Pray three Our Fathers.

It is recommended that this prayer be recited before the image of El Niño Fidencio, by placing a lit candle on your altar and a clear glass of water at the time you are petitioning spiritual work.

COMMENTARY:

Great faith compels persons to pray to a saint or folk saint for the saint's intercession with God and for there to be a favorable outcome for their petition. The saints and spirits must be propitiated with prayers and offerings. Many people suffer their entire lives from an assortment of problems with faith and prayer often their only available avenues to find solace. Additionally, it should be noted that our common prayers were first passed on orally, then, recorded in prayer books. Now, in the age of the Internet, these same prayers are transmitted electronically. Many prayers have been altered and have evolved as necessary for specific purposes. Curanderos have adapted prayers from a variety of religious traditions as they search for what is best for their followers.

7. NATIVE AMERICANS — *INDIOS AMERICANOS*

I have recently seen articles about El Niño Fidencio and am very much interested in his life and cures. I am a Native American and we have our own beliefs and they seem to be very similar to El Niño's. This is why it is very easy for Native Americans to embrace his powers.

I have been having a very hard time with my family, especially my daughters, and I feel that jealousy or ill will might make something bad happen to us. I pray for all my family and it seems that the more I pray, the more bad things interfere with our happiness. We smudge cedar in our home. Smudging is a belief of our fathers and their Native American medicine ways. This is how we rid our home of evil things. It needs to be done on a regular basis, too, because of unknown things that could follow you home.

I am asking that you keep us in your prayers.

Please note that smudging is the burning of sacred herbs such as sage, tobacco, or cedar, and using the smoke to clean the area, person or home of bad influences or spirits.

CURANDERO'S RESPONSE:

Thank you for your interest and your petition for prayer. We are interested in the healing spirits of light and other protectors. It is very probable that El Niño Fidencio was himself part Native American. We need to learn more about how all of the original peoples of the Americas are related and connected. We need to especially know more about Native American shamanism. We know very little.

In the Latino tradition, we burn incense to clear and clean our homes and family from negative and evil energies. We have to do that on a regular basis also. We take spiritual-healing baths, hold and partake of spiritual-healing rituals and cleansings to ward off evil spirits just like you do. We are more similar than we are different. I will most certainly pray for you. Did you know that Blessed Kateri Tekakwitha, an Algonquin/Mohawk was converted to Christianity by Jesuits near present day Quebec and is considered to be a patron saint of Native Americans and their connection to the Christian world? She is celebrated on July 14. You may also pray to Saint Turibius, March 29, who is also a patron saint of Native American populations.

COMMENTARY:

Before there was a border between the United States and Mexico, Native Americans lived and traveled freely across the border sharing their beliefs and practices. This is why Mexican curanderismo and Native-American practices are so alike. Today we witness a continual blending of practices and beliefs, especially in Latino curanderismo. It is not uncommon to see icons of Asian religions mixed with Native American and Afro-Caribbean beliefs all being practiced together. Please note that, the Bureau of Indian Affairs has attempted to persuade Native American tribal members, still living in Mexico, to return to reservations in the United States. They fled across the border in the 1800s to avoid bondage, enforced poverty and removal from their sacred ancestral homelands. In Mexico, they have intermarried with Latinos and other mixed Hispanic and Native Americans for over 200 years.

8. WE BELIEVE IN EL NIÑO — *CREEMOS EN EL NIÑO*

I see that you have been a Fidencista for many years. On your Internet page I see that you have given sessions, and have noticed that in the United States, the mentality of the people is very different from that of Mexico. In spite of the United States being a country that has liberty of belief, belief in the Niño Fidencio is seen by some to be a pagan rite or witchcraft. This includes some Catholic priests who accuse Fidencio of being a *brujo*, or a warlock.

Believe me; it makes me very sad that ignorant people who don't understand *Fidencismo* condemn us this way. I have met Catholic priests who do believe in the power of the Niño Fidencio, and, believe me; these priests are humble and take great care to spread the Gospel. They simply ignore those who condemn them. I have also noticed that there are Catholic priests who do not seem to have any vocation for the path they have chosen. Often, they take advantage of their positions for personal gains or worse.

You know that the path of the Niño is one of suffering, but it is also one of happiness, faith, hope and charity. Many, who do not understand *Fidencistas,* accuse us of believing that Fidencio is a god, but we know that is not true.

Many people give testimony about the miracles and cures they have received when all hope seemed lost. I know that we are nothing and that if we do this, it is because we feel this way and not to seek glory. We only seek to give thanks to God because He is the one doing the miracles not Fidencio. Fidencio is the messenger.

True believers, who are on the healing path of service through Fidencio, place their faith in the hands of God. We do this with great penance and suffering so that those who need His help will find it through the Niño Fidencio. There are those who abuse the path of the Niño and only exploit the people. The path of the Niño is one of humility and suffering and of never having enough for one's self. The path of the Niño is one of penance and great faith in God. Any person who seeks to follow the path of Fidencio must have great faith and devotion and, above all, must be humble and place all in the hands of God all powerful.

CURANDERO'S RESPONSE:

Everything you say is true. Liberty of belief does not come without liberty from criticism. I can also vouch that there is a Catholic priest who regularly attends the *fiestas* or pageants of the Niño Fidencio in Espinazo. On one occasion, three persons came to Espinazo; they presented themselves as Catholic priests and told us that a Catholic bishop sent them to gather information on the Niño Fidencio. Later the Catholic bishop of Saltillo, Coahuila, México actually journeyed to Espinazo to see for himself and praised the work of Fidencio.

The Niño also says that his path is full of thorns but at the same time satisfactory. Thank you for your writing and your friendship. Please, I invite you to continue to share your thoughts with this servant of God and the saintly Niño Fidencio. Your orations and his are always greatly appreciated. May God grant us permission to go forth and to suffer the weight of the Holy Cross, Santa Cruz, which we carry with devotion and sacrifice and offer up for the sins of man. Pray to San Martín de Porres celebrated on November 13 that he eliminates all discrimination from the world and especially from religious belief.

I offer you further greetings on behalf of the Fidencista hearts of North America, to all the Fidencista hearts of the Mexican republic. I remain always in prayer in the Spirit and love of our Lord and Creator of the universe and His servant the Niño Fidencio.

COMMENTARY:

This person is concerned about the evangelical church and the Catholic Church's intolerance of curanderos, in both the United States and Mexico. In reality, I have met many Catholic priests who are very tolerant and understanding of their flocks' cultural need to adhere to the beliefs and practices of their native folk saints and healing traditions. Recently, Catholic investigators visited Espinazo during the fiesta, collecting information on why their Catholic members have so much faith in El Niño Fidencio.

Additionally, the bishop of the Catholic Diocese of Saltillo, Coahuila, México has visited with the leader of the independent followers of Fidencio in Espinazo, Nuevo León. Many young Catholic priests, who are from native societies in Latin America and Africa, have incorporated healing rituals, and beliefs into their pastoral lives as priests in both Mexico and in the United States. They generally are not able to outwardly voice their beliefs and practices for fear of reprisals from their intolerant superiors.

9. HEALING MISSION — *MISIÓN DE CURACIÓN*

I am a Fidencista; we have our healing mission, with our own *materia*, or trance medium. I visit you once a year and I need to contact true Fidencistas like you here where I live. I have a small altar in my home in honor of the Niño Fidencio. I have great faith in him and am devoted to him. I have not been able to find many Fidencistas in my area so I feel alone and isolated. I go through moments of great loneliness because I don't have people to talk to who believe like me.

I thank God that I have no vices. But I am in a very bad way in my family relations. We have many debts, and now after once having had everything, I have nothing, not even my family left.

The Niñito has told me that there will be better times ahead. But I get desperate in my solitude and need a little money. What I earn is not enough to get me out of this situation. I have debts and my children distance themselves from me more and more. I pray to God and to Fidencito every day. I offer flowers and votive candles and yet I feel empty, without hope, with no desire or will to live.

I am a modest professional, but now I find myself in bankruptcy. I have not given up my desire to be successful. I am a Fidencista and as such I am a part of the family of *Fidencistas*. I love the Niñito and I plead to you for help.

CURANDERO'S RESPONSE:

There exist many thousands of true Fidencista followers. The popularity of the Niño Fidencio is concentrated in the states of northern Mexico, Nuevo León, Coahuila, Tamaulipas, and a few other places. Also, there are many Fidencistas in the United States, such as in Texas, California and throughout the Midwestern states. In your case, because it has gone bad for you with your family and you find no help from your *materia*, the medium of the Niño or from other Fidencistas, you must continue to pray and request three straight times by calling out the name of the Niño Fidencio in a crystal glass of water and soon he will help you. My friend, boil seven heads of garlic and take a bath with the water. Do this three straight times. I will light a votive candle on my altar for you. You will see, soon your fortune will turn around and your family will return to you.

COMMENTARY:

The Niño Fidencio movement is mainly located in the northeastern Mexican states and throughout the Mexican American population of the United States. Mexicans who have grown up in homes as followers of the Niño but have relocated to other areas of Mexico often cannot find practicing Fidencistas in their new communities. Followers from Mexico who live in the United States travel to Espinazo during the days of fiesta, and while there, they seek out Fidencista contacts in the states where they live. I have met many Fidencistas who live in the American Midwest or West and schedule their annual vacations to coincide with the Niño's fiestas in Mexico. *Knowing where the nearest Fidencista healing community is located is critical to their physical and emotional well being and health-support network.*

10. EL NIÑO ON THE INTERNET — *LA RED ESPIRITUAL*

Today I finally know that the spirit of the Niño Fidencito really exists. The truth is that my father is very ill and the doctors have already told him that there is no cure for him. He suffers from diabetic neuropathy. His nerves are shot and the diagnosis given by the doctors has no remedy. Through the Internet I have come to know the Niño Fidencio and also to know that you are his instrument that can heal persons.

I would like for you to help my father, and entrust all my heart to the Niño Fidencio. Is there is something my father can take since it is practically impossible for him to move around. Could you orient me to where the nearest Niño Fidencio healer is located because I would like to visit a healing mission, *misión de sanación*, as soon as possible?

I am grateful for your attention and in advance am very thankful to God and the Niño Fidencito. I have faith that my father will be healed.

CURANDERO'S RESPONSE:

I am glad that you have become aware of the Niño Fidencio. It could be that because of your faith and that of your father, through the Niño's mediation, God will grant your father a miracle. It has happened before. Thank God for giving us the healing Internet. I am very sorry for what has happened to your father. Even though his condition is irreversible, we must not lose faith; first God and then the Niño Fidencio will spiritually perform the cure he needs.

Also, maybe it would help your father to take herbs, including *matarique* and *tronador*, or a mixture of *mezquite*, *salvia* and lemon grass, or *zacate limón*. You can find these at your local herb store, *hierbería*. You mix them together in equal quantities. Mix one tablespoon of each herb in one cup of water. Boil the mixture and give your father one cup in the morning and another cup of the remedy after supper and let me know how he is doing in a couple of weeks.

COMMENTARY:

Today, young Latinos look to curanderismo for assistance with their problems more than ever before. This is primarily due to the fact that the health-care system does not provide for their cultural needs. This person writes that he is fearful about his father's health. The health-care system has written the father's life off. The fact that health care is difficult to access, combined with feelings of desperation and isolation, provokes persons to seek alternative health care modalities. Love for one's parents and concern for their well being enables them to contact curanderos for assistance. At the point that this family finds itself, faith and church and curanderismo are the only health-care alternatives available to them. It is significant and gratifying that this computer-literate petitioner has come to the Niño Fidencio via the Internet.

11. NIÑO'S HELPERS — *SUS AYUDANTES*

It has been a short time since I was chosen by my medium, or *materia*, to serve as the Niño's guardian while the *materia* is in trance. Since I have been appointed to this new and important position at my healing center, or *misión*, I am now collecting songs, or *alabanzas*, to Niño to sing during the healing ceremonies. I found one on your web page but I know that there are many more. We are very grateful that the *misión* of the Niñito extends to the United States and my only intention is to send you greetings and to ask for your help in finding more songs.

CURANDERO'S RESPONSE:

It is a great responsibility and a very necessary position of great importance to be chosen to be the guardian of the Niño Fidencio. As a missionary, the guardians can buy the Niño's spiritual music in Espinazo, Nuevo León, México, at the fiestas of the Niño. I will also help you as much as I am able to acquire the songs if you are not able to go to Espinazo.

Congratulations on having been placed as the guardian of the Niñito Fidencio. I am happy to know that there is still a desire in the people to study and learn about the spiritual path of the Niñito. It is a path of true love and spiritual surrender. It is an honor for believers and missionaries of the Niño to serve in positions of responsibility as guardians. It is a position of admiration for his faith and sacrifice that is required to give one's life to serve the Niño in his work for humanity.

There are a number of other items you will need to collect or make in order to help your *materia* set up her *misión*. These things can be made by hand and include a standard, or *estandarte*. The *estandarte* usually carries the name of your *misión,* its location, along with a very personalized and self-styled painting of the Niño or your *misión's* patron saint. The saint could be the Virgen de Guadalupe or the Santo Niño de Atocha or some other saint important to your healing *misión*.

Your flag or *bandera*, will usually be the tri-colors of the Mexican flag, green, red and white formed in a rectangle measuring approximately eight feet long by four feet wide. Finally, you will need an official registration book which carries all of the names and addresses of your membership along with any special office they might hold. This book becomes the official record of your *misión*. The Niño's very first *misiones* have standards, flags and books which date back to the 1920s. They are greatly protected and passed on from one generation of followers to the next in sacred ceremonies.

I pray that God and the Holy Spirit spread over you and your little group His charity and satisfaction of joy and happiness in song to the Niño Fidencio as he performs his treatments and miracles.

COMMENTARY:

Each trance medium or materia of the Niño Fidencio has a hierarchy of assistants beginning with the primary called a guardia or vigilant assistant. Since the materia is in trance during the healing session, the guardia is responsible for protecting and watching over the materia and assisting with whatever material elements the Niño requests. This includes writing down the receta or prescription that the Niño orders be taken. Since the trance medium will remember nothing that transpired during the spiritual healing session the primary assistant also plays the role of communicating to the medium any spiritual messages and other items of importance that might have transpired during the session. It is not uncommon for spiritual-healing sessions to last 12 hours or more.

Also, there usually is another helper in charge of leading the singing by smaller groups of followers present at both the beginning and conclusion of the healing session. Sometimes the same individual performs both tasks. All of the traditional Fidencista songs are available from other Fidencista groups or over the Internet for use by newly-formed healing centers. However, in most cases songs and rituals have been passed down from older Fidencistas to the next generation when they have proven that they are ready to serve faithfully.

Many of the older colonial Mexican towns and villages maintain socio-religious traditions or cargo cults in which there is an expectation that the sacred items associated with the town's patron saint are protected for one year by a person or family. Service to the confraternity or *cofradía* carries great honor in the town and is directly related to social and political status. The head of the activities for a year is often called the *mayordomo*, an honorific title harkening back to colonias days but still very important. The servants of the saint will take him out on his saint's day and show him his town or *rodearlo*. There will be processions or a *procesión* in which the saint is carried on the shoulders of the faithful from barrio to barrio and from sanctuaries to *santuario*. Each sanctuary is considered a mystical place or *lugar místico*.

The procession is intended to show the saint his town, for there to be a spiritual walk or *caminata* so that the saint or patron can enjoy seeing how much progress has been made by the faithful in the town and to allow those seeking miracles or performing penance or *penitencias* to complete their *promesa* or promise.

12. WAITING FOR A BLESSING — *ESPERANDO SU BENDICIÓN*

I bought my wife the Cross of Caravaca to wear around her neck and to protect her from harm, but now she says that it makes her face tingle at work. She thinks that it is doing something bad to her. We are waiting for a blessing from the Niño Fidencio and his holy helpers. I need your blessed help and that of the Niño Fidencito to look after my wife. At her work there are two persons who make her ill when they approach her. We think they are pure evil. Please help us to fight off their evil influence.

Also, I feel very bad and have a lot of back pain. It seems as if I have a thorn in my back and my feet burn a lot as well. I think I have picked up some witchcraft somewhere. I await your help, so that God may bless us. I feel that these two evil people are performing dark works on our humble, simple little family. We need you and Niñito to protect us from evil and to save our souls.

CURANDERO'S RESPONSE:

The Cross of the Caravaca, *Cruz de Caravaca*, is known to be miraculous and has the grace to flow light, love, health, power, protection, luck with money and peace for those who wear it on their body and who have great faith in its powers.

This reliquary cannot be tolerated by an impious spirit. It protects the person who wears it around their neck and will literally repel evil by throwing it backwards and away from the bearer. This is the case with your wife whose face tingles when she wears the cross around her neck. This is a powerful sign that there is an impious spirit in the body of the two people you fear.

I hope that the spiritual treatments will exorcise her body, soul, and save the life of your wife. I think that it is possible that these evil people have also caused an impious spirit to surround your wife's body.

However, these bad spirits are weakened by the power of the cross. In order to help her, you must boil the herbs *tumba vaquero*, *peonía* and *salvia* together and she is to take one cup of tea in the morning and another at night for seven straight days. This is to remove all the fluids that enable the spirits that persist in attacking her and which are attempting to live in her. Please advise me on how she is doing. Meanwhile, please pray Psalm 135 to live an honorable and protected life.

COMMENTARY:

In this situation, the petitioner refers to a common amulet called the Cross of Caravaca. Believers in curanderismo and spiritism commonly wear the Cross of Caravaca around their necks. The curandero recommended the petitioner's purchase of the amulet for his wife in order to protect her at work. The necklace produces a tingling in her face which leads the curandero to believe that it is a sign the amulet is performing its spiritual duty. The curandero has to reassure the petitioner that it is doing its job. The co-workers are envious of her and this has introduced an unclean spirit into her body or empowered an evil aura to enshroud her.

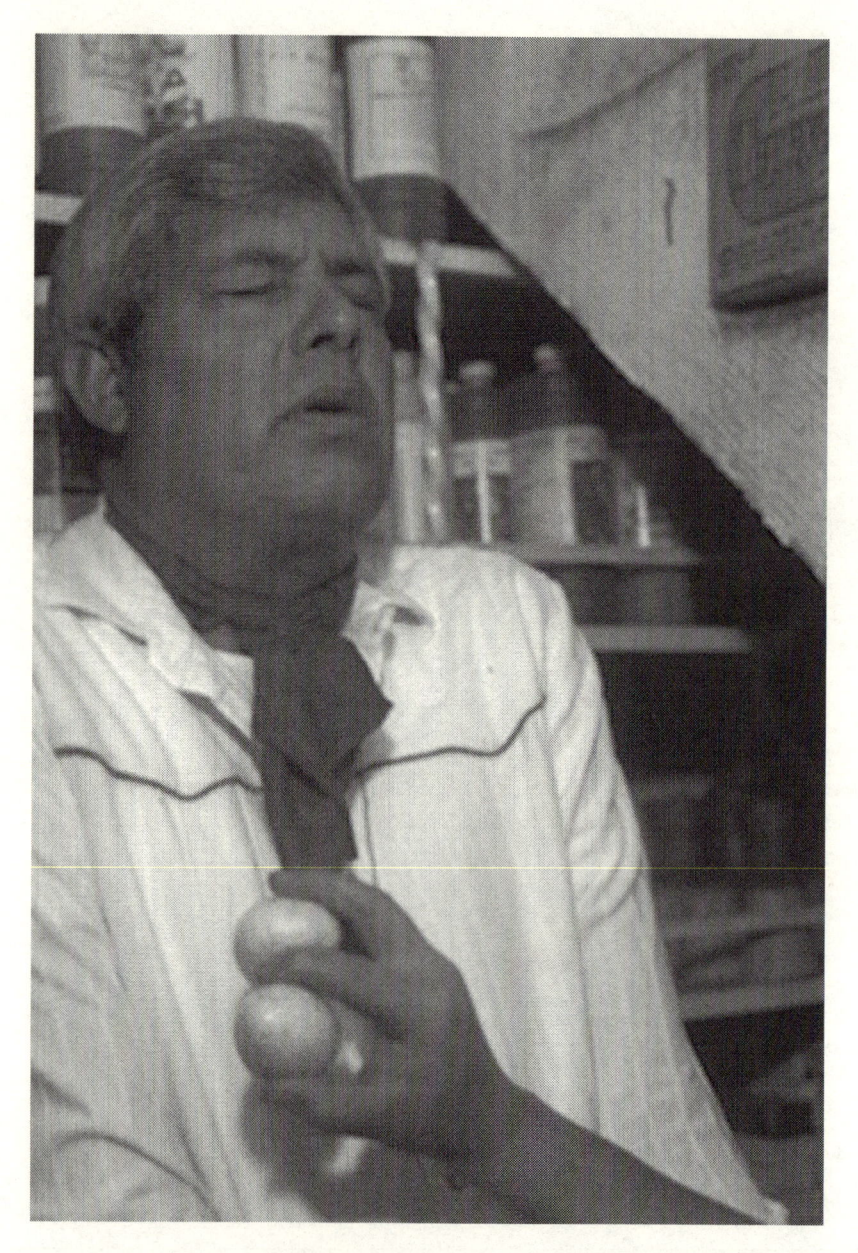

Author and *curandero* Alberto Salinas Jr. receives a spiritual cleansing or limpia with live turtle eggs at the Mercado Sonora in Mexico City. (Photo José M. Duarte)

PART THREE
CURANDERISMO:
The Healing Arts and Sciences

"Curanderismo is alive, and lives in the hearts, and in the minds and in the souls of our people. Curanderismo lives in our dreams and in our memories, and in the messages we receive from our parents and our grandparents who have gone before us."

—***Alberto Salinas Jr., curandero***

13. THE SPECIALISTS — *LOS ESPECIALISTAS*

I am writing to you because I found the El Niño Fidencio Curanderismo Research Project on the Internet and it is just what I have been looking for. I am a Latina high-school student and I have chosen to write my senior paper on *curanderismo* because I am told that long ago my great-grandmother was a *curandera*. I have always had this interest in the back of my mind like the spirit of my great-grandmother is urging me to find out about it. One of my aunts even says that I have her "gift." I have found a lot of material on the Internet but could you please help me by explaining how many different kinds of *curanderas* there are? Please respond as soon as possible because my paper is due in a couple of weeks. Thank you.

CURANDERO'S RESPONSE:

There are many different kinds of *curanderos/as*. Many are specialists in certain areas just like doctors. For example, the *sobador/a*, is a folk-massage therapist, and an expert in realigning bundles of nerves that can cause tremendous pain throughout the body and affected area. While not generally thought of as a *curandera*, persons who have the gift and ability to work with their hands are highly valued in a culture which has historically performed physical labor. The *sobador/sobadora* may also have other functions such as bonesetter, or *huesero/a*. Bone setting is, for all practical purposes, a lost art since emergency room treatment for broken bones is readily available most places.

There are many other specialties in *curanderismo*. *Hierberos/as*, or herbalists, are persons who identify the medicinal plants of the countryside, or *campo*, and know of their preparation and use. Specialists in this area gather and dry the plants and in some cases prepare *compuestos* or herbal mixtures very much like a pharmacist would before the advent of preprepared or patent medicine called *medicina de patente*. In fact, the folk pharmacy is called the *hierbería* or *botánica*. As in modern pharmacies, *hierberías* now sell a wide variety of items including, but not limited to, fresh herbs. Many medicinal plants used by our people are still very popular and are easily found in the mainstream grocery stores where there is a large Latino population.

There are lengthy catalogues containing the material sold in *hierberías* or the *materia medica* needed for the modern practice of *curanderismo*.

The naturalist, or *naturista*, is a modern term for the specialist who practices healing using all natural ingredients and is the modern form of the *hierbera*, or herbal specialist. Naturalists are often found in cities and practice right alongside medical doctors.

Another very important specialist is the midwife or *partera*. Midwifery is an ancient art and one that is highly revered and practiced in Mexico as well as other Latin American countries and throughout the world. For example, in Mexico, *parteras* were trained and licensed long before it was popular in the United States. This is why unsuspecting women from Mexico often seek midwives or *parteras* in the United

States expecting that they have the same training when they often do not.

Other important subdivisions of *curanderismo* include healers who only work with physical or material items; they are said to work *materialmente*. They include, for example, the *hierbera, sobadora* and *partera* who work with their folk knowledge and with physical items like creams, salves, and oils using their hands.

There are, however, *curanderas* who work on a higher plane, or with their minds, these are often called *mentalistas*.

Curanderas/mentalistas will concentrate their gaze on an object like a crystal ball; bowl of clear water or a religious icon and in their concentrated state of consciousness will look or "see" into the life of a questioner. Often they seem to be in a trance and are silent for a time; they "return" to consciousness with an answer or with a recommendation from the spirit world.

Ocultista is another term and form of *curanderismo*. Like the naturalist, *ocultista* is a modern term for a person who practices the hidden or esoteric arts, hence the use of the term occult or unseen. The different terms vary from region to region and from city to countryside.

Curanderas never think of themselves as *ocultistas,* although in the cities the term is not uncommon. Another practice of *curanderas* is to work spiritually, and, hence, the term *espiritista*. The *espiritista* is actually a trance medium who, while in a trance state, works with or brings down a spirit. The medium channels the spirit of a once-living entity which speaks and acts through the medium to bring about the healing through consultation with the spirit.

The term shaman is also well known and is used to refer to a native or indigenous healer. All shamans are healers, but not all healers are shamans. Shamanism is often associated with altered realities and supernatural states of consciousness. Basically, shamanism and *curanderismo* are similar and have very similar practices. Shamanism is a term adopted by anthropologists to describe medicine men and women in Native American and other populations. Both shamanism and *curanderismo* incorporate the material culture and the spirituality of native beliefs. It doesn't matter where the native people or cultures come from. Shamanistic beliefs are universal in the human population.

I have been very fortunate to meet and get to know, and even work with many shamans from many diverse North and Meso-American cultures during my career as a *curandero*.

There is basically no difference in the two terms and the practices of one are common to the practices and beliefs of the other. One of my closest companions is a Huichol shaman elder I met from the Mexican state of Jalisco. I met him on a spiritual journey to Real de Catorce in the Mexican state of San Luis Potosí about 20 years ago. He has taught me quite a lot, including the art of the *temazcal* sweat lodge, and how to conduct a *peyote mitote*. Both are healing rituals.

In Latin American culture, the card reader is a very important category of folk practitioner. A card reader is said to throw the cards or the *baraja*, usually they use the Spanish tarot deck. There are many different styles of card spreads and traditions which date back a thousand years. The more modern card readers are usually found in urban areas and may use the European tarot deck like the well known Rider-Waite deck while the more traditional card readers in the Latino community almost always use the Spanish tarot deck.

This form of divination called cartomancy, or card reading, continues to be extremely popular and pervasive in the Latin community today. Most card readers do not think of themselves as *curanderas,* while some may actually operate in both realms.

Just as there is a God and a devil, just as there is good and evil, there are persons who practice both good and evil traditions. Generally speaking, we think of *curanderas* as persons who aid their communities and who therefore do "good."

Curanderas, generally work in one of the traditions at a time. Good is said to be performed by using the right hand. However, there are those who are dedicated to the traditions and forces of evil and some are said to work with the left hand, and are considered sinister. Some work with both sides, good and evil. When this occurs they usually keep these practices separate from one another. They operate in different spaces or places, on different days and at different hours of practice. Doing witchcraft cannot be mixed with good.

In every Latino community, both practitioners of good and evil exist and are often active against each other; carrying on wars, *curanderas* vs. *brujas*, healers vs. witches, for decades. We call the people who practice witchcraft and whose job is to harm people or to make them sick, *brujos/as* or warlocks or witches.

Brujas, or witches, fall into many categories. *Brujas* may use completely indigenous traditions gleaned from active native groups in Mexico or other places. Or they may use traditions that have been popularized by mixing the ancient with the modern and the Eastern with the Western traditions.

Active in the country today, are many varieties of cults which have grown out of these traditions including satanic cults or devil-worshiping cults such as the ones with their origin in Catemaco, Veracruz. While cults are not a familiar part of Latino culture, recently notable sub-cultures have sprung up surrounding both real and imagined folk figures.

Most notable is the recent popularity of La Santísima Muerte in Latino culture. Sub-cultures and cults are generally regionalized and surround a popular folk figure, such as Malverde, Pancho Villa, Juan Soldado, and many others.

Curandero specialists no longer commonly include the tooth puller, or *sacamuelas,* the person who specialized in sucking out illnesses, or *soplador;* the enlightened healer or *alumbrada*; the *algebrista/huesero* or bonesetter; the *sangradora* or bleeder; and the person who prayed illness away or *ensalmador*. All of these specializations are included in today's common term of *curandero*.

COMMENTARY:

Where do curanderismo and popular religions emanate? In his book, The Church in the Barrio, Roberto Treviño states in speaking about the origin of what he calls "ethno-religion," and quotes from the work of Roberto Goizueta,

"The Mexican Americans in Texas and in the Southwest carried on this ethno-religion that, in the spirit of its medieval and Indian roots, made room for faith healing and other practices deemed superstitious by clergy; favored saint veneration, home altar worship, and community-centered religious celebration that blurred the line between the sacred and the secular. These are all important practices of curanderismo. Ethno-religious rites tended to simultaneously and selectively participate in institutional Catholic Church practices, yet hold the Church at arm's length. Ethno-Catholicism was essentially countercultural, as it represented an organic, holistic worldview...at odds with post-Enlightenment notions of time and space, of the material and the spiritual, and of the person's place within time and space, within the material and spiritual dimensions of reality." (p. 4-5)

For example, Saints Damian and Cosme are regarded as the patron saints of pharmacy and medicine and are celebrated on September 26.

The first Europeans in Mexico encountered a culture that was a syncretism or mixture of medical and religious beliefs that has passed down to curanderismo. Curanderos of today's America are not only lost in space and time, they are the agents of its interpretation. The male healer is the curandero and the female healer is the curandera. Curanderismo is a term coined by researchers and those who study curanderos/as. It refers to the practice or the art of folk healing in the Latino community. The curandero's response outlines the many specializations and practices that are ordinarily categorized under the title of curanderismo. The El Niño Fidencio Curanderismo Research Project web page is http://vpea.utb.edu/elnino/fidencio.html.

This website is the most extensive one currently on the Internet dealing with curanderismo and the phenomena of the Niño Fidencio movement and it contains articles, links and an extensive bibliography.

There is a new generation of Latinos and others, who want and need to know about the world of the curandero. If not for Alberto Salinas Jr.

and others like him who have a calling to teach, the esoteric information on curanderismo would be lost for ensuing Latino generations.

Ancient and modern books have documented through literature and votive paintings that the stock in trade of curanderos/as has changed only slightly since the arrival of Europeans in Latin America. Each curandero has his or her spiritual tool kit or herramienta espiritual. In her book, Pestilence and Headcolds: Encountering Illness in Colonial Mexico, *Sherry Fields states, "This is the world of the sick-room, both a physical space abounding with strange tonics and brews, bleedings and leeches, curanderas and barber-surgeons, and saints and virgins, as well as a cultural space complete with its own structures of meaning." Today, little has changed in the healing room of the curanderos/as of the borderlands.*

In Mexico, as everywhere else, there were always those who practiced the healing arts outside of the law. In colonial Mexico they were called intruders or intrusos. To an extent, this still exists today with many persons pretending to practice curanderismo while knowing little or nothing about it.

Cultural Competency: *This book contains material on the importance of the incorporation of cultural understanding in the health-care delivery system. Called cultural competency, this material is intended for training use from the clinic waiting room to the boardroom. Cultural competency resources number 1 and 2 in Appendix I, provide the reader with information on understanding the role that culture plays in the delivery of health care, the most important resource websites and bibliographic material.*

Resource material: *Many of the 190 questions, answers and commentaries in this book have Internet links and web page references for further study listed in Appendix II.*

14. THE FOLK PHARMACY — *HIERBERÍA -BOTÁNICA*

What is a *hierbería*, also spelled *yerbería*, all about? I am not Latino but I am married to a Latina. In the spring we moved to our new home near the Canadian border and in the winter we live in south Texas on the Mexican border. I have asked my wife several times about her visits to places called *hierberías*. Each time all she would tell me is that I would not understand. She doesn't want to recognize that I understand more about Latino culture and folk ways than she knows and that I would like to learn more.

I see some similarities and some differences between these *hierberías* she visits. I also notice that she always goes to these places after she has spoken to her mother or her sister on the phone. In some of these places they have card readers or fortune tellers who do readings for a fee. Most have herbal remedies of all kinds. Some stores seem to have all sorts of religious items such as candles and saint's prayer cards. I see these places everywhere we go in Latino communities, whether they are in Chicago or in the Rio Grande Valley of Texas. Some of these businesses carry *piñatas* and all kinds of Mexican products and curios of all sorts.

I see different cultural items such as medallions, candles, oils, perfumes, amulets, talismans, powders, spiritual lotions, potions, some alleged to have divine, magical, mystical or some kind of cosmic power. Some of these products sold at these *hierberías* raise many questions in my mind. In some of these stores I can't help but notice that the lady death or Santísima Muerte seems to be a very popular item these days. I have seen some products that are alleged to do good things and others that seem to be meant to do harm.

Just the other day, we went to this *hierbería* where they had a person my wife said was called a *curandero*. My wife said she needed a ritual cleaning or *limpia* ritual done on her. She and the *curandero* went into a room in the rear of the store where she says she had a consultation with him and that he performed the cleansing ritual on her.

In researching *hierberías* and *curanderos* on the Internet, I came across your website. Can you help me better understand what these places are, what their purpose is and what *curanderos* are, so that I may better understand that part of my wife's culture which I know so little about?

CURANDERO'S RESPONSE:

Historically and traditionally, *hierberías* started out being a place where freshly-picked medicinal and cooking herbs and spices would be purchased. *Curanderos/as* often give their clients a written prescription, or *receta*, to take to the *hierbería* to be filled. All medicinal and cooking plants were useful in the cultural home. Home remedies with the power to heal have been in the market places as trade products since ancient times. The original term in English for the pharmacy is apothecary, and in Spanish it's *botica*. The patron saint of the art and practice of pharmacy is Gemma, celebrated on April 11.

Mankind has a natural ability to evolve in infinite ways and throughout history has addressed life's ills, adversities, problems, situations and issues. The herbalist, or *hierbera*, is a specialist in the knowledge of healing herbs. Religion has always been associated with the healing arts and so it is common to find religious items of all faiths and different cultural beliefs in these important folk pharmacies. Ideologies based on the concept of good and evil and even the concept of the alleged power, both positive and negative, of the Santísima Muerte have found their ways into the modern *hierbería*.

Today's *hierberías* started out as small herb stands and have evolved into major Internet businesses. Additionally, because the *hierbería*, like any other business, is market driven, the items of material culture have mixed and combined distinct ideas. The reason for this is to produce remedies for the human condition with solutions to complex questions. This consists of persistent and annoying life problems with the *hierberías* offering spiritual options, and, sometimes, answers.

I thank you for your question. I get called on for my services as a *curandero* from many diverse ethnic groups and cultures. My clients are many different types of people walking on many different life paths. As a *curandero*, I have come to learn that the more I am able to understand my fellow man's cultural ways, the better I am able to live a life of service to others. You are doing well in trying to better understand your Latina wife's ways. I'm sure you care deeply for her. Let her know how much you love her. She will trust you more and will eventually confide more in you. Right now she is afraid that you will ridicule her beliefs. When she realizes that you will not, she will open up to you. You may not have been raised with the same cultural values that she was raised with but that should not matter. With increased love and trust between you, and with a willingness to understand each other, you will move in the right direction toward understanding and a happy future together.

Antonio Zavaleta and Alberto Salinas Jr.

COMMENTARY:

The indigenous peoples of the world have ancient traditions which identify the use of medicinal plants. The study of medicinal plants is so ancient that the Holy Bible lists approximately 60 plants used for medicines and spices, and all play roles in Latino culture. Sixteenth-century Catholic priests brought the biblical plants to the new world and incorporated them into clerical practice and rituals. These plants are listed in the border herbal in Appendix III. Additionally, all of the esoteric and magical materials that are used by the diverse practices and beliefs of Latinos are available through Internet-based hierberías and botánicas.

In her book, Fields points out that the concept of the pharmacy, or botica, is one that pre-dates the arrival of the Spaniards. They licensed and regulated them in 17th century Mexico. The pharmacist, or boticario, held a position of high esteem in the community, and was the "only establishment that was licensed to sell the public ready-made medicines or have a physician's prescription filled. The first Roman Catholic priests in Mexico regarded a certain representation of Mary the mother of God depicted as Madonna and Child as Our Lady of Pharmacy. This representation is believed to have had a German origin. In colonial Mexico, pharmacists were required to demonstrate a solid knowledge of the medicinal properties of several hundred plants, animals and minerals." (p. 61)

Today's curandero/a, retains ancient medical and esoteric knowledge, but on a much smaller scale. The oldest-known Aztec manuscript documenting an herbal in 16th century Mexico lists 251 plants while Sahagún, who studied folk medicine in colonial Mexico, identified 225 medicinal plants used by the Aztecs. Interestingly, the two lists contain fewer than 20 duplicates placing the total Aztec herbal at close to 500 medicinal plants. (Alarcón, p.29)

The Border Herbal: The vast amount of information in Appendix III is culled from literally hundreds of sources. The herbal provides the reader with the most commonly used medicinal plants on the border with English names Spanish names, and Latin names, and their uses. It is important for the reader to note that this material is provided as a resource and definitely not intended for medical use without a physician's supervision.

15. SPIRITS AND FOLK SAINTS — *SANTOS POPULARES*

You hear about so many different spirits and folk saints these days. I have trouble keeping them all straight. Who is who and which ones are good or bad? Can you help me understand all these spirits and entities and who and what they are?

CURANDEROS RESPONSE:

There have always been saints in the Catholic Church and there have always been folk saints like Pedrito Jaramillo, Santo Niño de Atocha and El Niño Fidencio. The saints of the church are tried and true and the primary folk saints are also known to be spirits of light. Recently, a whole new group of folk entities and spirits have appeared, that are popular in the media and at *hierberías*, and that is why you are confused.

The most popular folk saint and the most dangerous is La Santísima Muerte, or Holy Death. Others you see and hear about are Malverde, Juan Soldado, Pancho Villa, Maximón, Indios, gypsies, doctors and many others who are regarded as popular saints, or *santos populares*. The Niño Fidencio is generally regarded as a good folk saint of healing and basic human needs. My advice to you is not to get caught up in the cult, or *culto*, of regional folk saints and stick to what you know is good and time honored. Pray to Saint John Mary Vianney, August 4, that the Catholic Church and especially Catholic priests open their minds to the importance of understanding and tolerating multicultural beliefs. Santa Mónica, August 27, is often invoked to enlighten Catholics and to bring them back to the Catholic Church. Ask Santa Teresa de Ávila, October 15, to fill them with the grace of the Holy Spirit.

COMMENTARY:

Intense faith in folk saints is seen through belief that the spirits of the saints may be channeled, or "brought down" to earth by a trance medium for a consultation or consulta. Loyal followers maintain long-term meaningful relationships with the popularized folk saints; celebrating their birthdays and affectionately calling them by their first names in the diminutive. For example, El Niño Fidencio becomes Niñito and Saint Michael the Archangel becomes Miguelito, or little Michael. In addition to saints, invocations are recited over magical and/or supernatural entities such as *duendes*, or forest elves, and mythical spirits such as La Llorona, the weeping woman. Invoking child-spirit helpers is another common practice found in curanderismo, and includes the lost child or *niño perdido*, Aurorita, Tomasito, as well as many others.

The curandero wisely advises the questioner to stay away from many of the most recently-appearing entities and folk saints since they are usually associated with sub-cultural groups that these curiosity seekers might not understand. While his intent may be honorable, praying to these spirits could cause them great harm or put them in touch with persons who are unsavory or have bad intentions.

Many people in northern Mexico and south Texas have grown up in families where faith in folk saints like the Niño Fidencio is strong, such as faith in the Virgen de Guadalupe. Ordinary folks across the countryside assign popular sainthood, or *santificación popular*, to favored miracle workers, thaumaturge, or *taumaturgos*. This is perfectly normal since their faith fits into the parallel world of folk religion which is juxtaposed with institutional religion. As such, their faith and devotion to the Niño is comparable to Catholic saints and they most often claim to be Catholics. Often, innocent people are surprised to learn that faith in the Niño Fidencio is not recognized by the Catholic Church.

Acceptance of spirits and the supernatural is rooted in hundreds of years of tradition by Native American groups in Latin America combined with medieval Catholic beliefs and rituals brought from Europe. In today's practice of curanderismo, the traditions of Europe and the Americas have been combined and mixed with those from Africa and Asia in what is called syncretism.

16. LITURGICAL HOLY DAYS — *EL SANTORAL*

I regularly attend a Niño Fidencio healing center in my town and I am also a practicing Catholic. I have never had a problem doing both, although some of my friends don't understand what I believe. I cannot help but notice that *curanderos/as* celebrate many of the same holy days, saints' days and other liturgical *fiestas*, which we celebrate in my parish. It is mostly Mexican people where I go to church.

I'm interested in knowing more about the yearly cycle of celebrations in the church and that *curanderos/as* recognize, as well.

CURANDERO'S RESPONSE:

As a *curandero*, I am also a Catholic. I know that some people can't accept that, and some Catholic priests I know turn their backs on me. However, others support my healing mission completely and accept what I do. I believe that Catholicism and *curanderismo,* are two sides of the same coin, but sometimes narrow-minded people can't see that. As far as I know, the only *curandero/a* practice that the Church cannot accept, is spirit channeling. But spirit channeling is just a very small facet of what we do, and every spirit could be considered a variant of the Holy Spirit.

I have done my best to list below all of the special dates and saints' days that I consider to be important in what I do. You can see that most of these dates are Catholic saints' days or church holy days, in addition to *curanderismo.*

I hope this helps you. All I can say is don't let the beliefs of man keep you from opening your heart to the Holy Spirit in whatever form He appears.

Curandero's saints' days or the *Curandero's Santoral*

January	1	New Year's Day
January	6	Feast of the Epiphany and the Three Kings, or Reyes Magos
January	7	Saint Anthony Abad, or San Antonio Abad
Feb.	2	Candlemas or Candelaria
Feb.	14	Saint Valentine or San Valentín
Feb.	25	Ash Wednesday, or Miércoles de Cenizo (date varies)
March	4	Saint Casimir, San Casimiro

March	19	Saint Joseph, or San José as well as Fiesta del Niño Fidencio
March	21	Spring Equinox
March		Holy Week, or Semana Santa (flexible date)
April	25	Saint Mark, or San Marcos
May	1	Saint Joseph the Worker, or San José Obrero
May	3	The Holy Cross, or Santa Cruz also Jesús Malverde
May	15	Saint Isadore, or San Isidro Labrador
May	28	Saint Justice, or San Justo
June	5	Birth of Pancho Villa
June	13	Saint Anthony of Padua, or San Antonio de Padua
June	24	Saint John the Baptist, or San Juan Bautista
Also baths of San Juan the Summer Solstice and Juan Soldado		
June	29	Saint Peter and Paul, or San Pedro y San Pablo
July	3	Death of Don Pedrito Jaramillo
July	16	The Virgin of Carmen, or La Virgen del Carmen
July	8	Saint Elias the Prophet, San Elías el Profeta
July	14	Saint Camilo of the Sick, San Camilo de los Enfermos
July	15	Saint Bonaventure, San Buenaventura
July	22	Saint Mary Magdalene, Santa María Magdalena
July	25	Saint James, or Santiago
July	31	Saint Ignatius of Loyola, San Ignacio de Loyola
August	8	The Feast of the Assumption
August	11	Saint Clare, Santa Clara

August	16	San Roque
Sept.	8	The Virgin of Remedies, or La Virgen de los Remedios
Sept.	11	Saint Patient or San Paciente
Sept.	15	The Virgin of Pain, or La Virgen de Dolores
Sept.	24	Our Mother of Mercy, or Nuestra Señora de la Merced
Sept.	29	The Archangels, Arcángel San Miguel
Oct.	2	All Guardian Angels, or Ángeles de la Guarda
Oct.	4	San Francisco as well as Niño Fidencio and Fall Equinox
Oct.	28	Saint Jude or San Judás Tadeo
Nov.	2	Day of the Dead, or Día de los Muertos/La Santa Muerte
Nov.	3	Saint Martin of Porres, or San Martín de Porres
Nov.	15	Saint Albert the Magus, or San Alberto Mago
Nov.	27	Our Lady of the Miracle, or Señora de la Medalla Milagrosa
Dec.	8	Immaculate Conception of Health, or La Virgen de Salud
Dec.	12	The Virgin of Guadalupe, or La Virgen de Guadalupe
Dec.	16	The Posadas and Pastorelas begin
Dec.	24	Christmas Eve or Noche Buena/Winter Solstice
Dec.	25	Christmas Day
Dec.	31	New Year's Eve

COMMENTARY:

Loyal followers of Catholicism and its alternate form, folk Catholicism, recognize that there is a hard-and-fast liturgical calendar. The term folk Catholicism refers to the pseudo-religious beliefs, culturally-based beliefs and rituals that are practiced by the people but not sanctioned by the Catholic Church. Year in and year out, the religious seasons and holidays, saints' days and other special days are celebrated with common prayers, practices and rituals by both the Catholic Church and by curanderos/as. Regardless if one is in the church or in the home of the curandero/a, the practices are the same. This fact unites the two traditions in the minds of the faithful.

"Saints were patrons of various diseases, illness frequently took on moral tones, and medical books customarily included enormous numbers of prayers, novenas, and religious tracts for preventing and curing disease" (Guerra 1969:183). While not all curanderos/as do follow the traditional santoral or church liturgical calendar today, it is coming back into favor by the younger generation which wants to do things the way their grandparents did.

Through the centuries many of the Catholic saints have developed traditions, rituals and cult followings. In her book, Fields states, "in January 1737, procesiones and novenarios to various divine images were made through the streets of Mexico City. To ask for relief from the fiery epidemic that people are suffering from in this kingdom. The Mexican cult of saints has origins in the pilgrimage traditions practiced in medieval Europe" (See pages 80-81). The same traditions practiced in colonial Mexico are practiced by our curanderos/as today.

17. THE FOLK PSYCHIATRIST — *EL CURA MENTES*

I want to thank you for all you have done for me. You have been counseling me for two years now and with your help I have been able to lead a mostly normal life. I was diagnosed with paranoid schizophrenia when I was a teenager and for years I was not able to attend school or function normally, to hold a job or to have a lasting relationship.

My mother turned to spirituality in order to help me and eventually we were referred to you for help. Even though I take my prescription medications and see a therapist regularly, it was not until I began coming to you for counseling that I was able to keep my mental illness in check. My illness will never leave me but I know that you are protecting me from the evil spirits which surround me. Even though this torment will be with me for the rest of my life, through your support and prayers I am able to live. I thank you so much for always being there for me and for protecting me.

CURANDERO'S RESPONSE:

I thank you for your testimonial and have enjoyed knowing you and helping you during the past two years. Your stability has been remarkable and it should continue as long as you take your medication, see your therapist and place your faith in God. Together we have built a wall of spiritual protection which surrounds you, and your guardian angels will watch over you and keep you from evil. Continue your prayers and always have a candle burning on your home altar. This way you will maintain an impenetrable circle of protection around you.

COMMENTARY:

It is very clear to the reader that the curandero/a provides an important safety net to those who require an ongoing, and sometimes lifelong, cultural component in their treatment. Published in 1968, Ari Kiev's book Curanderismo: Folk Psychiatry was one of the first studies to deal with curanderismo in a systematic and scientific manner using experiences from a clinical setting. As a psychiatrist who worked in the San Antonio area for many years, Kiev theorized that a large percentage of cases presented to curanderos/as were directly tied to emotional, psychological and psychiatric issues. Today curanderismo remains an intriguing mixture of the spiritual, physical and emotional issues and remedies that all people face in the human condition. It is fair to say that curanderismo fills a void in the Latino culture where psychological and psychiatric counseling are not available in the same way we associate a society of insurance-covered, mental health care access.

It is advised that anyone working in the mental health area and who requires an appropriate diagnosis reference should consult Appendix I: Outline for Cultural Formulation and Glossary of Culture-Bound Syndromes, (pp. 897-903), of the Diagnostic and Statistical Manual of

Mental Disorders, Fourth Edition, Text Revision DSM-IV-TR, published by the American Psychiatric Association, 2000.

There is an ancient history in the Catholic Church, both in Europe and in colonial Mexico, concerning the origins and treatment of mental illness. It was commonly believed that a person's illness was caused by a misdeed or an act against God or a saint.

There are several Catholic saints who are patrons of the behaviorally and mentally ill. Saint Anthony is regarded as the patron of nervous disorders while Saint Cyriacus is the patron of mental disease. Saint Dymphna, is celebrated on May 15th and is generally considered the patron for the insane.

18. HOME REMEDIES — *REMEDIOS CASEROS*

Hi! I am a college student working on a project and my mother gave me your e-mail address so I could ask for your help. I am in an anthropology class and I am working with a team of students. Our class project is to re-create a list of household items and substances that the old *curandera* who lived in our neighborhood and our grandmothers and great-grandmothers used to heal us with when we were ill. That is, in a time when there were no pharmacies. My part of our project is to construct a list of things that our Mexican and Mexican American mothers used back in the day. Please let me hear from you.

CURANDERO'S RESPONSE:

Many people, not just Latinos, remember the old *curandero/a* home remedies our grandmothers used to use when the family was sick. The list is lengthy but here are the ones that I still use today that I know were also used in the old days: vapor rub; camphor; iodine; merthiolate; mercurochrome; fresh hen's eggs; lemons; alum rock; candles of all kinds; freshly cut herbs from the yard; castor oil; spider web; mineral oil; olive oil; cod liver oil; salt; sugar; fresh honey; laxatives; *piloncillo*; purgative; hot water bottle; soaps; *jabón de barra* or *jabón de la paloma*; *amarillo* or *blanco*; volcanic; *linimento blanco*; kerosene; rubbing alcohol; *parche Guadalupano*; ipecac; *cataplasma*; vinegar; chicken soup and broths; aspirin; sulfur; gentian violet; *estropajo*; three roses brilliantine; *agua florida*; lard or *manteca de puerco* or *manteca de coyote*; elixirs; tonics; ash or *ceniza;* incense; tobacco; ammonia; and pine oil for disinfecting. I am sure there are some I have left out, but this is a basic list.

COMMENTARY:

There are many websites where you can look up home remedies from a multitude of diverse cultures. It is remarkable how similar our health needs are, and therefore how similar our healing traditions also are. Grandma always knew how to settle an upset stomach. The curandero has listed the majority of those items that are used by our Latina grandmothers. Also, the many indigenous groups that are represented in the makeup of today's Latino population all had their favorite local plants, animals and minerals used for healing. For example, astringents are used to heal wounds, cuts and scrapes, coagulants or coagulantes, and styptics or estípticos, and vulnerary or vulnerarios for stopping bleeding, and are therefore some of the most common items in the curandera's medicine kit. Arnica and all kinds of citrus leaves and blossoms are used for this purpose as well. Germicides or germicidas, and disinfectants or desinfectantes such as sage and rosemary are also used to prevent or treat infection.

On the other hand, there are many household remedies in grandmother's medicine kit that are useful, such as tonics or tónicos, stimulants or estimulantes and restoratives or restaurativos, for fortifying and strengthen underweight children and the elderly.

Many of our beliefs in curanderismo have been handed down to us from a "culture of illness" derived from colonial Mexico and are still valid today. This is one of the principal reasons why curanderos/as are still necessary. They heal our cultural selves. Numerous authors have pointed out that native-healing traditions in the Americas were, and are, a conglomeration of magic and religion, with a prodigious knowledge base of medicinal plants. In the early days, historians attributed native knowledge of the "qualities" of food and medicine with European origins, but today most believe that the native populations of Mexico had developed a more comprehensive theory of disease than the fabled world of the Greeks and Romans. It has been said that "Unlike the mostly worthless Hippocratic and Galenic medicine brought to Mexico by the Spaniards, there was a strong empirical basis to the medical practices of the Nahuatl speakers of central Mexico. It is well known that the invaders trusted the treatment of their wounds to Aztec rather than their own doctors, as the former were far more adept as surgeons and curers" (Coe and Whittaker, 1986, p.38).

19. FAITH AND FOLK HEALERS — *DON DE CURAR*

I'm really upset with my family. I was raised to tolerate all faiths and beliefs. But now I feel that my parents and my brothers and sister are hypocrites because they refuse to understand or accept my beliefs. I was raised Catholic and we would go to mass and my mother would sometimes take us with her to see a healer or *curandera*. Now my entire family has converted to an evangelical church that moved into our neighborhood.

To make matters worse, the Latino preacher at their church told them that the old cultural ways are demonic and that all *curanderos/as* are satanic. I just can't believe it's true and I refuse to be changed by this person because I know in my heart that he is wrong. In their church, they have a healing ceremony they call laying-on-of-hands, which to me, is no different than the healing techniques my *curandera* uses. Don't the evangelical and the *curandera* heal with the same Holy Spirit? Don't they both derive their healing powers from the same God? Can you help me to understand the difference between what the *curandera* does and what the evangelicals do, if anything?

CURANDERO'S RESPONSE:

I am fascinated with your question about evangelical faith healers and the laying-on-of-hands in comparison to what *curanderos/as* do with their hands. People just like you ask this question all the time. I firmly believe that both the evangelical ministers and the *curanderos/as* use the same gift of the Holy Spirit described in the Holy Bible. The laying-on-of-hands for the purpose of healing is a gift to all people and not exclusive to any one religion.

Your family has been swayed by this new neighborhood church that practices faith healing. I have seen this so many times before because these little churches pop up everywhere like mushrooms after a rain. We must pray for them to be tolerant.

Your family shuns you and condemns you because their new preacher tells them to, and they are trying to please him with blind faith. Eventually, they will understand this is wrong but it may take awhile and the relation you have with your family will continue to be strained. I can assure you that seeing a *curandera* who gives you support in your cultural beliefs is not evil.

Your parents' laying-on-of-hands and your *curandera's* healing hands are one and the same. I believe that both derive their healing powers from the Holy Spirit. The two healing traditions are simply different cultural manifestations of the same spiritual power.

Evangelicals demand that you repent your ways in order to save your soul. I believe that their intolerance is what's wrong and that they should respect your beliefs as you respect theirs.

COMMENTARY:

Curanderismo is often condemned as the worshiping of false gods or paganism. In reality, the Holy Bible lists the Seven Gifts of the Holy Spirit, including the gift of healing and condemns the worshiping of false prophets. The Holy Bible does not speak of religion, so any culturally-based healing practice that calls upon God must be using the same power of the Holy Spirit; it is simply in a different cultural form. It should be noted that authentic curanderos/as always work with the forces of good against evil.

20. MISTRUST OF CURANDEROS — *LA DESCONFIANZA*

You know, it really saddens me when people within the Latino community put down *curanderos/as* because they feel that their religion is better than others and that the ways of the *curanderos/as* are evil or they think that they are too educated to believe in the ways of our grandparents. I hear this very often and I just simply do not argue with these people because, to be quite frank with you, it isn't even worth wasting your energy with them.

God manifests His Spirit in many different ways and I know for a fact that the *curandero/a* way is definitely one of God's manifestations. Just from the little that we know of one another, God has opened up my intuition even more and I can truly feel the change that has taken place in my heart since I started seeing a *curandera*. Nothing could be more important to me.

We are all God's children and He loves us all. And, yes, I am very aware of people who disguise themselves as *curanderos/as* and scam other unsuspecting people. I believe that this happens in all religions. Please let me know what you think.

CURANDERO'S RESPONSE:

All ethnic groups have their own particular brand of culturally-oriented traditional medicine. Many people of all cultures think that the shaman or *curandero/a*, is from the past but that is not true. El Niño Fidencio, Don Pedrito Jaramillo and others were very famous and popular *curanderos/as* when they were alive.

Originally, the healing traditions we now call *curanderismo* were ways of life based on cultural traditions. Today, *curanderismo* is mostly a mixture of traditions and no longer pure beliefs of one single tradition. It might be said that a new form of *curanderismo* is emerging. Now there is modern and Western medicine and more conventional ways of treating illnesses. As new generations of people have become knowledgeable and experienced in the ways of new and advanced methods of modern scientific medicine and health care, traditional *curanderismo* is frowned upon and seen as taboo by many. There is little or no value placed by most of society on *curanderismo*. These people have little or no knowledge of the ancient spiritual ways that still could potentially address the basic, physical, mental and spiritual needs of the human body and soul. Learn from this.

COMMENTARY:

The curandero's response is very common and quite correct. Most organized religions that Latinos are affiliated with today hold a very condescending and non-Christian attitude toward curanderos albeit their respective congregations seek them out whenever they are in need. Cultural realities are deep-rooted and not easily brushed aside nor forgotten when a person or family is confronted with difficult or tense situations. People frequently tend to rely on what they know best and draw from their personal life experiences, which are culturally based.

In colonial Mexico, the practices of the curanderos/as were considered suspect and operated outside of the Roman Catholic Church. Therefore, over the centuries Catholics have been taught to fear curanderos/as. Since curanderos "claimed to have unique intimacy with the supernatural," they were denounced by the church and mandated to practice underground or in the occult.

21. FAKE CURANDEROS — *CHARLATANES*

How can you tell if someone is a real *curandero/a* or a fake? We paid a woman $780 to help us with a family problem. She called herself a *curandera* and said the money wasn't for her, but was intended to purchase the material things that she needed to help our family like oils, incense and candles. She was going to buy eight sets of everything because she said that someone put a spell on my parents when they were younger to break up their marriage. That did not succeed because my parents' love for one another was true and strong. She said that because of the failure, the spell has spread onto we kids and that it was affecting us each in a different way. She seems legitimate to me, I don't get any bad vibes from her but I just want to make sure this woman is really helping us or is she just taking us for a ride?

She is not the only *curandera* that has told us about a spell being put on my parents. Another woman offered to help last year, but backed out because she said the warlocks or *brujos* that did it are really mean and she thought they would come back and do something to her. Basically she was too scared to take on our case. I wish we had learned about you sooner.

I know we could not afford to travel to see you, but with the miracle of the Internet you are now just a few keystrokes away.

CURANDERO'S RESPONSE:

Authentic *curanderos/as* do not ask for $780 to try to help someone in need. Good *curanderos/as* will try to help anyone in need whether they have money or not. I believe you have been sold a bill of goods and will get nothing in return from your investment. Always be wary of someone who wants your money. Real *curanderos/as* will accept your donation, but never ask for a fee.

COMMENTARY:

A general rule of thumb is to always question and think twice about an alleged curandero/a, who wants to charge an exorbitant amount of money for a cure. It is perfectly normal for curanderos with a need to purchase materials for a cure, but always do the math. A legitimate curandero serves the community and not his or her personal bank account. However, most legitimate curanderos/as will accept or expect some type of a donation since that is probably their only income.

Cultural competency: Resource numbers 3 and 4 provide the reader with recommended federal cultural competency standards, three through seven, and discuss the importance of linguistic competence in the health-care delivery system, see Appendix I.

22. SANTERÍA — *CREENCIAS AFRO-CARIBEÑAS*

I have contacted you before, wondering about spiritual matters. I was involved in Santería, an Afro-Cuban spirit religion. I had a reading done and the *santero* said I needed to have a male goat sacrificed for the spirits to keep me and my little girl alive. They wanted lots of money. Is this work evil? I am seeing my dead friends in my dreams. I have not talked to the *santero* again and don't plan to. I was told to pray to San Lázaro, but I don't understand why. What kinds of offerings does he like on his altar?

I suffer from a mental illness called schizophrenia and don't really know what to do. Is the Rosary good for protection against evil spirits? Do you recommend anything else I should do like candles or what?

CURANDERO'S RESPONSE:

I would advise you to not venture into something you are not comfortable with. Use your common sense and if it tells you something is not right, it probably is not right for you. I understand you did not give the *santero* lots of money, right? It sounds like he is just interested in your money! Remember, love of money is the root of all evil. Seek professional counseling in regard to your dreams and your mental illness and I will support you in the spirit realm. I am sure faith and prayer will benefit you spiritually, holistically, emotionally, mentally, and physically. I recommend you light candles to Saint Michael the Archangel, to the Guardian Angel and to the Niño Fidencio for spiritual guidance and protection. San Lázaro is the Christian version of the Santería Orisha, Babalú-Ayé, and his preferred color is violet and he is celebrated December 17.

COMMENTARY:

This person believes that illnesses are cured through the intercession of El Niño Fidencio. It is also obvious that this person has had contact with Santería, which is an alternate form of curanderismo practiced in Afro-Caribbean cultures. Santería and similar religions are found throughout the Americas and wherever these cultures have relocated. The reference to Saint Lazarus and the question, "what does the saint like as an offering?" is a direct reference to practices in santería and learned from consultation with the santero, or priest of santería.

Many Latino families keep home altars and make altar offerings to patron saints. This is not dissimilar to what Fidencio did during his lifetime; he would bless fruit and candy and throw them out to anxious throngs of people. He always said that they were medicinal and if a piece of fruit or candy hit someone in the crowd, it held a very special healing for that person. His faithful followers continue this practice to this day. Fully-initiated santero priests and priestesses are referred to as padrino or madrina meaning godfather or godmother, which are terms of high esteem. Their followers and those who seek initiation into the cult or culto are referred to as ahijado or godchild. Santeros use fruit and many other items in their spells, trabajos and rituals. An example of an offering to San Lázaro for good luck might look like this: place a bowl at the foot of the santo and add one penny a day for 17 straight days; each day add seven grains of rice; seven grains of wheat; seven grains of corn; honey; shavings of gold; shavings of silver; dry red wine; palm oil; and cooking oil. Recite aloud: with these grains I will receive wealth; with this honey, I will receive harmony; with these coins I will progress; with this wine I will be happy; and with this alum rock, all these will continue. Light the mixture with a match reciting a prayer to San Lázaro. Repeat the ritual for 16 more days. At the end of the 17 days offer the saint some bread and a cup of coconut juice. Finally, take the entire concoction and dispose of it in an open field.

Santería is a legitimate religion and should be respected as such. Every religion, sect and healing modality has its legitimate and illegitimate practitioners. Curanderismo and santería have both been plagued by unscrupulous individuals who attempt to make money at the expense of needy and desperate people. This is why we must always obtain word-of-mouth references from people who have successfully utilized the services of a specific healer, before we agree to pay for healings. The most common santería Orishias or saints and some corresponding colors are:

Olodumare: God or Supreme Deity, All colors

Obbatala: Saint Joseph, the figure of Christ crucified and others, white

Yemayá: Virgen de la Regla, blue/white

Aganyú: San Cristóbal, Saint Christopher, white, red and yellow

Oggún: San Pablo, San Pedro San Juan and others, green/black

Ochosi: San Norberto and San Humberto, lavender/black

Eleggúa: Santo Niño de Atocha, red/black

Changó: Santa Bárbara, red and white

Ochún: Virgen de la Caridad del Cobre, yellow/green or red

Oyá: Virgen de la Candelaria, Virgen del Carmen, maroon

Dada: San Ramón/San Lazaro, light blue

Babalú-Ayé: San Lázaro, light blue

Inlé: San Rafael Arcángel, blue, green and yellow

23. CARD READER — *LA BARAJA ESPAÑOLA*

Many of my friends are head-over-heels crazy about card readers, going to them for every little thing. In fact, where I work it has become sort of a game where people look for new card readers and then the whole office goes, guys also go to them. I am a Latina but even the white girls and the black girls love to do this. As a Latina, they expect me to know about it and understand how it works, but I don't. I didn't grow up with this. I don't remember my mother or for that matter, anybody in my family going to have a card reading. Where I was raised, there were no card readers and my mother never even remarked about it. Please help me to understand.

CURANDERO'S RESPONSE:

Tarot cards or Spanish tarot card reading, which is divination or fortune telling, is as old as the hills. Today there are many different kinds of tarot card decks and many different methods for "throwing" the cards or spreads and for reading them. For us Latinos our most commonly used deck is the Spanish tarot, but there are many others. You can buy one very inexpensively at any store which specializes in Mexican products. Ask for *la baraja* or for the *lotería*.

The following story provides us a glimpse of the personal life and development of a card reader and her gift:

When I was very young, back in the 1960s, I met a woman where I lived who was a renowned card reader. She was phenomenal. It seemed that everything she would tell me would come about. She would hit the nail on the head every time. I believe she had a very beautiful and powerful gift and she served her community all of her life and was very humble, and loved by everyone. My grandmother told me that she would tell which sons would return from World War II alive and which would not. Back in those days we all had a lot of faith in her because she was what they called a "good" *curandera*.

I have suffered from scoliosis of the spinal column and from polio since I was a child and my mother died when I was very young. I was just 15 when she died. But before her death, she told me that I had a special gift from God, the gift of prophecy. The card reader that we would see back then would always tell me the same thing my mother used to say and that got my attention: *"Mija, tienes un don, daughter you have the gift."* She also told me that my husband would have a gift as well and that we would lead very humble lives of helping others as healers and counselors.

In many cases a person may have something serious happening in his/her life that moves them to seek help, advice or to look for someone who might be able to provide some guidance. There are many different kinds of professional counselors with the intention of trying to help those in need. There are also cases where a person seeks help with the desire of finding answers and solutions to the questions and doubts in life, but does not need to see a professional. It is in exactly these cases that card readers can play a helpful role.

COMMENTARY:

Most people in the United States who are familiar with tarot cards are familiar with the European tarot deck. Years ago, the most common tarot deck was the Rider-Waite deck consisting of 78 cards, 21 face cards of the major arcana and 56 cards divided up into four sets of 14 in the minor arcana. The fortune-telling card deck (most commonly used in Spain and Latin America and by most Latina card readers) is the Spanish tarot, or baraja Española comprised of 48 cards organized into four suits with three face cards and nine numbered cards for a total of 12 cards for each suit: clubs, coins, cups and swords.

Having your cards read can be fun, but when it becomes an obsession it can really interfere with a person's decision-making process in life. In his book, This Saint's For You, Thomas Craughwell lists Balthasar, one of the Three Kings or Reyes Magos, as the patron of card players; he is celebrated on January 6th. (The authors thank Lydia Posas Salinas for her assistance with this contribution.)

24. INCANTATIONS AND RITUALS — *ENCANTOS Y RITUALES*

I finally got the candle Divina Providencia, Divine Providence, at the *botánica*. It's funny because my son and I went to buy food at a store nearby and I told him I needed to stop at the *botánica* and pick up a candle. Anyway, I asked the guy if he finally got the shipment of Divina Providencia candles in and he said he had. As a matter of fact, he received one shipment and it sold out and he had another shipment come in and he saved the last one for me, it was $2. That's a good deal and it was meant to be. How do I perform the ritual for prosperity?

Do I place my photo face up under which candle and what do I write on the note? Do I place coins by the candle also? Do I say a special prayer?

CURANDERO'S RESPONSE:

All you need to do is to say a prayer. Ask the Lord for help with your job, light the candle over your photo, face up and place a clear glass of water next to the candle. No coins are necessary but can be used.

You can write out your petition on parchment paper and also place it under your photo under your candle. It's essential that you also recite the Holy Trinity prayer or the prayer to the Divine Providence. Candles that come in glass containers usually have a prayer printed on the side and you could recite that as well. I usually request a specially-prepared candle that is one that has been prepared just for you and your special case with certain oils and essences. Candles which do not have glass containers should be used very carefully and prepared with oils. Always act wisely to avoid setting your house on fire.

One should never attempt to utilize candles in the form of a figure of a man or woman because they are used for witchcraft, and potentially very dangerous to the unsuspecting dabbler. Caution! Remember, a witchcraft spell will always come back on the person casting or ordering the spell in some fashion or another.

You probably noticed in your *hierbería* there is a book display and if you study it more carefully you will find, *El Libro de San Cipriano*, the book of Saint Ciprian and *El Libro del Rey Salomón*, the book of King Solomon. Books on performing magic, books on Psalms, medicinal plants, on candle rituals, different kinds of prayers, amulets and talismans, and ancient Aztec remedies are available to you to learn more. Some of these books are very useful and I will guide you on which ones to buy and which not.

COMMENTARY:

A layperson won't be very cognizant of the utilization of a candle, or how to perform candle magic rituals or how to recite incantations, or spell casting. The curandero who orders or recommends the candle, spell or ritual, should always be able to instruct the user in the proper use. The salesperson at the hierbería or botánica may know only limited information about these topics. Don't rely on them.

There is an enormous collection of literature of inexpensive books and pamphlets on a wide range of the incantations, spells, pacts and rituals used in the curanderos/as repertoire. The book of Saint Cipriano, a book on saints, on medicinal plants, and Psalms are useful reading resources and will assist the first-time seeker understand more about curanderismo.

Additionally, each Latino sub-group, including Puerto Ricans, Cubans, South Americans, Central Americans and Mexicans all have their favorite patron saints and folk-saint and pilgrimage shrines, and therefore, books specific to sub-cultures. I have collected books from hierberías and botánicas from all these locations and while the material is basically the same, there are many cultural and regional differences and subtleties you must be aware of.

25. AMULETS AND TALISMANS — *EL LIBRO DEL REY SALOMÓN*

Many of my friends wear all sorts of objects around their necks, place objects on their clothes, on their baby's clothes, in their yards and at their places of work. They use words like amulet or talisman. What are these things and should I have them also?

CURANDERO'S RESPONSE:

Many Latinos use a wide variety of protective devices called amulets and talismans. Some people would rather use a necklace of the Sacred Heart of Our Lord, the medallion of the Virgen of Guadalupe or their favorite protective patron saint on a chain or some other charm worn around the neck. For Latinos, our Lady of Guadalupe is always your best bet for protection. The feast day of the Virgen of Guadalupe is celebrated December 12. One of the most beloved items used instead of a regular amulet or talisman is the ever popular Holy Rosary. The Holy Rosary is the ultimate protective talisman when either carried in the pocket or around the neck.

The Caravaca Cross is also a popular talismanic symbol used to project against spells. Lately many have fallen for the fad of carrying the image of Saint Death, or La Santísima Muerte, in a gold medallion around the neck. There are many, many symbols used for specific activities, desires or fears. For example, the little Buddha is a favorite with many bingo players.

These symbols called relics, or *reliquias*, are comparable to the mojo bags, made and prepared by *curanderos/as*. Others are used to bring good luck, protection, or money drawing. Talismans and amulets represent a very important part of the faith of the believer and may be used to identify sub-cultural beliefs and sect participation of the bearer. Elephants with raised trunks, horseshoes, owls and many other curios in the form of statues, yard protectors, and jewelry are chanted over and blessed with the intention of saturating them with supernatural and magical energies. Other items like the *ajo macho*, or male garlic head, are also popular.

COMMENTARY:

Amulets and talismans are as old as magic and can be traced back to the Old Testament and to King Solomon's wisdom. Every ancient culture, whether Asian, Greek, Egyptian, Indian, Aztec, even European, all have storied histories with amulets and talismans. They are all used for the same purpose: protection in one form or another, and they are always self-styled to the bearer's likes and wishes.

26. DANCING WITH THE DEVIL — *BAILANDO CON EL DIABLO*

One of the first stories that my mother ever told me was about a girl who danced with the devil because she disobeyed. She told me she knew a girl in her town that danced with the devil, but now I'm hearing that this is very common story among Latinos. So, I'm writing to you to clarify it for me.

As the story goes, there was this girl who was very disobedient and her punishment was to dance with the devil. When my mother told me this story, I was too young to realize that she was training me to be obedient. Since I also loved to dance every chance I got, the story fascinated me when I first heard it when I was six.

The story goes something like this: The young girl was very pretty and loved to dance, but she was also very spoiled, *chiflada,* and did not obey her parents. She never obeyed her curfew and worried her parents to death. One time she went to a dance on a Friday night and did not return home until Saturday, and that was the last straw. She danced all night long until the early morning hours. Since she was very pretty and popular with the boys, her parents worried a lot. She was always able to attract the most handsome boys to her side. This final time, she ignored her parents' warning and they were sick with worry, but once again she ignored their pleas.

Having reached the breaking point, the following weekend her parents did not allow her to go to the Friday night dance. This was to be a very special dance, honoring an engaged couple in the town, *los novios,* but since she was such a disobedient child her parents absolutely would not allow her to attend.

Once again, this wayward girl disobeyed her mother and snuck out of her bedroom window and was off to the dance. When her mother realized that her daughter was gone, she had an uneasy and ominous feeling because she knew that girls like her were punished by a dance with the devil, and not all survive.

The mother wrung her hands and prayed that nothing would happen to her daughter that evening. She could only think of her daughter laughing in her face and saying, "I love to dance!"

The disobedient daughter danced the night away with the local boys. But just before midnight, a handsome stranger entered the dance hall. He was the best looking young man the girl had ever seen. He was tall with beautiful dark eyes. As he walked towards her, no words were needed; she was lost in his deep eyes as he placed one hand on her waist, and with the other, gently enveloped her hand in his. This was the young man she had been waiting for all her life. They danced one polka after another, forgetting the witching hour and that she had missed curfew once again. She was enraptured in his spell. The world had disappeared. Only the two of them existed.

She didn't want to let go of him, ever. "Will you be here next week, she asked?" He stared deeply into her eyes and then began to laugh. His laugh reverberated from deep within his chest, a dark, unnatural laugh. She tried to step back, but he wouldn't let her go. Instead, his hands became like steel, locking her in place, despite her struggles. As she chanced to look down, his feet had changed and instead of the shoes that were there before, one foot was shaped like a rooster claw and the other a goat hoof. They were large and red. How had she not noticed them before? Terrorized, she realized that her dancing partner was the handsome devil, *el diablo guapo*; her mother had warned her about. She screamed loudly not certain of the fate about to befall her.

Some say that she never disobeyed her parents again, others say that she went mad, or *trastornada*. Still, others say that she died engulfed in flames or that she simply disappeared having been taken to hell by the devil. Maybe it was just a dream. The townsfolk still talk about her to this day, and mothers still tell their daughters to obey and to never dance with handsome devils, pick ordinary boys like their fathers.

CURANDERO'S RESPONSE:

It's a fascinating story. You are correct, this story is almost everywhere there are Mexican Americans or Latinos. This story urges us to obey and that is always a good thing. My wife also knew a disobedient girl in her town that danced with the devil. In her case, she was consumed by fire and died with the sin of disobeying her parents on her soul. Who knows how she was judged by God. The disobedient young girl in this story must pray to Saint Cyriacus for the rest of her life. Saint Cyriacus is believed to keep the devil at bay. Celebrate Cyriacus on August 8.

COMMENTARY:

Indeed, the tale of dancing with the devil is commonplace in Latin American folklore, especially among Mexican Americans. Everyone has heard this story and almost everyone knows someone who claims to have physically witnessed a similar event. The tale is intertwined with complex variants which convey a variety of messages and teach vital values to our children. This is a classic morality/cautionary tale used in child-obedience training in Latino culture. (This story was submitted by Rachel E. Barrera.)

27. THE PASTORELA AND POSADA—*FIESTAS NAVIDEÑAS*

This past year our prayers were answered and we were truly blessed. As we began the year, we had so many problems that seemed insurmountable. Our family has been consulting with you all year and you have never let us down. Each prayer you gave us, each remedy, *remedio*, and with each spiritual cleansing, *limpia,* we slowly resolved our family issues, and our situation improved. We are truly grateful to you, to the Niño Fidencio and to all the forces of good, which assist us in overcoming evil.

For the first time in many years, we have returned to our Catholic faith and traditions at our neighborhood parish. I especially enjoy singing and performing the *pastorela* and walking the *posada*. There are many religious figures and symbols represented in the plays and I'm not sure what each means. I believe that somehow my family got disconnected from our culture and I think that is why we got sick. So many bad things happened to us. How can we learn more about the symbolism in the *pastorela* and *posada*?

Could you help us with a little explanation or pointer on where to look for more information? My family is even talking about getting more involved next year and that's very exciting. It feels like we are coming home to our cultural roots.

CURANDERO'S RESPONSE:

Years ago, every Mexican American *barrio* had a *pastorela* and a *posada* during the Christmas holidays. That has changed now, and it is only in the rarest of Mexican neighborhoods or *barrios* Mexicanos, that you find these customs still practiced. This cultural "soul loss" is very sad. (See Rachael Barrera's testimony.)

Simply stated, the *pastorela* reenacts the story of the three kings, or Reyes Magos, Balthazar, Melchor and Gaspar, celebrated on January 6, following the star of Bethlehem and the Archangel Michael's battle against the devil.

There are both short and long versions of the *pastorela*. The shorter versions tell the story of the Holy Family, the shepherds or *pastores,* and the Three Kings, Reyes Magos. Some versions include Saint Michael's battle against the devil, but many do not. The feast day of Saint Michael the Archangel is celebrated on September 29. The shorter *pastorela* is usually reenacted in about two hours. The more complex *pastorela* includes San Miguel, the hermit, *el ermitaño,* the *pastores,* the Holy Family, the three kings and as many as a dozen devils. This more complete *pastorela* varies in length with some plays taking several days and nights non-stop to complete.

The *posada* commemorates the Holy Family searching, from door to door, for safe haven. There is much to be learned about both traditions.

In some places, people still commemorate the *posada* by placing a nativity scene depicting the Holy Family in front of their home and having family and friends over on Christmas Eve, *la noche buena.* They pray the Rosary and sing, distribute candy to the children, and celebrate with a traditional meal consisting of *tamales, buñuelos* and hot chocolate or another traditional drink called *champurrado.* In some households, all go to the Midnight Mass or *misa de gallo,* at their neighborhood parishes.

With people like you, our cultural traditions will make a comeback. It takes family unity and devotion, as well as strong leadership from the neighborhood and parish priest to keep our beautiful traditions alive.

I thank you for your kind words and I am elated that your problems are being resolved. Pay back your good fortune by renewing your cultural traditions and fulfill your promise, or *promesa.* Get a hold of a liturgical calendar and rediscover all of the celebrations for the entire year and practice them. (For the liturgical calendar see #16.)

COMMENTARY:

Latino and other ethnic groups are rediscovering their valued traditions. It is refreshing to witness a community exercise its ancestral traditions. While not all traditions are associated with religion, many are. Traditional American holidays such as Easter, Halloween, Thanksgiving and Christmas have become primarily commercial holidays with their religious significance and origins lost. In many cases, they are being taken back by people wishing to teach their children about the true meaning of these important religious cultural holidays.

28. EX-VOTOS — *MILAGROS PINTADOS*

This year, we were finally able to save enough money to complete our promise, *promesa*, to the Virgen, and to make the pilgrimage to La Villa de Guadalupe in Mexico City on December 12th.

It was a magical experience; one our family will never forget. One thing we noticed was that there were many persons selling little metal figures of children, and heads, and arms and other body parts. There were even cats, dogs and trucks. The people called them little miracles, or *milagritos*. People buy them and then take them into the *basilica* to be blessed by the Virgen as they passed under her gaze on the conveyor belt, or by a priest who was there just to bless items to be taken home. People place them on their home altars to remember the miracle they received in their family. Would you please explain to me what they are and how they are used? We bought several and want to be sure to use them correctly.

CURANDERO'S RESPONSE:

You can get little metal miracles, called *milagros,* at most *hierberías,* or at a Mexican product store near you. They take almost any form, especially the form of parts of the body or of children or animals. They literally represent the body part or object that is being prayed for or which received the healing. They are called a *milagro* because each one represents a prayer answered or a miracle received. People bring them to my healing altar all the time. The use of *milagritos* is an ancient and beautiful custom of giving thanks for prayers answered. The *milagro* was first brought to Mexico by Catholic priests from Spain. The tradition is ancient in Europe and endures in Mexico to this day as they serve as a physical symbol of the thing or body part healed. The belief is that it is important to give something back for something received.

There is also a written or painted form of the *milagro* scene called an *ex-voto*. The written and visual testimony of an event in one's life is commemorated on tin in the form of a painting. In Mexico, as in Europe before, the people would hire a local artist to paint the story of the event and miracle on tin which was then taken into the church and dedicated to the saint or Virgen. The painted story included a written description, usually at the bottom of the painting and the folk art item is called an *ex-voto*. You and your family are wise to ask about this and to re-introduce these traditions in your family.

COMMENTARY:

The milagro's legacy is to take the object symbolizing an event and a miracle received on a pilgrimage to the shrine of the patron saint whose intercession was sought and to pin the milagro to the saint's garment. The ex-voto is also left at the shrine and the major shrines have thousands of these objects dating back several hundred years.

The tradition of the painted ex-voto is quickly fading. There are fewer and fewer artists who make their living painting ex-votos than ever before. At one time, it was a viable profession. When the family whose prayers were answered traveled to their respective saint's shrine, the detailed painting was commissioned and a professional ex-voto painter produced the object on the spot and it was left at the shrine. The tradition is still carried on at the major shrines in Mexico, but most of the older ex-votos painted long ago have become valuable folk-art collection items and have been sold to collectors or dealers. An ex-voto I once saw in Espinazo at the shrine of the Niño Fidencio read as follows, "Doy gracias a Dios y al Niño Fidencio. Ya dejó un poco de beber mi esposo y le pido que ya no tome nada." (S.L.P. 29-11-83) That is, "I give thanks to God and to the Niño Fidencio. My husband is drinking less and I ask that he not drink at all." It was dated 1983. (Name withheld, from a wife in the Mexican state of San Luís Potosí. See page xxii).

Fields points out that "The Catholic Church is one of the most important cultural agents in the evolution of Spanish American medicine" (p.158). This is why in the 21st century, illness and health cannot be separated from religious and supernatural beliefs practiced on the one hand by the church and on the other by curanderos/as.

29. THE HOME ALTAR — *EL ALTAR FAMILIAR*

I have started to set up an altar in my home and sometime back I sent you a photograph of my altar. I know that home altars are very important in Latina culture and my mother, my two grandmothers, and all of my aunts have home altars. Now that I have my own home, I want one as well. I know that it will be the center place of spirituality in my home and that from that sacred place I will make all of my petitions, and it will have very special supernatural powers. The home altar is a living thing that hears and sees what is going on in the home. To begin my own home altar, what should I place on my altar to have spirituality enhance my life?

CURANDERO'S RESPONSE:

Thank you for your updated letter and your question in reference to your altar. I pray things keep getting better for you. Please use a large clear glass container for the spiritual water you keep on your altar. The spirits of light hear your prayers through the water and it becomes a powerful blessing. In fact, it is your medium to the spiritual world. The spirit manifests through your glass of water for healing and blessing purposes, just as your prayers are sent to heaven by the burning of candles on your altar along with any incense or *incienso* you burn on your altar. It is also a good idea to place a clear glass of water under your bed at night and then throw it out in the morning. The water will protect you from evil by absorbing and neutralizing it before it attacks you. Do this especially when there is trouble in your life, but not every day. Remember that evil is believed to arrive in darkness, or *las tinieblas*, and the vessel of water protects you and your family members from the unseen.

For healing purposes, please place a fertilized hen's egg, a head of garlic and a lemon and alum rock, or *piedra alumbre* on your altar.

Whatever you leave on the altar overnight will be ready for the next day's spiritual healing rituals. You might say it will be fully charged with the spirit. The next day, use these blessed objects to clean, or *limpiar*; give your loved ones a spiritual sweeping, or *barrida*. Do this by rubbing the egg, the lemon or the garlic head over the body of the one being cleansed while saying one "Our Father," *Padre Nuestro*, the Lord's Prayer, and by making your petition. Do this in front of your altar. It can be done any day at any time. Dispose of what you use for your cleansing ritual by throwing the materias outside of your home or yard. Be sure to dispose of them where they cannot hurt anyone else.

Religious artifacts are important symbols of faith and powerful articles that influence the soul, transforming emotion into spirit. It is always important to use objects as symbols of your faith, hope and prayer. Chanting, sacrifice and penance also open pathways to the spiritual world. Use these methods as one's journey through life. It takes personal resignation and discipline to help make a home altar. The remaining objects on your altar may consist of the photographs of loved ones with your offerings of love, understanding and devotion to almighty God. For spirituality to work, you must have faith.

Always dress up your altar with a bowl of water, and with an offering, or *ofrenda*, of a fresh bouquet of flowers, fruit, and with candles, oil and incense. Most importantly, you must offer your life and your soul to God on your sacred altar. If you do these things, your altar will take on life and serve as a direct conduit to the supernatural and your prayers will be answered.

COMMENTARY:

Constructing a home altar is a surprisingly-delightful family ritual that promotes spirituality in the home. All may participate and maintain a personal precinct on the altar with special intentions, petitions and personal patron saints. The home altar is a mode of encouraging faith and religious beliefs in our children to have the same beliefs perpetuated into their adult lives. Always include your children in anything that concerns the altar because it is their lifeline as well.

Home altars are crucial because they are basically designed and maintained by the women of the family, who are primarily responsible for the family's faith, devotion and spirituality.

30. PROMISE AND PILGRIMAGE—*PROMESA Y PEREGRINACIÓN*

I saw a story on the news the other day about a little girl who promised not to cut her hair until it reached the ground if her sick little brother received a miracle cure for his cancer. The story went on to say that the brother was in remission and that his sister grew her hair to floor length and then cut it with great ceremony and solemnity. The long braid was then taken to the Basílica of San Juan, Texas, to be offered to the La Virgen de San Juan del Valle. The story said that she completed her promise, or *promesa*, by making a pilgrimage to the shrine in Texas. Her four-foot-long braid was dedicated to the Virgen and left at the shrine in the miracle room. Can you explain to me what that is about and how I could make a promise?

CURANDERO'S RESPONSE:

It is because of a family or personal crisis, and at the hour of great need, when a loved one is very sick, or when there is impending danger that a promise, *promesa*, is made. One petitions a patron saint or the Virgen to intercede with God on behalf of the sick or needy person. A solemn promise is made that if the miracle, or *milagro*, is granted, the petitioner and beneficiary will complete the spiritual contract, or *manda,* by making a pilgrimage, or *peregrinación,* to the saint's sacred site. Once at the site, an offering, or *ofrenda,* or a token, or *prenda*, is made by leaving some special object at the foot of the saint. By doing this, the promise, or *promesa,* and the burden, or *manda,* are fulfilled.

The person making the promise makes an offering at the shrine and by doing so, the spiritual contract is fulfilled. When a miracle is delivered, completing the promise and spiritual contract is a very important task. It is an obligation which cannot be forgotten or overlooked. There is no time limit to complete the promise; the petitioner has a lifetime to fulfill the spiritual contract. However, not to complete one's promise may result in dire consequences as all broken promises with God are eventually punished. Here is one example of a sacred promise. A couple tried for many years to conceive a child with no success. They asked, through their faith and prayers, for the intercession of La Virgen de Guadalupe. The couple promised the Virgen that if they had a baby, they would make the pilgrimage to her shrine in Mexico City to present the baby to the Virgen. Their prayer was answered and it took them five years to save the money needed to make the trip, but they fulfilled their promise. Today, both the parents and the child are happy and healthy through the intercession and protection of their patron saint.

Some people even name their children after patron saints. In this case, it could be Mary, Mario, Guadalupe or Lupe depending on gender.

Gestures of gratitude and devotion include taking flowers, monetary offerings, lighting a candle or delivering a little miracle charm, a *milagrito*, in the form of a baby to the shrine. It could also involve the promise to deliver your hair or some other item of great personal value like a driver's license to the shrine. Most importantly, is the presentation of the child to the patron saint and giving thanks.

In some cases, if there were serious risks and complications during the pregnancy, a promise is made that if the child is born healthy. The child is then said to "belong" to, or be dedicated to the intercessor. In this case, the child is taken to the pilgrimage site by a method of great sacrifice and penance such as traveling the last hundred yards to the shrine on one's knees.

The child could be carried on the backs of the parents for great distances and eventually they crawl on their backs; carrying the child on their chests or bellies as they enter the holy shrine. By doing this, they fulfill the promise introducing their child to the patron saint; making a public demonstration of thanks and delivering the child into the spiritual realm of lifelong divine protection and guidance of the patron saint. It is not uncommon to have a special devotion to a patron saint or Virgen passed on in a single family for generations.

There are as many patron saints as there are needy people. There are many very popular Latino saints and *virgins*, including: the Virgen de Guadalupe; the Virgen de San Juan de Los Lagos; La Virgen del Chorrito; San Francisco de Asís at Real de Catorce, celebrated on October 4, San Luis Potosí, and the Santo Niño de Atocha at Plateros, Zacatecas, celebrated on December 15 and often on the same day as the Los Reyes Magos, January 6. There are many others. All these locations are major Catholic pilgrimage sites, mostly in Mexico. For Mexican Americans, pilgrimages most likely require a return to the mother country.

There are also many folk saints, who have pilgrimage sites such as El Niño Fidencio in Espinazo, Nuevo León, Mexico, celebrated both in October around the 19th and in March on his saint's day of March 19, and Don Pedrito Jaramillo in Falfurrias, Texas.

COMMENTARY:

Each Latino sub-culture, including: Puerto Ricans; Cubans; South Americans; Central Americans; and Mexicans, have culturally-preferred Catholic saints and folk saints according to their respective beliefs and each has a pilgrimage site and shrine. These locations are key destinations especially during the saints' holidays or days of fiesta. Both Catholicism and folk Catholicism require a penance be carried out to receive mercy or misericordia from our suffering. In this, the miracle that has been requested is seen as merited.

For example, a saint or folk saint of almost universal popularity throughout Latin America is the Holy Child of Atocha, Santo Niño de Atocha. The Christ Child of Atocha is a Spanish representation of Christ as a child in the form of a pilgrim. This devotion was brought to the new world in the 16th century. The reverence for the Child of Atocha and the belief that he is a miraculous figure still remains strong today with the main pilgrimage shrine located at Plateros, Zacatecas.

A very beautiful tradition rarely practiced in the United States but still popular in central and southern Mexico, is that of the taking on the saint's responsibility for a year of service. Sometimes called the cult of cargo, in the towns and villages which have maintained this tradition families wait decades for their turn to protect and care for the saint. They are called mayordomos and usually belong to confraternities, or cofradías, or even third orders dedicated to the saint. At the beautiful ceremony of transferring responsibility after a year of service, the parish priest presides over the accounting of each of the saint's clothing and objects which are passed from one family to the next in line.

During the saint's days of festival, icons are paraded through the streets of each barrio in the town or village. The saint is said to see his town and his people and is proud of their accomplishments.

A walking procession in the accompaniment of the town's patron saint is an ancient ritual. The entire process is considered sacred and all involved are believed to benefit spiritually. The walk or caminata brings tranquility or tranquilidad and relief or alivio from both physical and emotional burdens. The walking procession also represents sacrifice and often people faint or experience mareo. The religious procession represents both the hope, esperanza, faith, fe, and charity, caridad, of the population. The procession is led by the chaplain or capellán, followed by the devoted or devotos and by confraternities or cofradías in the town or region. Through this sacred process which may initiate an entire week of festivities, both the people and their town are blessed.

Antonio Zavaleta and Alberto Salinas Jr.

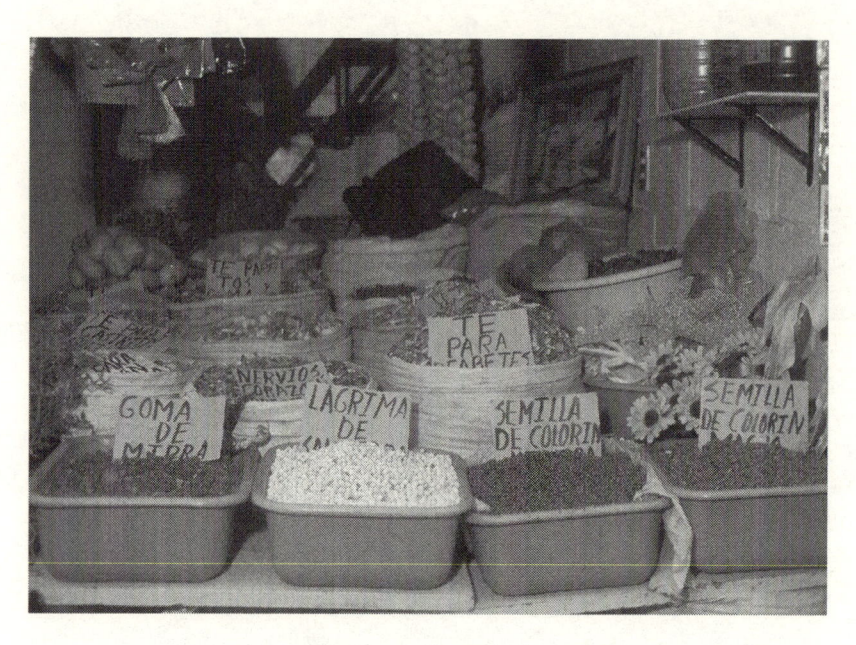

Medicinal plants are displayed by a vendor at the
Mercado Sonora, Mexico City.
(Photo by José M. Duarte)

PART FOUR

CURANDERISMO:
Healing the Body's Aches and Pains

"Curandero Conversations helps us to understand our Latino and curandero religious healing heritage and to have empathy and compassion for these practices that are often either misunderstood or missing all together from the health care system."

—*Miguel Alemán, M.D.*

31. COLDS AND FLU — *LA GRIPA Y RESFRIADOS*

Hello again. I am the college-educated Latina that spoke to you last year. I asked you what you thought about me having my baby delivered by a midwife at home the way our grandmothers used to. You advised me to look for a certified nurse midwife (CNM), and I did. I didn't even know they existed. Today, thanks to a midwife and my local clinic, I have a beautiful, happy and healthy six-month-old baby girl.

Lately, I have been hearing so much on the news about how the children's cold and flu medications are actually dangerous for kids and do little for their symptoms.

Can you help me to know more about our grandmothers' remedies because I know there are many ways to treat cold and flu symptoms without store-bought medicine? My pediatrician agrees, and believes that the cold and flu viruses that kids get should be allowed to play themselves out without doping the kid up with a lot of chemicals. So I hope you can point me in the right direction.

CURANDERO'S RESPONSE:

I do remember your letter about helping you to find a midwife and I admire what you are doing, and how you are thinking. It is through young people like you, that our traditions will be preserved and live on.

In fact, there are hundreds of home remedies for treating the symptoms of colds and the flu, what we call *la gripa*. I will share with you just a couple to put you on the right road. Most stuffy little noses can be helped by rubbing Vicks® below the nostrils and on the child's chest. At night, vaporizers help them to breathe and sleep through the night.

For fevers, give a tea made of *sauz*, or the willow tree, or *borraja*, the herb borage, or *cardo santo*, blessed thistle, or *epazote de zorrillo*, called wormseed, all heal or *valeriana*, castor bean or *higuerilla*, pennyroyal or marigold or *calendula*, *caña fistula*, ginger or *jengibre,* honeysuckle or *muicle*, and many others. All will reduce fever. See which one works best for your child. At the *hierbería*, there are prepared herbal mixtures called *compuestos* which are ready to use to reduce fever.

For sore throats and persistent cough, give teas prepared with lemon, onion, garlic, cloves, eucalyptus and honey. Medicinal plants you can give for cough and sore throats also include bay leaves or *laurel,* borage or *borraja*, clematis or *barba de chivo*, marigold or *calendula*, mallow or *malva*, mulberry or *mora*, pomegranate or *granada,* elm or *olmo,* and sumac or *zumaque*. Saint Quentin is the patron saint of coughs and is celebrated on October 31 while Saint Blaise protects the throat. His day is February 3. If an upset little tummy is part of the problem, prepare a gentle tea made from *manzanilla* or chamomile.

Breathing and respiratory problems and congestion have dozens of remedies that can be used including lavender, *lavándula*, borage, or *borraja*, mustard seed, licorice root, agrimony, *arbol de la cera* or bay berry, bay leaves or *laurel*, sour orange tree leaves, called *naranja agria*, bold or *boldo*, camphor weed or *arnica Mexicana*, common juniper or *enebro*, cudweed or pennyroyal or *poleo*, and many many more that are available depending on your location.

You could even start your own home medicinal plant herb garden. For example, basil, mint, rosemary and many other common medicinal plants are available year round and can be used in teas. Rosemary, or *romero*, works well with chronic coughs.

Always prepare a chicken soup for your sick little ones, and collect the remedies that work for you, and you will have your grandmother's medicine chest right there in your home and she will look down upon you lovingly.

COMMENTARY:

More and more people are gradually withdrawing their family members from toxins. There are many marvelous medications for serious illnesses that do save lives. However, there is also a plethora of home remedies for minor and simple ailments which can, and should, be used. Willow, or sauz, is a well-known analgesic, or analgésico; meaning it has an active ingredient to relieve pain. Increasingly, pediatricians and family-practice physicians are attempting to wean entire families, especially children, off of unnecessary drugs. If a cold or flu degenerates into a respiratory infection, an antiasthmatic herbal tea will often be given, such as acacia. In the case of mouth pain like toothaches, the curandero will prescribe poleo, a mint or the toothache plant, from the compositae family. Head colds and flu also create congestion in the nasal passages and sinuses, in which case an herbal expectorant of basil, or albahaca is used.

Medicinal plants that are used for making soaps and detergents such as the root of the century plant, or maguey are used in keeping bedding clean and germ free.

Neither the authors nor this book endorse ignoring prescribed medications. Always listen to, and follow your physician's advice, but also be culturally savvy.

Cultural Competency: *It is critically important that health-care providers understand the importance of incorporating concepts of culture into the organizational structure of the health care delivery system. Everyone from medical intake workers to clinics and hospital board members must be sensitive to the cultural realities of their clients. Cultural Competency resource number 5 in Appendix I addresses federal government mandated standards eight through 12. Cultural competency resource number seven in Appendix I examines essential principles of cultural competency as developed by the Commonwealth Fund.*

32. FALLEN FONTANEL — *MOLLERA CAÍDA*

My mother says my baby may have *mollera caída*, also commonly called *caída de la mollera*. My baby is 10 months old and has been crying day and night for about a week and does not stop being irritable. The doctor checked her out and wants to see her again tomorrow to give us the results of the tests she did on her. Could it be true what my mother says, that my little girl could have *caída de la mollera?*

We tried praying over her and did an egg healing on her for evil eye or *mal de ojo,* and for fright sickness, or *susto,* but nothing has worked. What else can we do? Please help us and keep us in your prayers.

CURANDERO'S RESPONSE:

With all due respect to your mother, your baby does not have a *mollera caída*, a fallen fontanel. Your baby is 10 months old and therefore cannot have this condition because her *mollera* has already closed. At birth, there is an area about the size of a quarter on top of the skull above the forehead that has yet to close the soft spot, or fontanel.

After birth, it takes the skull bone four months to completely enclose the soft spot. After this occurs, there is no longer a soft spot and so there can no longer be a *mollera*, or fontanel, to fall.

COMMENTARY:

Mollera caída, fallen fontanel, is a common folk symptom in which the fallen or sunken fontanel is associated with an irritable and/or hungry baby. This condition is usually called *caída de la mollera* but that is technically incorrect. It's actually vice versa, an infant who is sickly, dehydrated and not nursing adequately, will lose body weight and water weight causing the fontanels to sink or fall.

A mollera caída is usually seen in a baby suffering from intestinal dysentery or another illness which causes the infant to not breast or bottle feed. The hungry child becomes extremely irritable and refuses to respond to nursing. Folk beliefs hold that the fontanel, or *mollera*, must be reset, and "pulled" outward to its normal position. This is a common "folk illness" and is generally achieved by holding the baby upside down and tapping gently on the bottom of the feet while pressing gently down on the palate with one's thumb. If the pressure "pops" the fontanel back to its normal position, then the baby is once again able to nurse without pain. An infant that refuses to be nursed and has diarrhea, must be taken to a medical doctor immediately.

33. THE MIDWIFE - *LA PARTERA*

Dear Mr. *Curandero*, I am writing to you because I want to ask you about my choice to have my baby delivered by a certified nurse midwife (CNM), or *partera*, at a birthing center instead of a hospital. My mother tells me that all of my brothers and sisters born in Mexico were delivered by midwives, *parteras*. They are all fine and all of my brothers and sisters born in the United States were also delivered by *parteras*.

There are *parteras* where I live but all of my friends are horrified that I would think to have my baby delivered by a *partera* and not at a hospital. I want to honor my cultural heritage and know what you think. Is it safe?

CURANDERO'S RESPONSE:

The majority of Latino babies have been delivered at hospitals, however, many have also been delivered by midwives. In Spanish we call the midwife a *partera* referring to women who attend the delivery, or *parto;* literally the separation of the baby from the mother. In Mexico, there is a long tradition of midwives being certified to practice by the government so women who come from Mexico are familiar with the system and believe that women in the United States who call themselves parteras are also certified. Be careful because that is not always true.

Please get the spiritual and the supernatural involved with both your pregnancy and the birth process. There are three saints you can pray to for a normal pregnancy and a healthy baby. San Ramón Nonato celebrated August 13, Saint Gerard celebrated October 16, Saint Cecilia and Gabriel the Archangel celebrated September 29, Saints Marina and Margarita July 20, Saint Anne is the patron saint of infertility and she is celebrated on July 26, and Saint Catherine of Sweden protects against miscarriages and is celebrated on March 24. Any of the patron saints mentioned above protect our pregnancies, birth and the perinatal period.

It was not until recently, that programs in Certified Nurse Midwifery (CNM) have become available. FQHC's, Federally Qualified Health Centers, and Migrant Health Clinics have used certified nurse midwives to deliver babies.

Many states have also adopted laws that regulate the practice of midwifery, but one must always be cautious to choose a midwife who is certified and supervised.

There are many plant remedies you can use for different issues during pregnancy. Be sure to check plant references for more about their uses. Basil or *albahaca*, corn silk or *barba de maíz*, *perejil* or parsley, *damiana*, desert broom or *hierba de pasmo*, pennyroyal or *poleo*, fennel or *hinojo*, feverfew or *altamisa,* chamomile or *manzanilla,* Mexican oregano or *oregano*, and *sasafrás* are just a few that are used as teas, baths and douches.

COMMENTARY:

Choosing to have a baby delivered at a birthing center or by a midwife is an increasingly common and time-honored cultural event. Always be sure to check in your community to verify that the person or clinic you choose is staffed by certified nurse midwives and/or certified lay midwives and that they have a direct relationship with a medical doctor and a hospital in case of emergency complications during the delivery. Not all curanderas are midwives, but those who are serve as very important resources in their cultural communities and should be called upon for help as well.

Mexico has a long history of training and certifying the practice of midwifery. Midwives, called parteras and matronas, were assisted by "gossips" and by tenedoras, another class of birth helpers. Pre-Columbian rituals and practices were prevalent when the Spaniards arrived. Later, they began overseeing the delivery of all indigenous infants born in the urban areas.

Cultural Competency: *This section contains a number of well-known folk illnesses in Latino populations. The appropriate delivery of health care requires an understanding of the culture that is served and, as such, knowledge of anthropological theory is important. Cultural competency resource six outlines the major components of the Kleinman physician-anthropologist model of cultural competency.*

34. STOMACHACHES — *EMPACHO, CÓLICO, Y LATIDO*

Can you help me with my child? He cries a lot and is very uncomfortable. He seems to have a bulge in his stomach and he has not had a bowel movement. He does pass gas, but nothing else comes out. He is starting to look, as they say, a little green. He has been like this for three days in a row and we are very worried about him.

We took him to the doctor and he gave him some medicine, but he is not getting any better. My grandmother says that he has a blocked stomach or is *empachado* or has *empacho*, but I'm not sure what that is and how to treat it if he does not get better. He is only four years old.

Prior to this, he has had a lot of stomach problems, diarrhea, and fever and vomiting. Everything he eats disagrees with his stomach. Do you think that he may be allergic to something? He has not been doing well going on three days now. What should we do? Please help us. We are desperate. Should we take him to the emergency room at the hospital?

Antonio Zavaleta and Alberto Salinas Jr.

CURANDERO'S RESPONSE:

You may need to take your child to the emergency room if he does not respond, but it might just be a bad case of *cólico*, or colic. For *cólico*, the best remedy is *té de manzanilla*, or chamomile tea. You could also give him a tea made from *hierbanís*, or anise, or *epazote de zorillo*, or wormseed. Since he might have an intestinal obstruction called *empacho*, give the child a teaspoon of olive oil with a pinch of salt on the tongue. I see all kinds of digestive disorders and there are numerous home remedies for them. For example, you could take agrimony or *agrimonia*, almond or *almendra*, aloe vera or *sávila*, wormseed or *epazote*, anise or *anís*, bay leaf or *laurel*, bitter wood or *cassia*, black cumin or *comino negro*, blessed thistle or *cardo santo*, mint or *poleo*, cinnamon or *canela*, giant hyssop or *toronjil*, horehound or *marrubio*, *limón* or *lima*, Mormon tea or *popotillo* and numerous others.

Under no circumstance should you ever give your children a substance called *greta* or *azarcon* (100% lead oxide). These yellow powders are readily available at *hierberías* and are considered to be useful remedies for all kinds of stomach problems in children. However they have been found to be almost 100 percent lead and will poison your children causing mental retardation and eventually kill them. Don't let that happen to you.

It is much safer to call upon and pray to the saints who assist us with colic and stomach problems: Saint Agapitus for colic; Saint Erasmus for colic and intestinal disorders; and Saint Timothy for stomachaches, especially in children. Pray to Saint Bonaventure to resolve problems of the stomach and intestines. Celebrate Bonaventure on July 15.

Next, rub the abdomen gently with olive oil for three minutes. Turn the child on his stomach and rub olive oil on his lower back for about three minutes. Place a towel on the lower back and gently pinch the skin using both hands, side by side, using the towel to pull outward until the skin pops.

Repeat this procedure moving lower down the back each time. Pulling and popping the skin on the lower back of the body is the action that causes the *empacho*, or intestinal obstruction, to successfully be dislodged from the intestinal tract, and the digestive system will then begin to function properly.

You may try this procedure as a complementary treatment. But first and foremost, always take your physician's advice.

COMMENTARY:

Intestinal aches and pains, including blockage called empacho, are some of the most common ailments that curanderos treat. Empacho is a term used to describe a condition resulting from an intestinal obstruction caused by a clump of undigested food lodged somewhere within the digestive system. This stomach condition is due to something that the person ate which remained in the intestinal tract or by something consumed that was spoiled. Contamination of the food or rejection of the food usually occurs because it wasn't sufficiently cooked or was spoiled. This folk ailment, which is very common in children, can occur in adults as well. All types of stomach and intestinal problems were frequently treated by our grandmothers with an enema, or purga. Most Latinos raised in traditional households are familiar with this preventative enema. There are many herbal products such as flax seed that serve as antidysenterics; antispasmodics such as calamus or sweet flag, or yarrow; emetics to induce vomiting and nausea like las habas de San Ignacio; called purgantes, or purgatives, and/or herbal laxatives such as Epsom salts and many others.

Cólico and latido are familiar stomach and intestinal problems that curanderos/as are asked to treat. Simply speaking, colic translates as stomach gas commonly called indigestion. Latido literally means throbbing, but also refers to the symptom of nausea in the folk lexicon.

Because stomach and intestinal problems are so much a part of our human condition, there are literally hundreds of remedies for them passed on generationally. Geography also dictates cures, depending on where medicinal plants grow wild. In some cases, stomachaches can be reduced by a tea made of yarrow or of lemon, basil, chamomile, mint and many others.

35. BACK PROBLEM POULTICE — *EL PARCHE GUADALUPANO*

I write to you to see if you are able to help me. I was in an accident two years ago and suffered injuries to my back. What has resulted is that now I cannot stand the pain in my back. I have suffered for two years. I have visited specialists, doctors and chiropractors, but they have not been able to make me well. I am a true believer of the Niño Fidencio; this is why I ask for your help. I would like to know if my illness is good or bad. What is my prognosis? Can you recommend a good *sobadora,* folk-massage therapist?

CURANDERO'S RESPONSE:

What type of accident did you have? By chance, did you fall, or did you suffer an automobile accident or some other type of serious accident? What type of therapy have you had? What other treatments or operations have you had? Have you had massage therapy? Are you allergic to any medications?

Always remember that God is first, and with His help we will try with faith and goodwill to help you as well. One proposes and God disposes. You should ask San Tomás the patron saint of back problems whose feast day is celebrated July 13, also Saint Lawrence for back problems in general to help you.

I know that they have probably told you that it was some ill placement, *malpuesto* or *brujería,* or witchcraft, but I see spiritually that your accident came naturally.

I think that part of your problem is from an old scare or *susto pasado.* It is possible that you may be relieved significantly of your pain. If you can, let us know when you may come to cure you of *susto,* a past *susto,* a trauma, fright or pain. You are going to need a total realignment of your back as well as your spirit, so let me know when you can visit me.

Meanwhile, you may boil *salvia* and lemon grass together and drink one cup of tea in the morning and another at night for 40 consecutive days. General aches and pains are among the most common physical ailments I treat and there are a wide variety of medicinal plants or *plantas medicinales* that can be used. The plants can be taken as teas, or prepared as saves or ointments and rubbed on the body part that hurts. Some of the most commonly used are, aloe vera or *sávila*, ambrosia or *hierba amarga*, angels trumpet or *florifundo*, black mustard, or *mostaza negra*, boneset or *eupatorium*, burro bush or *hierba del burro*, camphor or *alcanfor*, camphor weed sometimes called *arnica*, Indian plantain or *matarique*, nutmeg or *nuez moscada*. Commonly, I ask people to take one garlic capsule and two aloe vera capsules, in the morning and at night, the same for 40 straight days. Pray Psalm 3 for headaches and backaches.

COMMENTARY:

In the Latino healing community, there are specialists called bonesetters, or hueseros, and massage therapists recognized as sobadoras. These folk specialists often have the uncanny ability to redirect nerve bundles and to soothe strained muscles. They should always be used to reinforce or complement medical advice. Often, back problems and bone and joint complications are caused by inflammation. Anti-inflammatory and antispasmodic or antiespasmódico and linimento, or liniment, such as volcanico and arnica, are prescribed by curanderos to reduce inflammation. Kidneywood or palo azul is one of the best-known hierbas used for reducing swelling. Lemon grass, or zacate de limón, is taken as a tea and used to reoxidize the blood. An agent which reintroduced oxygen to the blood is called an antioxidant or in Spanish, antioxidante. A common antispasmodic is yarrow, or milenrama.

36. EARACHE FUNNEL — *EL CUCURUCHO*

I don't have a clear recollection of my third or fourth year of life, but I do clearly remember that I always had ear infections. In fact, at least some of my hearing loss today can be attributed to the fact that my ears were always stopped up and infected. I have a clear memory of an old woman coming to my home and rolling up a piece of newspaper in the form of a funnel and placing it in my ear and lighting it on fire. Now, as a parent, one of my co-workers has recommended that I use this same technique to my child. Have you ever heard of this? Can you please explain it to me?

CURANDERO'S RESPONSE:

Earaches can be very painful and there are a number of things that can cause them. Most commonly it is air, *aire*, or water in the ear. Foreign objects and stopped up ears from colds and influenza can also cause earaches. In older persons, often high blood pressure or sinus problems cause ringing in the ear. So, as you can see, there can be any number of causes of earaches. It is always recommended that you consult a doctor especially where infections are present and children are involved. Young children are particularly susceptible to chronic ear infections that if left untreated can cause them lifelong hearing loss.

One of the most common home remedies is to place olive oil in the ear or an *unguento*, or unguent, paste made from pig lard covered with a plug of cotton. Other medicinal plants that I commonly use for earaches include, bay leaf or *laurel;* coriander or *cilantro;* marigold or *calendula;* red sage or *mirto*; and rue or *ruda*.

For generations, *curanderas* have been treating earaches with the funnel, or with the *embudo*, method. This method is based on the belief that the earache is due to an imbalance of air pressure within the ear. The *curandero* forms a funnel shape usually from newspaper, placing the narrow end of the funnel slightly into the ear cavity, and then lighting the fire around the edges of the newspaper of the large open end of the funnel. This remedy is as old as the hills and many of us had this remedy applied to us as children by our grandmothers or aunts. Our grandmothers usually would also light a candle to San Mauricio, whose feast day is celebrated September 22 and to Saint Cornelius on September 16 as well as to Saint Louis asking him to cure diseases of the ear.

However, it is not safe for the funnel procedure to be performed by a novice and it is never recommended that anyone who is not an expert attempt it. For example, this procedure must never be done without a container of water handy to dip the lighted paper into to put out the fire. And it should never be done inside a house. Once the funneled paper is lit, the fire will burn gradually getting larger and requiring more and more air to burn. If there is any excess air causing pressure on the ear, the fire will suck it out causing an audible pop. Seeing the paper in flames is very impressive, but dangerous. If performed properly, the person should have immediate relief from the pain.

If immediate relief does not occur, air pressure is not the cause of the ailment and the person should see a physician. We do not recommend anyone try this procedure at home. Another common home remedy used by *curandera*s for earaches is to place camphor oil on a cotton ball and to place in the ears for three straight days, or to heat the gel from the leaf of the aloe vera, or *sávila*, and to place gently on in the outer ear for a few minutes. This remedy usually solves the problem in cases where the earache was not caused by infection.

COMMENTARY:

Earaches can be traced to a multitude of causes. Both allergies and ear infections cause accumulation of fluids in the inner ear; creating a buildup of pressure and pain in the ear. This is very common among children. Many cultures acknowledge that fire sucks out oxygen and air from a higher gradient of pressure to a lower gradient to relieve pressure. If air is captured within the inner ear and unable to escape, a paper funnel with the small end placed next to the ear opening with the paper's large end lit, it is thought to draw the air out of the ear; restoring ear-pressure balance, which results in diminishment of the pain.

37. CARING FOR FATHER — *CUIDANDO PAPÁ*

I was writing to see if you could tell me what is wrong with my father. He has been sick for over a month and I am just now finding this out because he always keeps it from me.

My husband is a real jerk and he hardly ever lets me spend time with my father. I am trying to gain the strength to get a divorce, but my husband keeps telling me about how he will kill me if I ever try to leave him for good. I am really scared and I just want out of this horrible marriage. Can you help me?

I am taking my father to see my doctor so that he can examine him. He is not taking his diabetes medicine and has not gone to his doctor in a very long time. He has been having stomach problems with everything he eats. He really gets an upset stomach or vomits. I am just really scared for him.

CURANDERO'S RESPONSE:

I do not understand why your father will not tell you what is wrong with him. Will his doctor tell you? I will pray for him. I will also keep you in my prayers so that you will have the strength and valor to go on with whatever you need to do to find happiness in your life.

Light a San Alejo candle and a San Ignacio de Loyola candle with a glass of water over your father's picture between the two candles. Also, Santos Cosme y Damian are celebrated September 26 and are the patron saints of men's health problems. Pray to them for your father. God bless you. I am praying that your father does not have something worse wrong with him.

COMMENTARY:

This woman is simultaneously concerned for her father's health and resentful of her husband and terrible marriage. If we dig deeper into this case we find that this woman already lost her mother and she clings to her father. Additionally, she neglects her marriage and this may be why her husband reacts negatively to having been abandoned emotionally by his wife. There are always at least two sides to every story that the curandero must investigate.

Threats or fear of threats of violence are not helpful and serve to further compound his wife's fragile emotional state. Simply stated, she is terrified of losing her father and perceives that she would then be all alone in the world. A continued conversation with the curandero in this case provides a calming effect as the curandero takes on the role of the marriage counselor.

Cultural competency: *Resource number eight provides a model developed by Georgetown University entitled, The Cultural Broker Program. This program is designed to assist the health-care delivery system and subsequently develop outreach to the cultural communities that they serve. This could include community health workers, migrant camp aides, and most recently, promotoras de salud, or lay health workers, in colonias or outlying settlements.*

38. GRANDMOTHER'S RHEUMATISM — *LAS REUMAS*

I just wanted to know if there is anything that my grandmother can do to relieve the pain in her legs. Yesterday after you prayed for her and swept the pain from her right leg, it seemed to go away. As we were walking away from your place, she said that she felt better and felt that she could move her leg a little easier.

But once we left and were halfway home, she started rubbing her leg and said she was starting to feel a little pain in her knee. We told her not to worry that the pain was going to go away. At times, she says it feels as if though her whole body and all of her joints hurt and she cannot control her legs. She feels that her legs want to take off by themselves and move. At night, she cried again because not only the right leg was hurting, but her left knee was starting to hurt as well. She has been using an ointment, but it takes a while to work, and when it does work it's only for a short while. What else can we do for her? It really hurts us to see her suffer this way. If its arthritis, I don't know why the over-the-counter creams and the medication the doctor gave her don't work. Is there any remedy that she can take for this pain because she doesn't get much sleep at night?

We also wanted to know if some of this pain isn't being caused by someone trying to hurt her by using evil. Yesterday I forgot to show you the scratches that appeared on her arm for no apparent reason. Could this be evil? We appreciate any help you can give us. We are also saying a prayer that we found on the Internet to the Niño Fidencio. Please pray for my grandmother and Niñito Fidencio that her pain may be relieved and that she be able to sleep at night. I also need a little help to feel better because caring for my grandmother is getting me down.

CURANDERO'S RESPONSE:

Thank you for your e-mail and for keeping me informed. It seems to me that your grandmother is suffering from *reumas*, that is, arthritis, or rheumatism and there are many remedies for these ailments, but this is a normal part of aging and will never completely go away. Many people swear by the copper bracelet. You can buy one fairly cheaply. I would also recommend that you prepare a tea made from garlic cloves simmered in milk. Have her drink the cup of milk for nine consecutive days, especially when she is suffering.

By the grace of Our Lord and in the name of the Holy Spirit we pray for your grandmother. Have her rub lemon juice on her leg and knee, then rub egg white on her leg when in pain.

She may also try a tea made from lemon grass, *zacate de limón*, and of *salvia* or sage. Have her drink a glass of tomato juice with her meal and then apply tomato juice on a paper towel and place the towel over the knee and painful area while praying over her. Do this once or twice a day for nine straight days.

Additionally, have your grandmother drink cherry juice. Give her an ounce in a glass of water a day for three straight weeks. Get an extract of *nopal* or cactus leaves, and *linaza* or flax seed from your neighborhood pharmacy, or *hierbería*. If you can't find these ingredients, ask for *linaza* fiber. Use one or the other putting one teaspoon of the fiber in a glass of water. Mix well and give it to her to drink once a day for two straight weeks.

Pray to San Francisco whose feast day is October 4 to relieve your grandmother's leg pain and to Saint James the Greater on July 25. Prayers to Santa Mónica, the protector of women, on August 8, are in order as well.

Just to be safe, cleanse your grandmother's home. Pass a fertile hen's egg over her body. The hen's eggs must be prepared for three days by placing them in a triangular form and by sprinkling or spraying them with perfumes for health and strength. Cleanse her body with the prepared egg every Friday for seven Fridays in a row and her health will return. Cleanse her home by performing a *sahumerio* or smoking cleansing ritual, and by speaking that all evil and negative forces be cast out of the home.

COMMENTARY:

Many Latinos, especially the older generations, have many chronic health problems which aren't being treated by doctors because of their inability to pay, lack of insurance or simply due to noncompliance. The long-range results of untreated chronic heart disease, arthritis and diabetes will ultimately result in system failure which is the primary cause of death for diabetics. This is probably the primary health problem among all Latino populations. In this case, grandmother must see her doctor. Taking her to the curandero at her insistence is at best a temporary relief.

Problems with arthritis and rheumatism are common in all elderly populations and each person has a favorite remedy. In the traditional Latino populations of the United States-Mexico border, a favorite remedy is to ferment a small amount of leaves of the marijuana plant inside a bottle of green alcohol. Cloves are often added. This concoction is a kind of topical anesthetic, or anestésico, or an anodyne, anodino, which is believed to relieve mild pain by numbing the nerves. Lemon grass also serves as an antirheumatic. Place this mixture at her bedside for the massaging of her aching joints.

39. HELP MY LITTLE SON — *AYUDA MI PEQUEÑO*

My son is 10 years old and has been seeing doctors all of his short life. The condition he has is called cerebral palsy. As far as we know, the doctor says he is doing fine every time he goes to the doctor's office. But it seems that his seizures are more frequent and the doctor keeps changing his medication to see which one will stop his seizures. I hope this little bit of information can help you to determine what we can do in the spiritual world to help him. It all seems strange to us because he scares so easily.

CURANDERO'S RESPONSE:

His condition is natural, not supernatural or evil. Prepare a tea made by boiling *hierbanís*, anise, and *tumba vaquero*, or morning glory and have him drink one cup of tea a day for seven straight days. Then stop giving him the tea and let me know how he is doing.

There are a number of different illnesses and conditions that deal with the brain and nerves and each requires a different *remedio*. Some of the most common plants are black mustard or *mostaza negra*; mistletoe or *injerto*; night blooming jasmine or *huele de noche*.

Please send me his picture as well. Light a candle on your home altar to San Bartolomé, the protector of the nervous system and to Saint Valentine who protects us against paralysis and epilepsy. I will buy candles to burn on my altar for you and your son as well.

Sometimes I will have to suck an illness out of a person or *soplar*. Finally, pray Psalm 9, which is used to cure male children. Saint Willibrord is often consulted on issues of epilepsy, and seizures, his day is November 7, and Saint Felicitas on July 10, is the patron saint for baby boys.

COMMENTARY:

The curandero must allay the fears of each and every person who wish to affix a supernatural origin to problematic life situations. While some persons may want to blame witchcraft and/or evil origins to every situation they encounter, it is unrealistic to believe witchcraft is responsible for every negative happenstance in our lives. While the curandero realizes this and attempts to keep the petitioner in balance, the curandero, however, will always check for viable evidence of witchcraft. Often, this is accomplished without alarming the client until it is necessary.

Curanderos/as will often use a number of personally, acquired and developed, healing techniques. These include both actual and psychic surgery, as well as blowing into the body, sucking out of the patient's body and spiritually transferring illness or objects from a patient to the curandero. Curanderos/as can often be taken ill through these processes and will go through a period of rest and the cleansing of their bodies before they may return to their practice.

40. LIKE OTHER CHILDREN — *COMO OTROS NIÑOS*

I have a nine-year-old daughter who was born with spina bifida. The nerve endings to her bladder and bowels are damaged. She has no feeling when she goes to the restroom. I use a catheter for her four times a day. This is the first year she attends school and the situation is hard for her. She understands that she is different from others, but they are very cruel to her and she doesn't understand why. She constantly asks me why she can't be like the other children and why they are mean to her.

Last year, she had major surgery augmentation of her bladder and she is a little better now but one of her kidneys still does not function well, so all of the stress is on the one good kidney.

I have done a little reading on El Niño Fidencio. Do you think you can ask him to help my daughter?

CURANDERO'S RESPONSE:

My prayers are with you and for your daughter's health and well-being. If you could, please, make a tea of boiled corn silk, or *barbas de maíz*, and have her drink a cup every morning for 40 days in a row. I have an ointment called *pomada del Niño Fidencio*. I want you to rub it on her back over her spinal column near her kidneys to see if it helps her to get better. Kidney function can often be helped by alfalfa; almond or *almendra*; borage or *borraja;* creosote bush called *gobernadora*; corn silk or *barbas de maíz*; kidney wood or *palo azul*; thistle or *cardo santo*; and pink windmills called *hierba de la hormiga*.

One should always petition the Creator for good health in the home and for all of its occupants, especially children. Sometimes one should actually mention the organs, such as the heart, the eyes or the kidneys.

It is always important to voice your petitions to the Creator out loud and to San Andrés who protects children against illnesses. His feast day is celebrated November 30. Saint Nicholas, celebrated on December 6 is the patron saint of children and Blessed Margaret of Castello, April 13, protects persons with disabilities.

COMMENTARY:

The curandero can offer precious little to this exasperated mother other than hope and prayer. Since they are true believers, the fact that the curandero prescribes a receta or written prescription, isn't harmful. This simply sustains hope in a trying situation. This child requires medical care for her entire life, and combined with the curandero's lifeline, the family will have a continuous support system for many years.

41. ANGRY LITTLE BOY — *ENMUINADO Y ENCORAJINADO*

I have a request for Niño Fidencio. My grandson is five years old and is seeing a doctor about his stomach problems. His stomach gets very bloated. The doctors have done a series of blood tests and have not found anything wrong with him. Another problem is that he's very angry all the time. He starts fights with other children at his daycare and at home with his little sister. His grandmother has tried curing him with an egg and on the third day we broke the egg into the glass of water and the egg looked black and evil. It looked as if it exploded into the glass of water. His mother is wondering if he should have a cleansing by the Niño Fidencio.

CURANDERO'S RESPONSE:

Thank you for your prayer request. There are so many things that make children angry. It might be his diet which has too many "cold" foods and is causing his *bilis*, or bile, to rise. It could be that he is not getting enough attention at home or is jealous of his brothers and sisters, in which case we say that he is *chipil*. To treat *chipil,* place a small coral beans necklace around the neck of the child. The coral bean is known as the *colorín* or whistle tree. If the beans lose their bright red color the child is diagnosed as *chipil*.

Have you tried giving the child chamomile tea? *Té de manzanilla* is proven to work for colic. You may also wish to have him swept by the Niño Fidencio. I shall invoke the spirit of Niño Fidencio and San Basilio and petition in a prayer request that he spiritually visit your grandson and perform a healing through the grace of the Holy Spirit. The ugly egg yolk in the glass of water indicates the possibility that the child needed to be cleansed to remove an unclean spirit. Bathe your grandchild with Holy Water from a church once a day for seven consecutive days. The child should be fine after you perform this ritual. If not, please write to me for further examination.

Uncontrollable anger called *coraje* or *muina* is often treated by the doctors with medications which are sedatives and that is not always good for him because it changes his behavior. You could also give him a citrus tea which includes a mixture of various citrus products. This should have a naturally calming effect. Three consecutive *barridas*, or *limpias*, with *pirul* are also important. You can do this yourself at home.

COMMENTARY:

The ancient Aztecs believed anger was caused by a combination of natural as well as supernatural forces. A personality viewed as angry is most often attributed to the intervention of the devil and treated with a variation of incantations or prayers. This child could be suffering from empacho, an intestinal obstruction. The diagnosis and treatment for a folk condition would not ordinarily be addressed by a doctor. An undiagnosed condition could explain the child's continued outbursts. The parents and the curandero should not rule out medical conditions that fuel temper tantrums such as, ADD and ADHD, if this is a long-term behavioral pattern. The child should always be treated by a physician who should always be informed about the medicinal teas that are taken. This is especially true when treated children cannot verbalize their symptoms. It cannot hurt to take him to the curandero to be cleansed, but he must also see a doctor. This family has already attempted to treat him for mal de ojo with no result.

When encountering anger-management problems, called muinas or corajes, the first course of action curanderos/as usually take is determining if the bile, or bilis, is out of sync. This is a direct reference to 16th century Mexican medicinal beliefs.

Cultural Competency: *Resource nine is designed to assist the entry-level, health care provider to understand the reality that culture plays in health care. This material was developed by the American Medical Student Association for the training of future physicians. (See Appendix I)*

42. PRAY FOR US — *REZA POR NOSOTROS*

I am requesting your prayers for my eldest son. He has been in intensive care for a week and has a lot of complications right now. Both his kidneys have stopped working and, at this very minute, they are doing a catheter and then they will do a blood transfusion. The doctors wanted to wait until tomorrow to see if some of the infection clears up, but I just got a call from my sister and the doctors can wait no longer. They have given him a 50/50 chance of living. Please pass this along to all your family members and friends and your Niño Fidencio prayer circle so that you can help us pray for him and his wife and three children. And of course, pray for our whole family in our hour of need.

CURANDERO'S RESPONSE:

Family, remember this: Our Lord, hear our prayers and may His mercy be with this family. We pray for His miracle healing and for His blessing for the family. Protect the family home by planting aloe vera at all four corners of your yard. Over the front door and rear door place a red and green ribbon along with a lodestone, or *piedra imán*, with iron filings, three high John the Conqueror seeds, male garlic heads, red and white coral, three copper coins and three seeds of wheat, rice, corn, coriander, star anise and black and white mustard seeds. This magic will help all matters within your home. For difficult health problems, always pray to San Judás Tadeo whose feast day is October 28.

Be certain that your son immediately receives the sacrament of Extreme Unction, the last rites of the Roman Catholic Church.

COMMENTARY:

I always recommend the work of Dr. Larry Dossey, "Prayer is Good Medicine" and "Be Careful What You Pray For," on the efficacy and the power of prayer in seemingly hopeless medical cases. Prayer is always the gateway to God's miracles. Curanderos are called upon to minister in all life's rites of passage. This is especially true when death is imminent for our loved ones. Curanderos/as often request that their clients consult a Catholic priest to perform the last rites of the Church if they believe the death of the family member is near.

43. VERY SICK LITTLE GIRL — *LA ENFERMITA*

Last night, my aunt called to tell me that the doctors have diagnosed her two-year-old niece as either having kidney stones or failing kidneys. When she pees, she pees blood. The doctors said that if her kidneys are bad, they would have to do a transplant. My aunt would like to know if you and El Niño can help this sick little girl. They would also like to know if there is anything they can give her for the tremendous pain she has?

CURANDERO'S RESPONSE:

It is critical that you follow the instructions of your doctor and to tell the doctor if you are giving her any type of herbal tea. Have your aunt give her tea made from *hierba de la hormiga*, ant weed from the four o'clock flower family. You could also try creosote bush or what we call *gobernadora*, and/or a tea made from kidneywood, or *palo azul*. Give her one cup of tea in the morning for nine days in a row. Blend *salvia* and *zacate de limón* in a tea for the blood and pain. Be sure to offer a candle on your home altar to San Marcos the patron saint of childhood illnesses. His feast day is April 25. Santa Marta is the patron saint for healing of kidneys, celebrated July 29. Please be sure to keep me up to date on her condition and when she improves. Most importantly she needs plenty of prayer. Pray Psalm 33 to keep children healthy.

COMMENTARY:

In this, or in any other situation where a person is being treated by a medical doctor and also taking medicinal teas, it is critical that the physician is cognizant of which teas are being consumed to determine if there are any active ingredients which will react negatively with the doctor's prescription. There are many medicinal plants believed to have properties which assist the urinary tract and kidneys. To list just a few, they are: bee brush or quebradora; bilberry or arandano; birch or abedul; common juniper or enebro; cranberry or airela; dandelion or diente de leon; evening primrose or hierba del golpe; horsetail or cola de caballo and wild olive or anacahuita.

44. PREGNANCY AND BIRTH — *ENCINTA Y DAR A LUZ*

I read about your illness and hope you are doing better. I am a young Latina who has grown up in the United States. As such, I have very little knowledge of Mexico and the old folk ways. It is a great advantage for me to have all of the older women of our family around me. We have a united family, guided by strong women, and they were all born and raised in Mexico. They keep tradition alive in our family. The women in my family include my mother, many aunts, my two grandmothers and even one great grandmother. They are all treasures of folk knowledge, remedies and beliefs. Additionally, they are all deeply religious women combining folk remedies with Catholic saints.

The women in my family believe it is important to pass on their knowledge about pregnancy and birth to me and I embrace that. I was wondering if you could share some of the things you know so that when I talk to them I can surprise them with what I have learned and won't seem so uninformed to them.

I have a college education but not a cultural one. Please help me!

CURANDERO'S RESPONSE:

You are very fortunate that you have strong women in your family and that they are united in their beliefs and that their customs will be passed on to you. I will try to help you with what I have heard and learned over my years as a healer. Because I am male, I am at a slight disadvantage, but because pregnancy and birth are so important, I have learned from many others including my own grandmother, mother and wife.

One of the most important issues in every family is the ability to get pregnant. Sometimes it is very difficult and couples endure years or a lifetime without being able to produce a baby. This causes great stress in the family, especially with the couple's parents who want a grandchild. So when conception does not occur, it is common for the wife's mother or her mother-in-law to recommend that she see a *curandero/a*.

It is believed that the female reproductive organs must be "heated" in order for conception to take place. In Mexico, people learn that illness and many health conditions are caused by imbalances in the body; the by-products of improper diet of foods with hot versus cold properties. In my practice, when people come to me who can't have a baby, the first thing I do is prescribe a tea composed of hot herbs like *damiana* or *turnera diffusa,* and others which should be taken in the morning and at night for 40 consecutive days, the length of Lent. This usually does the trick, the reproductive system is heated and the woman gets pregnant quickly in most cases. Special massages with olive oil or other specially prepared oils are usually required of the lower abdomen area as well. This is to make sure that all of the organs are in their proper location as well as to heat them.

One of the by-products of pregnancy is the production of gas in the intestines and this may be controlled with a tea made from sage or yarrow. This *carminativo*, or carminative, will also reduce the abdominal discomfort. Many old *curanderas* would also treat pregnant women with olive oil which acts as a cathartic, or *catártico*, purgative used to clean out the digestive system.

The husband usually wants to determine the gender of the baby and there are many beliefs concerning the determination of the sex of the unborn baby. The women of the family will hold a red string with a needle dangling over the belly of the expectant mother. If the needle rotates clockwise, that indicates the baby will be a boy and if it rotates counterclockwise it indicates a girl.

Protecting the unborn and developing baby from outside negative forces is very important. For example, the unborn baby should never be exposed to an eclipse because this is believed to most certainly cause a deformity. Talismans and amulets are worn under clothing to protect the developing baby.

These are just a few of the hundreds of remedies and beliefs that exist and that we utilize during the various stages leading up to pregnancy, during pregnancy, during and after delivery.

Remember that San Ramón Nonato and Santa Cecilia are patron saints of developing babies and births, and Saint Camillus de Lellis is the patron saint of nurses and nurse midwives. I am sure that this is enough knowledge to impress your grandmothers and to generate a great conversation.

Pray Psalm 128 for a successful pregnancy and birth. And never forget that when a mother is pregnant, it will affect the behavior and moods of existing small children who will become jealous of the new baby, especially when and if the existing children are removed from their mother's breast. When a baby is sad, he or she is said to be *chipil,* which means that they are jealous of the new baby who displaced them. Good luck.

COMMENTARY:

Conditions surrounding pregnancy and birth are among the most common and important within the human sphere. Curanderos/as learn early that they must be prepared to treat these conditions with all of the time-tested remedies. Herbal teas, massages, magical protections and prayers to the appropriate saint are all necessary to ensure a positive outcome of pregnancy and birth. And these things are just as important to all female family members as they are to the expectant mother. There are many herbal teas recorded that assist pregnancy and/or induce abortion. Many also are used to assist the reproductive system in flushing lingering menstrual fluids. This is called an emmenagogue, or emenagogo. Yarrow or milenrama is commonly used for this. Pregnancy also causes water weight gain or edema. Curanderos often prescribe diuretics, or diuréticos, such as creosote bush for treating liquid retention.

An entire category of medicinal plants exists, such as borage, or borraja, used to promote the generous flow of breast milk after birth. These herbs are called galactogogues, or galactagogos, because they promote and enhance the production of breast milk.

Ailments and illnesses come and go. It's trendy to attribute a cure to a medicinal plant or a prescribed medicine. One must be careful! In addition to all of the popular folk medicines, the curandero should always refer a person to a physician or clinic which specializes in nurse-midwife assisted births. Regarding pregnancy and birth the person should inquire of both the doctor and the curandero.

45. THE FAMILY IS SICK — *ESTAMOS ENFERMOS*

Thank you so much for your prayers. I am sorry it has been so long since I've written. I haven't been as devoted as I should be. Please keep praying for me.

I just got married, and as a new wife, daughter and sister, I am having such a hard time. I am angry all the time and it is about the stupidest things. I feel depressed a lot. I was injured at work recently.

I fell and hurt my back. I am having a hard time just doing things around the house. Please pray for my body to heal and for my energy to return. I am overweight and really need to start exercising and get healthy. Please pray for me.

My mom wanted me to let you know that my younger sister has a bone abnormality. She has to have a CAT-scan (computerized axial topography) every year to make sure things are okay with her bones. She also has a bump on her head. She has always had it, but it looks like it might be getting bigger. We are really scared about it. She is so young and very precious to us.

My mom has been trying to qualify for disability, but she has been denied twice. This is her third attempt and she is worried. Her lawyer let her know that this is her last chance. If she is denied again, she will lose all of her benefits. She has had a constant pain in her body for a long time. The bones in her feet, her back, her shoulders, her neck and her entire body hurt. Please pray for her disability claim to go through.

At one time, my aunt called the disability office and claimed that my mother was making her pain up. She thinks that is why she is having a hard time being accepted. She really isn't making it up. She knows in her heart she isn't going to be able to work, and that is fine with her. She really needs to be accepted for this disability.

She would like you to pray, send her a prayer or two, and names of some candles she can light. Thank you so much for you support and prayers! We love you so much. God bless you.

CURANDERO'S RESPONSE:

Your entire family must pray to Saint Joseph the Worker, the patron saint of the family and home problems. His feast day is celebrated May 1. Your sister may drink a cup of tea made from *golondrina,* or euphorbia herb. Have her drink one cup of tea any time of day for four consecutive weeks. Then, she should take a cup of tea made from *boldo* or bold, also for four consecutive weeks.

I am sorry to learn of all your family's health problems. It can be very stressful. It can also be very confusing as you say, especially when the physician does not take the time to explain. And when the physician does explain, one sometimes has to have a degree in medicine to understand. I understand what you are telling me and that is one reason, as a healer, I care deeply and sincerely for those who come to me for prayer and comforting in their times of need. Sometimes just being there for someone to listen to and to hear them out can bring great relief. I am happy to be here for people of faith in spiritual healing.

Yes, I will pray for you and your family. I shall continue to keep you in my daily prayers. Please light the Niño Fidencio candle for a period of 40 straight days. Place a clear glass of water next to your candle. Call on the name of Niño Fidencio three times and take three drinks of water from the glass on a daily basis for the 40 day period and make your petitions to the Divine Spirit of Light. Meditate for spiritual inner peace. Pray to Santa Juliana the patron saint of chronic illnesses, she is celebrated on June 19th.

You already know what you need: inner peace. You also have faith in the power of prayers. I will chant for you and I will send my spirit with the best intentions for you, and you will receive it in good faith. I will pray for justice for your mother's disability claim as you have asked.

COMMENTARY:

It is clearly evident from these examples that the "system's" definition of disabilities is not conveyed. This is often the case with Latino families, especially when English is the second language. It is incumbent on the physician or other social service agencies to ensure that the patient/client fully understands the condition, the treatment and the consequences.

It's routine for people to pass through phases in which everything seems to be coming unglued. Family members are sick, work is not going well, and pressing financial problems and marital problems can quickly unravel life's daily rituals. Highly complex situations like this one require ongoing consultation and a support network. In the Latino community it is usually true that the only functional support network is that of the curandero/a. This is why people make regular visits to curanderas. In a case like this one, it is important that a legitimate curandero/a, be located who acts as a helper and not a commercial enterprise.

There are many plants that are used for the aches and pains of life. Some are taken as a tea while others are either rubbed on the skin, just a few include: acacia; aloe vera or sávila; ambrosia or hierba amarga; avocado or aguacate; bear grass or sacahuista; black mustard or mostasa negra; camphor or alcanfor; arnica; cottonwood or alamo; and milkweed or lechona.

46. HERBAL REMEDIES — *LA HERBOLARIA*

I am writing to let you know I went to buy the medicinal tea leaves you requested, but I could not find *malabar* that you asked me to get for the regulation of my digestive system. At the *hierbería* they told me they do not sell *malabar* in the United States because they are no longer available here. Can I still take the tea without that one ingredient or should I keep looking for it? And also should I grind the leaves in my blender so I can know how much to put in a cup of tea? Or is it one teaspoon of each? Or should I mix all of them together in the blender? I really don't want to sound ignorant, but I just want to get it right.

CURANDERO'S RESPONSE:

I am glad you found the herbs you were looking for. You say you did not find the *malabar kino*. We can proceed with the recipe using the other herbs, blending the *marrubio blanco*, or white horehound, with them so as to be sure you receive a proper treatment for regulating your digestive system. You could also take a tea of wormwood, or *ajenjo*, for stomachache. If the stomachache involves vomiting, take a tea of white horehound, or *marrubio*. If you can, try to grind the different herbs and then mix them well. Use one teaspoon of herb per one cup of water. Take one cup of tea in the evening before bedtime for three consecutive weeks.

COMMENTARY:

In this book's Appendix III, there is an exhaustive list of the most commonly-used medicinal plants in Latino curanderismo. Always consult a medical doctor before taking an herbal supplement, especially if you are simultaneously taking a prescription medication. Also, please consult the listed websites for information on medicinal plants. For example, malabar kino is a tree resin used in medicine which produces a reddish black juice. It is harvested from trees in the genus Pterocarpus.

47. HOT-COLD-WET-DRY—*TEORÍA HUMORAL*

I hear people at the company where I work talk about hot and cold food. They talk about what should be eaten and what should not be eaten at certain times and that to make a mistake could cause serious illness. I really don't understand what they are talking about. I was not raised in a family where our mother taught us about this sort of thing. Is it real? Should I be concerned about hot and cold foods, and what I eat? What exactly is a hot food or a cold food? At first, I thought they were talking about the temperature of the foods, but then I quickly learned they were not. They are talking about the classification of the food and its properties. Where does all this come from? I don't want to make a mistake that could cause me an illness.

CURANDERO'S RESPONSE:

I am sorry that I don't have the knowledge base to explain it to you completely, but I will try my best. Most ancient peoples, certainly people from Europe and the Indian cultures of the Americas, have traditions and beliefs that both health and illness are caused by the balance or imbalance of food and the environment. That is, our ability to maintain the balance of the internal body functions with the external environment and especially what we consume is critical to maintaining health or promoting illness.

Foods, including most meats, grease or lard, eggs, corn are considered to have hot properties, they promote growth and they accelerate body functions. Sometimes this is good and they are needed, but other times not. Cold foods include most fresh vegetables and fruits, either eaten fresh or in the form of a soup, dairy products, fish and chicken. The temperature of the soup does not influence that the food is a cold or hot food.

Outside conditions are also very important. If a child is affected by rapid changes in temperature by going from hot to cold without protection, they will develop a runny nose and possibly a cold. We call this condition *pasmo*, and we know it is not a virus and can be resolved by administering hot foods like chicken soup, or *sopa*, and protection from cold floors and walls. If the child has a fever along with the runny nose, then a tea of *borraja*, or borage, or *muicle*, also called Mexican honeysuckle, or a variety of other fever-reducing plants will work to reduce the fever. Remember, a feverish person must be brought back into balance before they can recover. There are prayers that are also believed to assist our balance. Pray Psalms 49 and 50 to maintain a balance of health in your family.

COMMENTARY:

Understanding the concept of balance in curanderismo is of utmost importance. Curanderismo's underlying belief system is derived from a mixture of Greco-Arabic medicine brought to the new world by the first European settlers; especially Catholic priests. The native cultures they encountered in the Americas had a very similar belief in balance, and so, over the course of time, the two systems meshed together easily into what we have today. This complex, yet elegant, belief system has been handed down through the generations to this day. For hundreds of years, physicians as well as native healers practiced these beliefs every day but 20th century germ theory transformed medicine and took it in another direction.

In his "Historia Natural," Francisco Hernández demonstrates that, like 16th century European medicine, Aztec medicine also prescribed foods and medicinal plants on the basis of their hot and cold, as well as moist and dry properties. The European motif is attributed to both Hippocrates and Galen as described by Siegel 1968 and Andrews and Hassig 1984, "...health was thought to be a balance of the four principal humors: yellow bile, black bile, blood and phlegm. These resulted from the combination of the four contraries (hot, cold, moist and dry) in the human body: blood was hot and moist and was associated with the elements of air along with spring and summer; phlegm was cold and moist and was associated with the elements of water and winter; black bile was cold and dry and was associated with the elements earth and autumn; and yellow bile was hot and dry and was associated with the elements of fire with summer and fall. Thus, health was primarily a balance of these four humors within the body, and healing was the process of reestablishing the disrupted balance by the use of food and medicine possessing the opposite qualities. (Siegel, 1968, p.17-19) These prescriptions, however, were not absolutes, they are also affected by the patient's personal makeup or nature; whether he is sanguine (blood-dominant); phlegmatic (phlegm-dominant); melancholic (black-bile-dominant); or choleric (yellow-bile-dominant). Diagnosis didn't merely identify the specific illness with a corresponding remedy, but balanced the humoral disruption by calculating the introduction of remedial amounts of contrary elements. This includes the factors of essential personality and season being taken into account." (Andrews and Hassig, 1984, p.31-32)

Today, the native healers including curanderos/as are the keepers and practitioners of this essential ancient wisdom. Often, we find that curanderos/as will prescribe a remedy of balance for an illness that the doctors can't cure, only to be amazed that the folk cure actually worked. They only need to dig out 17th century medical books to discover that the cure has been around forever. For example, people with fevers need to be cooled down and so they are prescribed antipyretic agents for fever reduction. Common medicinal plants like the mints hierba buena, or spearmint, are given in cases like these.

48. OLD-FASHIONED GRANDMOTHER — *ABUELITA ANTICUADA*

Ever since I was a little girl, I remember my grandmother telling me about foods that we can eat and cannot eat at different times in life and I really never understood why. In fact, I'm not sure she understood why. She said that where she was from in Mexico, everyone believed this. My grandmother raised me because my mother was not around and I don't want to offend her so I listen, but I don't want to just obey; I want to understand. When I was in school, I asked my teachers about my grandmother's beliefs, but they just shrugged their shoulders.

Now I am going to have a baby and I asked my doctor about what my grandmother is telling me and they just say these are crazy old wives tales from Mexico. They don't understand either. I still live with my grandmother and she simply won't let me eat certain foods because she says they will harm the baby. I want to respect my grandmother, but I also want to understand her beliefs. Is that unreasonable of me?

CURANDERO'S RESPONSE:

No, it's not unreasonable at all. You have every right to understand. Both my maternal and my paternal grandmothers had large families, and I am the eldest of 10 in our family. All my aunts and uncles also have large families. Being raised around large families, I know very well of your grandmother's advice regarding food. I have heard it my whole life and people frequently ask me about it.

She is telling you about how to be careful with what are called the hot and cold qualities of foods not the temperature of food. In our culture and in others, there are many beliefs about what foods should be eaten or avoided during pregnancy. From grandma's and my curandero's view, foods prepared in vinegar or with any kind of chili, hot sauces or spices are thought to have hot qualities and are not appropriate for pregnant women. Also, some meats like pork should be avoided because it is hot while chicken is cold. These foods, which raise the body's temperature, are not believed to be good for the baby or the mother.

Likewise, when the body is hot from illness or fever, it is thought that you can bring down the temperature by giving bland or cold foods. A vegetable soup, for example, is cold. There is no harm in any of this and if it makes your grandmother happy, then why not "humor" her?

Always consult your physician and ask him or her to tell you about hot-and-cold food taboos and humoral theory. Be sure to go to your prenatal checkups, but you are correct to ask questions and expect helpful answers.

COMMENTARY:

Grandmother is not necessarily old fashioned, but she is operating in another cultural mode that should be comprehended, and most importantly respected. There are many world cultures today that continue the practice of food taboos associated with pregnancy and birth, as well as with different disease states. These taboos frequently find their ways into the United States health-care delivery system. In Latino culture, it is widely known that women are told to eat bananas and avocados during their menstrual cycles in order to ease distress. It's medically documented that diet influences endometriosis which may be linked to different types of cancer. Many cultures know this from untold generations of word-of-mouth experiences passed down from mothers to daughters.

For a full discussion, see the work of anthropologist George M. Foster, whose study of the concepts of hot-and-cold food taboos in Latin America is published in the Journal of American Folklore in 1953 (this is the classic starting point for the seriously- interested researcher). More recently, María Santos-Torres published, "Food Taboos among Nursing Mothers of Mexico," in the Journal of Health and Popular Nutrition (2003). See author Jamie Sams' medical website as well: http://www.emergingworlds.com/ch_stories_detail.cfm?Content=46

49. ADVICE ON MY CONDITION — *PIDE CONSEJOS*

I called you because my sister couldn't connect me to her e-mail. I do not know how to consult with you by the Internet so she is helping me.

I am worried about my health. I have high-blood pressure and regular migraines and the pain in my head is intense. I feel weak and my legs feel heavy. Forgive me if I am overweight, but I have tried to reduce so I can feel better, but it just never seems to work for me. Please give me some good advice.

CURANDERO'S RESPONSE:

You must see a doctor immediately. Do not even consider alternative treatments without seeing a doctor. Begin to immediately pray to Santa Catalina de Siena, April 29, and to Saint Acacius, May 8, the patron saints of headaches and persistent illnesses. Saint Andrew, November 10, is the patron saint of strokes; if the headaches become more persistent.

High blood pressure is usually treated with several capsules of garlic always following the instructions. This is if you do not suffer from gastric ulcers or indigestion. I treat headaches with numerous plants and combinations of plants. For example, the ash tree or *el sauz*; but also, aspen or *alamo*; feverfew or *altamisa*; honeysuckle or *muicle;* marigold or *calendula*; hibiscus or *flor de Jamaica*; kidneywort or *hepática*; mint bee balm or *oregano*; and purple sage or *cenizo*, are just a few. Most commonly, I ask my people to take *toronjil*, Mexican giant hyssop, tea, one cup a day for 40 consecutive days. For your migraines and all headaches, you may regularly drink a tea made of hackberry bark, *palo blanco*, or from willow or *el sauz*. Do this also for 40 consecutive days. Find the tea of this sacred bark to clean your digestive system with the corn silk and the *hierba de la hormiga*, ant herb, or pink windmills, to wash out urinary ducts. After detoxifying your body, nourish yourself with the most correct diet and take vitamins and minerals for strength. What is positive is that you are aware of your ills and don't put off doing what I recommend.

There is a saying, "God helps he who helps himself." This is very true and you must take it to heart. It is also said "the one who does not speak, God will not hear." Pray to El Niño Fidencio so that he will speak to God on your behalf.

COMMENTARY:

The danger of combining medicinal plants along with medications is omnipresent. A doctor must always be consulted before combining herbal remedies with prescription medicine. For example, the active ingredient in willow tree bark or el sauz is salicylic acid which is the active ingredient in aspirin. Most curanderos/as possess only regional and limited knowledge of plant names because medicinal plants change geographically by region and so do their names. Plants may have one name in New Mexico and another in south Texas. In this case, the physician must be consulted and an expert on medicinal plants must diagnose the ensuing effects of plants prescribed by the curandero. Except in emergency cases, all hospitals in the United States forbid any type of vitamins and herbal supplements at least one week prior to surgery. This is highly recommended since they may produce excessive bleeding during operations or even reverse the anesthesia's intended effect.

50. MY DAD HAS CANCER — *CANCEROSO*

I write to you to see if you think that you can help my dad. He has cancer and it has spread to some of his organs. He has a broken hip and now must use a prosthetic leg. He can't walk anymore. He often has severe pain. We did not take him for chemotherapy because we thought the powerful chemicals would kill him. We did treat him with alternative medicine, but he does not have any health insurance.

I've heard many good things about spiritual healings and wonder if you may be able to help us. It is very difficult to take my dad out of the house, but if you think you can help him and if we must take him out, please let me know and I will do my best to get him to you.

CURANDERO'S RESPONSE:

My prayers are with you and your father. I believe it is best that he continue to see the doctor. Let me know what the doctor determines and I will keep all of you in my prayers, especially your father.

Light a Niño Fidencio candle and a white wax, seven-day candle. Place a clear glass, full of water, over your father's picture between the candles.

Call on our Lord and say the Holy name of San Rafael Arcángel as well as Santa Agueda, and Cosme y Damian; say the name of El Niño Fidencio three straight times and make your petition. In order to ensure that the last rites of the Catholic Church be given pray to Saint Stanislaus on August 15.

In Mexico people regularly use powder made from sharks and from rattlesnakes to treat cancer but there are also many plant remedies that are used. For example, you could make a tea for him from *arnica*, *alhucema*, or lavender, *perejil*, parsely, lemon grass and *salvia*. Blend them all together and boil them in two gallons of water. Give your father one cup of tea in the morning daily and a cup of tea in the evening for two consecutive weeks. Apple or *manzana*; black cohosh or *cohosh negro*; blood root or *sanguinaria*; fava beans of several types called *habas*; and regular wheat called *trigo* may also be used in teas.

I will continue to pray for him to receive the miracle of spiritual healing. Always be sure to refrigerate herbal teas, then, re-heat them. Do not leave them sitting out.

COMMENTARY:

The most common reason for a person to consult an alternative or complementary- care practitioner is desperation; having exhausted all other curative means. Many first-time visitors go to curanderos/as, as a last resort, while many others who visit curanderos are regular visitors. The regulars have developed long-term therapeutic relationships; additionally, they truly believe in miracles and ensuing evidence proves that they are eventually granted.

51. WHEN THERE IS NO CURE — *DESAHUCIADO*

I have three brothers and one is very ill. About three months ago, my brother began to feel ill and spots and welts began to show on his face, ears, knees and chest. He did not look well, and little by little he began to lose weight and his body began to ache in his joints and bones. My mother took him to the doctor and to the hospital, but they couldn't find anything wrong with him. Finally, they admitted him into the hospital and he was there about two weeks, and, according to the doctors, they could not find anything until they finally diagnosed lupus. According to the doctors, there is no cure, but there is treatment. My mother raised all three of us, but since I am the oldest I see how my mother suffers. If it were up to her, she would have preferred to have this happen to her instead of to my brother.

I am a believer in God and in the Virgen of Guadalupe and I have great faith. I would like to know if you could pray for my brother and ask the Niño Fidencio to help him with this terrible disease and also with his emotions. Sometimes he feels as though it's hopeless and that he is going to die. Sometimes he gets depressed, but my mother has long talks with him and sometimes he understands. I would like to know if you make home visits or do you only consult on the Internet? I have already been looking at your webpage and it looks great. Can you please help us? I know that we all have similar problems, but please help my brother.

CURANDERO'S RESPONSE:

Your brother has an illness in his blood and that is probably why he became anemic. The popular belief is that the red blood cells consume the white blood cells. But that is not the case. His body is not properly nourished and his diet is not balanced with vitamins and minerals. With the lack of iron in the diet, the body will not produce sufficient or healthy white blood cells.

Consequently, his immune system is weakened and it develops illnesses like that of lupus. Your brother needs to strengthen his blood by drinking a tea made from *salvia*. He should drink one cup in the morning and another at night for 40 consecutive days. It would be very beneficial to give him a tonic of vitamins including plenty of iron.

Also, please give him a ritual cleaning and sweeping using a handful of *gobernadora*, creosote bush or fresh *perejil*, parsley.

There are a number of plants that I use to fortify the blood. Agrimony or *agrimonia*; candlewood or *ocotillo*; eggplant or *berengena*; fenugreek or *fenogreco*; nasturtium or *tomillo;* Mexican thistle or *cardo santo;* nettle or *ortigilla* are just a few.

Do this on Fridays for seven consecutive weeks. How old is your brother? Do you all live in the same room? Who is assisting or looking after him while he is ill? It is important for me to know these facts.

Finally, pray to San Alejo to take the illness away from him. San Alejo's feast day is celebrated July 17. People with chronic illness should pray to Santa Juliana on July 19. Failing all else, pray that Saint Stanislaus, August 15, ensures that your loved ones receive the last rites.

COMMENTARY:

Here the curandero is providing the client with vital information concerning diet and nutritional supplements which may be useful whether the patient actually has lupus or not. Please note that the curandero is not qualified to issue medical advice or to accurately comment on causation of maladies. Clearly, if the doctor's diagnosis is accurate, then the family is in store for a lengthy, and possibly, terminal illness. It is good to establish a long-term consulting relationship with the curandero, which includes prayer but never abandon the support of the medical community.

52. DIABETES IS EATING ME — *ME ESTÁ COMIENDO*

I desperately need your advice. I never thought I would be contacting a *curandero*, but you have been recommended to me and here I am. I am a diabetic man and I take three medicines twice a day, but I need more help. I need a different kind of help; the kind past generations would have used. Many of my friends have told me that I should keep seeing my doctor and taking my medicine, but that I should find out if there are any traditional remedies and if they can help me. That is why I am writing to you and hope you can give me some cultural advice.

CURANDERO'S RESPONSE:

Ask San Pantaleón for help with your diabetes. He is the patron saint of all kinds of illnesses especially those difficult to cure like diabetes. He is celebrated July 27. I appreciate your faith in me and I will try my best to help you. Diabetes is such a terrible disease for those afflicted and their loved ones. I agree with your friends that the old knowledge and ways of your culture can help you. Diabetes has always been with us, but it was controlled by diet, exercise and herbal medicine. So let's go back to our roots. Catus leaf, or *nopal*, is the most common plant that I ask people to take for their diabetes, but there are many more. They include, artichoke or *alcachofa*; bricklebush or *prodigiosa*; fenugreek or *fenogrecco*; Indian plantain or *matarique*; sarsparilla or *zarzaparrilla*; and tree spinach called *chaya*.

If you are having trouble controlling your blood sugar and you are taking three medicines, then you are not doing enough exercise. In the old days, work and exercise were the same, but that is not the case today. You have to get off the couch and walk, walk, walk!

Secondly, you eat too much of the wrong things. In the old days, the portions were much smaller than today. Force yourself to eat less and then walk. Eat fewer carbohydrates, less corn, potatoes, bread, pasta and beans. Eat fruits and vegetables, small portions of meat and very little carbohydrates. Eat what your grandfather ate: rice and beans with corn tortillas. If you adhere to this and regularly drink a tea of cactus leaves, or *nopales,* and *matarique,* and *chaya,* which you can get at your local grocery store, or *hierbería,* you will lose weight, feel better and your blood sugar will go down. I guarantee it, and your grandfather's spirit will help you and smile upon you.

COMMENTARY:

Type II diabetes is one of the fastest growing diseases in the United States and is widespread within the Latino population. Remarkably, diabetes is controllable in many cases through a combination of medication, behavior modification and cultural support by the family. The most usual reason for diabetes to spin dangerously out of control is that the afflicted person is noncompliant.

The advice that the curandero offers the diabetic will, if precisely followed, align the patient onto the path to blood-sugar control. One has only to want to do it. Finally, in order to conquer diabetes you need the support of the entire family.

53. MY BABY IS SICK — *BEBÉ ENFERMITO*

I am a young mother and my baby is only six months old. I am far away from my family, my mother, my aunts and my sisters, and I feel lost and abandoned. I only have a high school education, but I do have a computer and I know how to use it. My baby has been a little sickly lately and I have so many questions to ask, yet I don't know who to ask about my baby's health. I was given your e-mail address and told that you would understand and could help me. I simply need a contact person who will listen to me about my baby's health and give me good advice.

For example, my baby is a good baby, but he has been crying lately and has these white patches in his mouth. Please help me.

CURANDERO'S RESPONSE:

Thank you for contacting me. I will do everything in my power to help you to answer your important questions about your baby's health. If I can't answer all your questions, I will find someone in your area who can. Actually you are not alone, there are people all over the United States who care about you and your baby's health and are available to assist you. I will help you reach out to them. Judging from what you have told me, your baby could have a serious strep infection or maybe simply the baby has what we call thrush or *algodoncillo* in Spanish. This is a fungus that can be easily treated. Take your baby to a clinic or a doctor. They will help you immediately. There are many other plant remedies that I use to treat fungus, including, blood root or *sanguinaria*; rue or *ruda*; celandine or *celedonia*; cedar or *cedro*; and tarbush or *ojase*. Meanwhile, try feeding your baby some yogurt sweetened with honey. Give your baby a little bicarbonate of soda to rinse out his mouth and the cotton mouth should clear up soon. Babies have many issues with their mouths because they will put anything they can in their mouths. Some of the medicinal plants I use for mouth issues include, blackberry or *zarzamora*; sage or *salvia*; flax or *linaza*; oak or *encino;* and orange or *naranja*. Always pray to the Holy Innocents celebrated on December 28, for petitions to make babies well also, petition San Marcos to heal your child. His feast day is celebrated April 25.

COMMENTARY:

Curanderos always look for both natural and supernatural causes in all childhood illnesses and conditions. Since children are innocent, their illnesses are sometimes thought to be caused by a transgression of the parents. Illnesses occur when the child's fate or luck is altered by something bad the parents did. The child is innocent, but suffers the consequences. The curandero/a, is called to reverse bad luck or fortune which will bring about the child's healing. One or both of the parents can become salted, or salada, and when this happens their children may be stricken with an illness as a consequence. There are many wonderful resources for child-health issues. Don't hesitate to search on the Internet for this helpful and revelatory information. Check government and hospital sites first. Locate a community or migrant health clinic that is a Federally Qualified Health Clinic (FQHC) in your area. They will have pediatric-resource and outreach workers ready to assist you.

54. BODY RASH AND ITCHING — *COMEZÓN Y RONCHAS*

I'm writing this letter to say hello, and wish you the best. I first of all thank God and then you for all you have done for me. My uncle and I consulted you on our illnesses. I had a horrible, itchy rash all over my body and you recommended baths with tomato juice and *arnica*. Thank God Almighty and you that I was able to get rid of the rash on my body.

The itch on my head returns every once in a while, but now it is only very moderate. I do continue using the tomato juice, and have faith in God. I know all of my problems will go away little by little until they are all gone, if I keep up my faith.

CURANDERO'S RESPONSE:

I'm glad that the baths have given you relief for the terrible itch on your body. To continue moving forward with your well being and to get rid of the itch on your head, you'll have to make a tea with parsley, lavender, *arnica*, lemon grass and common kitchen sage. Another tea you can take for nine consecutive nights contains cinnamon, or *canela*, with lemon and honey. Prepare a paste made with baked tomatoes and a small amount of liquor, then, rub it all over your body. A boiled liquid made from borage, or *borraja*, can also be applied by rubbing on the skin for sores. You could also rub coyote lard, or *manteca de coyote*, mixed with sulfur on the sores.

When you pray, be sure to pray to San Gil, patron saint of skin illnesses and to Saint Lazarus for skin, he is celebrated on June 21 and Saint Marculf on May 1, for all sorts of skin problems.

COMMENTARY:

There are many folk therapies and over-the-counter remedies for irritated, scratchy skin. Rashes and skin issues have many different origins and causes including emotional stress. Always consult a doctor or pharmacist first before you attempt home remedies. Curanderos will often prescribe that the body be rubbed with an antibacterial, antiseptic or antiseptic agent. There are many plants containing these properties including: common radish; and most of the mints or *hierba buena*; all heal or *valeriana*;

ambrosia or *hierba amarga*; creosote bush; parsley or *perejil*; dandelion or *diente de leon*; desert bloom or *yerba del pasmo*; horsetail or *cola de caballo*; myrtle or *mirto*; and the two trees, *anacua* and acacia or *huizache*. Unguents, or *ungentos*, constituted of barley, or *cebada*, achieve the same goal, a soothing, healing salve.

55. BARE FEET — *LA FRIALDAD*

My children love to run around outside without shoes on. So, the other day my neighbor came over to warn me that they could get sick doing this, that it was a dangerous practice. I thought that she was talking about cutting the bottoms of their feet or stepping on a bug, but she said that there were many illnesses that enter the body through the feet, especially when the ground is cold and wet. Should I listen to her? Is she correct about this? Because sometimes my children do get fevers and colds, coughs or other common childhood illnesses for no reason that I can determine. I know they pick up a lot of sicknesses at school as well.

CURANDERO'S RESPONSE:

Frialdad, or coldness, is an illness believed to have entered the body through the bare feet. This is also believed to be one of the causes of bedwetting in children and even in some adults. *Frialdad* is also a concept believed to be one of the reasons that some women are not able to conceive. This type of coldness is referred to as *frialdad de la matriz*, coldness of the uterus, and is an illness believed to have entered the body through bare feet. When this is a diagnosis by the *curandero* the uterus has to be heated.

Always pray to Saint Peter who assists us with fever and our feet and illnesses contracted through the feet. His saint's day is June 29. It is also believed that supernatural illnesses can enter through bare feet and even sometimes through covered feet.

Many Latinos attribute illnesses, misfortunes, suffering and all sorts of problems to having inadvertently stepped on or walked on witchcraft objects which were deliberately placed in their path. Illnesses or spells are believed to be transferred to the hapless person who touches or comes into contact with contaminated materials that have been used in cleansing healing rituals, recklessly left behind. As a *curandero* and a practitioner of ancient methods of dealing with certain ailments, such as bedwetting, one would take the urine from the one with the condition, and pour it onto hot-clay bricks or red-hot coals. The urine vaporizes onto the bare feet of the bedwetter who is sitting next to the hot coals. This breaks the coldness, or *frialdad,* in the bladder and brings about the end to bedwetting.

Bedwetting is believed to be a condition that could have come about by the body being exposed to cold temperatures as well. However, drinking excessive fluids near bedtime, or after a trauma, fear, or stressful condition can also cause it.

Coldness of the uterus is usually treated by massaging the *vientre,* or womb and lower abdomen, with warm olive oil for seven to nine days consecutively. Supernatural illnesses brought about by contact with unclean, demonic, evil spirits and negative energies which have entered the body through the feet will, in all likelihood, require the attention and cleansing of a reputable healer or a reputable exorcist if the case warrants it. Many times people have a fever which is one of the symptoms of *frialdad*, they should pray to Saint Domitian on May 7 for the cure of fever.

COMMENTARY:

In pre-industrial societies it is ordinary for people to believe that illness enters the body through the feet. Because this theory is partially true, it has persisted and is passed on generationally. Additionally, it is a common belief that getting wet or walking in water allows illness to enter through the feet.

Many children innocently pick up worms, especially if there are pets in the yard. Do not rule out having a medical doctor check children for pinworms or hookworms via a stool sample. These are common parasites and enter through bare feet; especially in areas where farm animals coexist. People who live in rural areas around farm animals generally eat pumpkin seeds, or semilla de calabaza, a well known preventive against intestinal parasites or anthelminic, or antihelmíntico.

56. MEDICINAL PLANTS — *PLANTAS MEDICINALES*

What is basil used for? Several stores that I have gone to don't sell the type of tea you requested. They say that it is used for abortions or for urinary tract infections. I don't know if this is true or not, but today I'm going to look for the tea and the candle. Thank you very much for your prayers. I am also confused about the fact that the same herb is called by different names. Can you explain that to me?

CURANDERO'S RESPONSE:

Basil has various qualities, uses, virtues, faculties and powers. It has also been used as a spice for cooking, as an herb for making tea to calm the nerves, tea to help you sleep, used also as an aromatic fragrance, used in cleansing the spirit, to cure the soul from fright, past fright, or trauma. It's also used in spiritual baths to rid negative energies, for good luck against bad currents and to draw money, as an extract, as perfume, as oil used to massage injuries, and also used as incense for self-cleansing and cleansing businesses, and your home. In many ways, it is one of the "master" herbs, but basil does not have ingredients or chemicals to provoke abortions. If you have a urinary tract infection, take a tea made from ant herb, or *hierba de la hormiga*, and corn silk.

There are about 500 most common medicinal plants that we always use but they are known by many different regional names. Always double check to see what you are getting when you ask for a plant by name. Thank you for consulting me and for your question.

COMMENTARY:

Albahaca, or sweet basil, is one of the herbs mentioned in the Holy Bible and is used, as the curandero suggests, for cleansing and as a tea. As the curandero points out, there are hundreds of medicinal plants known by thousands of names. The names are regional and also have folk names and indigenous names in native languages. For example, altamisa, ajenjo and estafiate may all be mugwort or wormwood or may not. Be sure you have a knowledgeable and reliable source for medicinal plants. If you have a Mexican products store near you they will have a pre-packaged section with the most common medicinal plants, or plantas medicinales, so you don't have to worry about what you are getting. The package will be labeled and in most cases they are reviewed by the United States Department of Agriculture.

57. CANDLES HELPED US — *LAS VELAS SIRVEN*

The candle of the Holy Trinity that you asked us to get for our health problems is already half gone. It's only been two days since I turned it on and already we feel better. The top part of the candle is pretty smoky, the flame measures about an inch tall. It looks like it's going quickly. Do I have to light another candle after the first one is gone until we are completely well?

CURANDERO'S RESPONSE:

It is always best to keep replacing candles until they no longer smoke. While the candle smokes, it is doing its job of cleansing and healing. I thank you for your meticulous attention. It's okay that the candle burns fast and has a high flame, and that it is smoking. Be very careful to not let the glass crack and cause a fire. Keep it in a dish with a little water just in case it breaks or burns all the way down, so that it won't cause a fire in your home. Also, if there is a price tag on the bottom of the glass, remove it. This is one of the fire hazards when the candle burns down. Always remember, when lighting a candle to thank the patron Saint of candle makers, Saint Bernard of Clairvaux, August 20. This was more traditional when candles were homemade but we should remember him, he will like that.

COMMENTARY:

The curandero suggested a Holy Trinity candle for universal maladies. However, a candle should be chosen solely on the basis of the particular petition. There are different candles and saints specializing in the particular ailment. More than likely, the curandero will prescribe a specific candle with an itemized preparation, ritual and prayer. Hierberías sell pre-prepared candles.

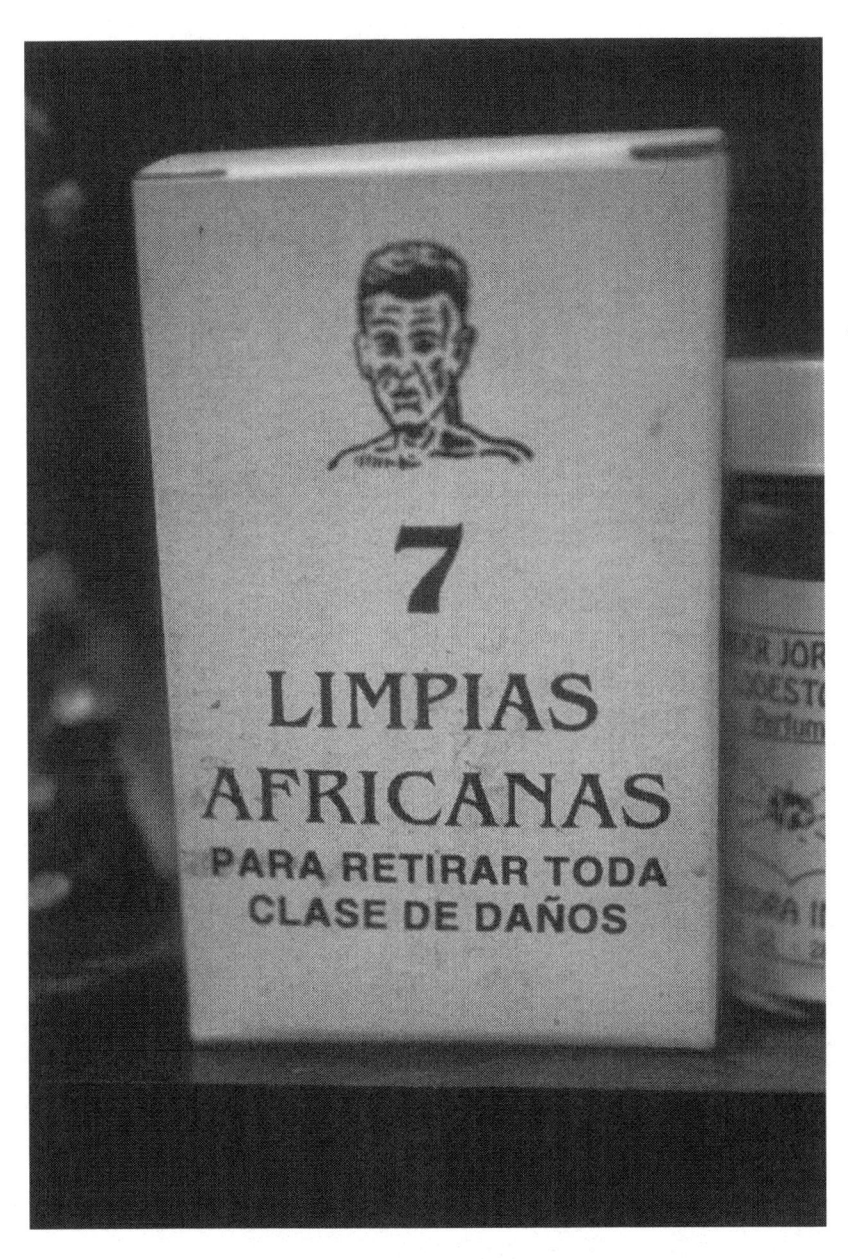

A pre-prepared spiritual cleanser intended to remove or prevent evil and witchcraft spells is displayed for sale at the Mercado Sonora in Mexico City. (Photo by José M. Duarte)

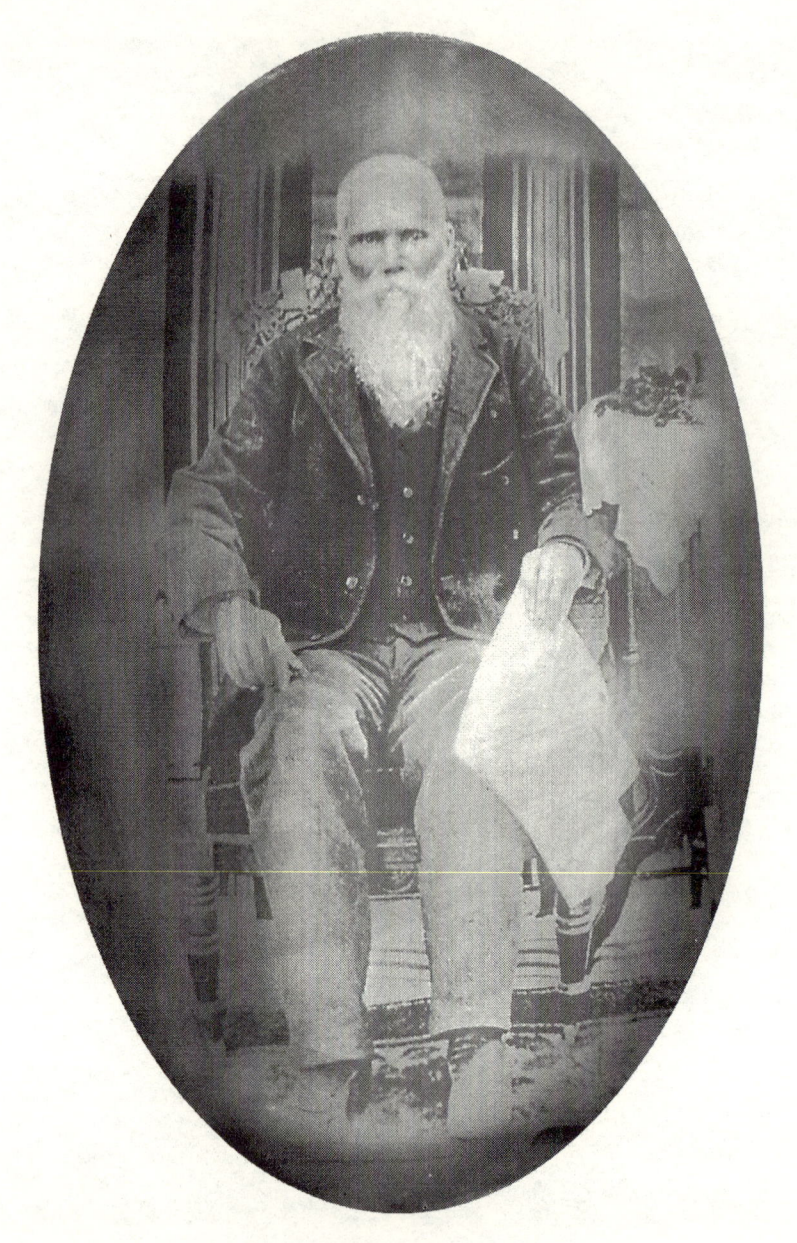

Don Pedrito Jaramillo "The Healer of Los Olmos." His shrine is located in Falfurrias, Texas.
(Photo from Zavaleta collection)

PART FIVE

CURANDERISMO:
Healing the Frailties of the Mind

"I am a curandero as were my father and my father's father. We are men of the people. God has entrusted us with the gift of healing. This precious gift was granted to us solely for the purpose of helping those in need. Our people are poor and sometimes desperate, and they come to us for help. If we violate their trust, God will revoke his gift to us."

— †*Don Perfecto Rodríguez, curandero*

58. BOGUS HEALERS — *EL ENGAÑO CUESTA*

Hoping you and your family are in good health at the arrival of this note. Well, you asked me to explain my motive for seeking you out. Like I told you, I have gone to see many other psychics and healers and card readers, and they have just taken my money and done nothing for me. One required $200, but before that, another one came to pray over my house "for things to go better for us." This same man owns a store that sells herbs, candles and things used for cleansing the home, and he told me that it would cost me $250 to cleanse my home. I paid him $100 to do the cleansing. After cleansing my house, he asked me to go to his store and every time I went I would end up spending at least $50. He told me that I needed perfumes, candles and other things to remove bad luck from our family. I ended up spending $2,000 and I still have a bad curse on me and he kept my money!

CURANDERO'S RESPONSE:

Well, there is no doubt you are certainly cursed and are full of bad luck and you make very bad decisions as well. I advise you to not throw your money away on *curanderos* that only trick you with lies. Stop paying them now! I have sent you the prayers of El Niño Fidencio. Print them, then pray them, and ask in faith for your petitions to be answered. If you have been taken by an unscrupulous *curandero,* pray to Saint John of the Cross, December 14, to mediate for you and to help to get your money back. Bathe with water collected from the morning dew; river water; well water; rain water; holy water from the church; coconut water; and/or goat's milk for seven straight days. Pray and ask the Lord to answer your petition while taking the bath. I am thinking that you are the source of your bad luck and not some witchcraft curse like you think.

COMMENTARY:

Many times the mind is swayed by faith with overriding beliefs. What the mind intrinsically believes then is combined with desperation. An individual's actions and judgments become incomprehensibly irrational and the person is no longer thinking clearly. True curanderos NEVER charge exorbitant prices for their spiritual assistance. It is reasonable that the necessary accessories must be purchased from a hierbería. Depending on how serious the situation is these items can easily cost several hundred dollars but only in the most extreme cases. They should NEVER cost thousands of dollars. That is an engaño, or swindle. This is simply an unscrupulous person who is taking advantage, or aprovechándose, of desperate and faithful followers. To modify an old adage: Buyer, believer, beware!

59. LOST THE WILL TO LIVE — *QUIERE MORIR*

My sister has had cancer twice and has had two below-the-knee amputations, lost a finger, had a mastectomy and is on dialysis. All of her problems have been brought on by diabetes which she does not take care of. She is a firm believer in God and states that God has spoken to her and told her that it is okay for her to die. She also says she does not want to be a burden on her family and is tired of living as only half a woman. She used to be very outgoing and happy. She enjoyed life and had a lot of self esteem. She has a daughter and son. Her son takes her to her doctor appointments and shopping. Her daughter tends to her personal needs and takes her to dialysis. Her husband tends to the home and makes all the meals.

What can we do to convince her that she is still a valuable resource to the family and that we love her just the way she is? Is there any prayer you can offer that will give her hope? She is refusing to go to her dialysis appointment and right now they only give her one to two weeks to live. What should we do? Can you help us?

CURANDERO'S RESPONSE:

Light a *Sagrado Corazón,* Sacred Heart candle, a Niño Fidencio candle and a candle to San Expedito, patron saint that expedites urgent cases, and ask that she be given back her will to live. Even though she has given up psychologically, her family and loved ones cannot give up on her. Place the candles on her home altar with a glass of water next to each candle. Make a special petition to Santo Josemaría Escrivá, patron saint of diabetics.

Be sure to check that your sister is not anemic as this is a common problem with people whose zest for life is reduced. I usually ask people to take an alfalfa tea with other blood-fortifying herbs included. You could include in the alfalfa base, croton, black cherry, *palo de brasil,* and *prodigiosa*. All of these healing items should be available to you at your local *hierbería*. In the alfalfa base tea, add one ingredient a week as you are able to acquire them to see how she tolerates it and if her constitution gets stronger.

When the candles finish burning down, take one of the glasses of water and sprinkle the water at the entrance of her house on the outside. Add the other glass of water to a bucket of Holy Water then bathe her with it.

Try to convince her that she is a benefit to her family and she will come around. Surround her with children and grandchildren and loved ones to hold her up to the Lord. Have everyone come together around her and pray the Holy Rosary. I will make a very special petition to the Niño Fidencio and ask him to come to her aid and to be her special spirit guide to wellness. Pray Psalm 13 to protect her from suffering and an unnatural death. Please keep me informed. The following is an example of a typical prayer to El Niño Fidencio

A PRAYER: OH NIÑO FIDENCIO CONSTANTINO

Hear my prayer, oh powerful Spirit of Divine Light that descends from the heavens to strengthen and enlighten those who find themselves in the valley of tears. I am your humble servant full of unbreakable faith and of great love for you. I call upon the miraculous Niño Fidencio, I invoke you in the name of God, to ask that, with the power of the Supreme Being, you grant me the gift that my sister get well and live a long and productive life.

COMMENTARY:

When there are life-threatening illnesses in a family, especially when children and the elderly are stricken, family members turn to curanderos for help. Most Latino families maintain a home altar to venerate the family's patron saint or saints. Prayer and faith are the underlying basis of a curandero's practice. In this case, the life of the petitioner's sister was spared. For example, in this case curanderos very often prescribe plants with a recognized stimulant, tonic and restorative properties.

60. FRIGHT SICKNESS — *EL SUSTO*

I will be having knee surgery for a torn ligament in my left knee very soon. I also have very bad arthritis in my right knee. I am not a person who can keep still. I hope this surgery comes out well and I can get my life back.

I prayed to God to send me a person who would be able to fix my knee and take the pain away and I pray that God has chosen my surgeon well.

Can you tell me how to cure *susto*? My seven-year-old granddaughter got frightened by a dead snake and now she is afraid all the time and doesn't want to sleep alone in her bedroom.

CURANDERO'S RESPONSE:

Thank you for your letter. Cut a lemon in half, then rub, squeezing the juice on your knees. Do this for five minutes. Afterward, rub the knees with egg white until the egg white becomes dry and sticky. Leave the egg white on and do not wash it off until your next bath. Repeat for nine consecutive days. Take tea made from *salvia* and *zacate de limón*. Boil the two together and drink one cup of tea for nine consecutive days.

In order to cure your granddaughter's *susto*, sweep the child with a *piedra alumbre*, or alum rock which you can buy at any *hierbería* or Mexican products store. Use this same rock to do the sweeping, or *barrida*, for nine consecutive days. Set the rock aside each day in a safe place and do not allow anyone to touch it because her *susto* could easily be transferred to an unsuspecting person. Perform this ritual the first thing each morning by praying to Santa Lourdes, and be sure to honor her on February 11. Ask her to protect you and your family.

Give the child a cup of spearmint, *hierba buena*, or basil tea for the same nine days you sweep her. After the ninth day of sweeping, start a fire and burn the alum rock on the hot coals. This will cure her of *susto*. Bathing the child with Holy Water will also help cure her *susto*.

COMMENTARY:

The petitioner is requesting a cure for fright sickness, or susto. Susto is one of the most recurring folk illnesses and may be treated by sweeping alum rock known as piedra alumbre over the body of the child or person who is scared, or asustada. Usually, this ritual sweeping is repeated for three to nine days in a row.

A person will recognize that they or their loved one was scared or startled. The scare triggers the usual symptoms of fever and sleeplessness. If nausea accompanies the fright sickness, the curandero often advises that an antiemetic herb, antiemético, such as wormseed, against throwing up be given such as wormseed.

The Apostles' Creed, or Credo, must also be recited while doing the ritual sweeping. At the end of the ritual, the rock used is burned outside the home over hot coals. Many believe that they can see the evil burned into the stone. It's also believed that the image of the person or entity which caused the initial susto or soul loss is reflected in the alum rock.

Severe cases of susto or fright sickness are called desasombro and can occur in both the waking and sleeping states. This severe case of fright is believed to cause the patient a fever, loss of sleep, desperation and should be treated by a curandero/a immediately. There are believed to be even more severe cases of susto called, susto pasado or susto meco. (Eliseo Torres, 2006, p.16)

61. ENVY AND JEALOUSY — *ENVIDIA Y CELOS*

I send you greetings and I expect that you are probably in Espinazo, Nuevo León this time of year. I am hoping that you will be able to help me with a problem that I have due to many people who are envious of me. I have seen lots of people, so-called healers, and asked them to help me, but so far they have taken my money from me. No one has been able to really help me. I am not sure why there are thousands of people who are out to get me. Maybe it is a holdover from a past life. I hope to hear from you and I am hoping to know if you received my previous e-mail. Are you the one to finally help me? With kindness and wishing you good luck, may the Father of all creation cast His blessings over you.

CURANDERO'S RESPONSE:

My dear friend, I believe that a good cleansing is in order for you. That would do you a world of good. Start with cleansing your person and your home by burning incense such as myrrh, *copal,* and storax or *estoraque*, from the sweet gum tree, also known as liquid amber, mixed with ground coffee beans and a little bit of brown sugar and dry rosemary. Add a few drops of essences of *narciso negro,* tobacco or rose oil, and then grab a handful of the mixture and drop it on the hot coals to cause lots of smoke. With that, you will begin the ritual of cleansing your home and yourself, which will work in removing all the bad and negative around you. Be sure to use *narciso negro,* or black narcissus, and mustard drops on the inside of each window and door in your house as protection against envy. I am sure that once you pray on it you will realize that thousands of persons are not envious of you. A few may be, but not that many. Your emotional state concerns me and we must have a further conversation about that but first things first.

I appreciate you writing to me. The power of faith and prayer will protect you, keep you from danger, and keep you from all that is bad. It will open the doors to true happiness so that you will be content and satisfied. I wish you health, money and love. I know and understand what you are explaining to me and I can believe how you feel frustrated and feel like the hope and spirit is diminishing. That's the result of the envious people around you. With what I have asked you to put together you will be rid of the negative energy that surrounds you and you will continue to be protected from all future envies. It is important that you believe this and have faith.

You can also make an amulet against envy by using green cloth. On a Monday, place nine drops of a combination of perfumes against envy, *contra envidia*. Get the recommended perfumes at your nearest *hierbería*. They will sell perfumes to protect you against envy. Carry the prepared, *preparada*, green cloth amulet on your person for best results. Also, get a specially-prepared white candle from the *hierbería* and every morning before you go to work pass it over your body, saying your special prayer against envy. Burn a candle on your home altar every evening when you return home. Do this in honor of San Cipriano, the patron saint who protects us from all types of evil. His feast day is September 16. Say your prayers to Saint Elizabeth of Portugal, July 4, to take away jealousy and pray Psalms 52 and 137 to protect you, your loved ones and your home and business from the negative influences of *envidia*.

COMMENTARY:

True curanderos/as establish a meaningful long-term relationship with their clients. Over the years they can become very close and dependent upon each other. They share information about family and friends and look forward to the occasional visit in person or over the Internet. With a lengthy relationship such as this one, the curandero does not let the petitioner who is suffering from a mental illness to sink deeper into paranoia.

Cultural Competency: *Resource number 10 is adapted from numerous sources including, Quality Health Services for Hispanics: The Cultural Competency Component. This material is intended to augment the health care provider with an understanding of the key cultural and social elements of Latino culture. Understanding how the Latino family functions both internally and externally in society is critically important in understanding illness and wellness. (See Appendix I)*

62. STRONG DREAM MAN — *EL SOÑADOR*

I am a candidate for a local political office and the campaign is getting dirty. When I first announced my candidacy, I told everyone that I would run on my merits, and not say anything bad about my opponent, leaving the decision to the voters. But now, I have been warned that my opponent, who is part of the local political machine, has hired a witch or *brujo,* to not only defeat me, but to harm me and my family.

Quite frankly I'm worried about this because I want to do the right thing and I don't want any problems. My opponent fears my popularity and my honesty. I have been told that there is a "strong dream man," a noted *curandero*, living near me who can help me to reverse any witchcraft spell that has been done to me.

Last night, a white dove appeared in my dream and landed on my hands and I felt that was a good sign. My kids found something ugly in our yard and, then, today one of my campaign workers suggested that I contact you. This is happening so fast, can you please help?

CURANDERO'S RESPONSE:

I know the *curandero* you are talking about and he is good. I highly recommend him because I know he works with the spirits of light and not of darkness. Your dream of a white dove landing on your open hands is a revelation of the gift of the Holy Spirit. The Holy Spirit is anointing your hands with the Divine healing power of God. You can expect that you will receive many more spiritual dream messages, and that over time they will reveal a spiritual path for you to take in

Curandero Conversations

your life. You will win your campaign, but you will have to always be protected spiritually from here on out. Evil never forgets.

During your campaign keep a journal by your bed and write down each dream you have. Before long, a pattern will emerge telling you what your opponent is trying to do to you.

I sense that you are indeed being worked and that you need spiritual assistance from the strong dream man. He is a renowned shaman who will go into a trance and with his spirit out of his body he will fly to where they are working you and literally see what is being done to you. Then he will tell what you have to do to reverse it. Often the outcome of elections is disputed and Saint Chad, March 2, is the saint to pray to and politicians should pray to Saint Thomas More, June 22. Also, pray Psalm 22 to keep misfortune away. Let me know how I can help you in the future as well.

COMMENTARY:

In the Latino community, practitioners of the supernatural are frequently used by opposing political candidates as well as by sports teams for assistance in reversing consequences of events in their favor.

Dreams are spiritual windows to the subconscious mind and many have symbols or abstract meanings that must be interpreted. While receiving treatment or counseling from a curandero, you should always have a dream book by your bedside. Upon awakening, write down the primary themes and symbols from the previous night's dreams. Witches, who are also shape shifters known as Naguals, are believed to fly around at night changing their shape into an animal or other nondescript entities in order to carry out their evil spells. This is a common belief and often influences people to not leave their homes after dark.

I am reminded of a story I was once told by a brujo in Mexico, who finally ended a decades-old war of witches by trapping and capturing a lechuza at night then hanging it from a tree. The next morning his long time rival warlock was found dead, hanging from the tree where the bird had been. The war was over, but later he told me that he missed his old rival.

63. PRAY FOR MY SOLDIER — *ORACIÓN POR MI SOLDADO*

I just wanted to ask you to put my son on your prayer list. He left for the army three weeks ago and he is struggling with his training. I don't know if you remember, we visited you recently. He joined the army right after our visit. I am proud of him, but I need your help to keep him motivated and safe. He sent me the saddest letter yesterday and I pray he gets better in his training. Please send the Niño Fidencio to him to make him strong and proud and to graduate with his army class.

CURANDERO'S RESPONSE:

Yes, of course I shall keep your son in my prayers. I suggest that you say prayers to Saint Michael the Archangel and recite the prayer of the guardian angel. Please also light the Saint Michael the Archangel candle as a special petition for his welfare and well being. We will pray for his strength, valor and happiness.

There are many patron saints for the protection of soldiers. You could choose one or all of the many. Saint George, Saint James, and Saint Joan of Arc, protect soldiers. The Immaculate Conception who is celebrated on December 8 is their special protector.

You may also say the prayer to the Niño Perdido, "The Lost Child," who is a little known but powerful patron saint of military personnel who go off to war. As far back as World War I, Mexican American mothers began praying to the Niño Perdido to protect their sons and daughters at war. Recite Psalm 60, to keep soldiers out of harm's way.

COMMENTARY:

Latinos have played major roles in our U.S. military, dating back to the American Revolutionary War. All of the major Latino sub-groups have distinguished themselves in battle and service to our nation. In fact, as an ethnic group, Latinos have one of the highest numbers of Congressional-Medal-of-Honor winners.

In spite of this, our women mourn their young men leaving the household and have established a long tradition of prayer and vigilance for their safe return.

The little-known shrine of El Niño Perdido just south of San Antonio, Texas in the small town of La Coste is an example of how prayer and vigilance have developed a following for this folk saint. Unfortunately, in 2007, the shrine, by then in extreme disrepair, was demolished by the landowners. It is not known if any of the shrine materials were preserved. The actual mystical figure of the Niño Perdido has been missing for some time.

64. A RUN OF BAD LUCK — *LA MALA SUERTE*

We would be ever so grateful if you could give us some advice on what to do with the sudden black cloud that we have hanging over us. As I told you, my husband broke his left wrist, and went back to work on light duty, then a few weeks later he broke his right ankle and has been out of work since then. He goes back to the doctor to be checked out soon.

We need help financially. We have bills to pay and we need better health. I have heard rumors from people who work at the plant where he works, and they say that the company is not planning to give him his job back. I don't see how that can happen, but I guess it can. The woman that he works with is very evil and I think she is causing all this because he would not sleep with her. No one knows what she is capable of doing to us.

I am severely depressed. I don't even feel like getting out of bed every day. The joy has gone out of my life. I am living one day at a time. I don't mean to be bothering you so much, but have you had a chance to confer with El Niño Fidencio? If you have, what did he tell you about us? Is there any hope? Something is seriously wrong with me; I have no energy whatsoever. One of my friends told me this is a symptom of depression. Is it?

Please don't forget to ask the Niño if he thinks my sisters are going to help me pay for the balance of our father's funeral costs.

CURANDERO'S RESPONSE:

Niño says there are still negative energies around you, which have caused someone to be jealous of you or to envy you, *envidia*. Niño recommends that you boil rosemary, basil and rue, and to strain the herbs from the boiled water and then to add one-half cup of honey to the water and for both you and your husband to bathe in the water.

Say a prayer to San Cristóbal and Saint Jude and make your petition. Niño said he would try to help your relatives pay their share of your father's funeral. But he doesn't think that they are able to at this time and that you should understand that.

Finally, Niñito says that you are going through a spiritual trial and that you should not give up hope, you will emerge from this. Your husband will change jobs and for the better. The woman you mentioned is "working" him but not to worry because it will come back on her.

COMMENTARY:

Bad luck is construed to be brought on by various ways. A person can develop a "run" of bad luck because of misbehavior or by breaking a promise to a saint. Bad luck can also be brought on by witchcraft or by a spell being cast on a person because of envy or for many other reasons. Knowing that there are persons who are capable of doing harm makes people fearful of others.

As the curandero states, there are persons who work with "negative energies" and some are more evil and dangerous than others. In order to ward off these dark forces, people place or keep items, on their person or in their purses like amulets and talismans. Protect your home as well.

65. THE PRODIGAL SON — *EL HIJO PRÓDIGO*

I have a son who is a recovering drug addict and alcoholic. He rarely works, but has quit all his addictions. But because he doesn't work, he is always asleep or in a bad mood. I think that he is in a deep depression. What can I do to help him, what do you recommend? I know he is in God's hands but I also believe that it is my responsibility to seek spiritual help and corporal healing for him, and that our Lord Almighty will help him not to give up on life. I know that God has charged me to continue to support my son, but I need your help so I can help him.

CURANDERO'S RESPONSE:

Esteemed sister, there is no doubt that you are a saint. God will continue to give you strength, health, and valor so that the cross you carry won't be so heavy. Please boil creosote bush or *gobernadora*, and bathe with the water for seven straight days. Be sure to immerse your entire body including your head.

You can also treat your son's depression with *plantas medicinales* such desert anemone or *hierba mansa*; persimmon or *nispero;* linden or *tila,* and rue or *ruda*.

I also ask you to pray the prayer of the Lost Boy which is from a little boy who appeared in the Mexican state of Guanajuato many years ago. He is different from the boy Jesus who stayed in the temple. There are no books about the Lost Boy or Niño Perdido, only an *estampa* or holy card. Give yourself a healing spiritual bath with the water of *romero,* or rosemary, for seven consecutive Fridays. Sister, God will give you valor and patience. Then, give your son a spiritual cleansing with a crucifix and a handful of fresh herbs of *albahaca*, basil, *pirul,* California pepper, *romero,* rosemary, and *ruda,* rue. Also, give yourselves cleansings with herbs for seven straight Mondays or Fridays. Do this, while you pray asking God and the Niño Fidencio to fulfill your wishes. Give yourselves baths with water of the spiritual cologne of the black narcissus for seven straight Mondays and pray to San Bibiana the saint who protects against drinking. Her feast day is celebrated December 2. Also, Dominic Savio, March 9, and Saint Matilda protect prodigal children, March 14. They are the patron saints of juveniles and their protection. Please inform me how you are doing. I am very sorry about your son, but don't give up hope. His life depends upon your strength. I understand your suffering, your anguish, the pain you feel and your needs.

In all of good there also enters evil. I am very happy to know that your son has abandoned the repulsive vices of drugs and alcohol. You must continue with your spiritual healing. It is also possible that he is traumatized by some past shock or some other ailment. You may have to treat him for *susto*. We need to struggle on through life because where there is bad, there is also good. Someone once said, "For a mother there is no bad son." Pray Psalm 28 to fight against envy.

COMMENTARY:

Scant factual information exists about the Niño Perdido (The Lost Child). There is a popular tale about a child who lost his mother. At some time in the early 20th century, the followers of the Niño Perdido moved the image into the barrios south of San Antonio, Texas. It has survived there to this day. The Niño Perdido has become the Tejano patron saint for mothers; mostly for those with sons and daughters who are away at war. Prayers are offered to the Niño Perdido to return a son or daughter safely home from war.

66. FAMILY ISSUES — *PROBLEMAS FAMILIARES*

I have a terrible situation in my family. It seems that for as long as I can remember, my family has been feuding. The situation is so bad that it has ruined lives. Our children are confused, and they act out in negative ways. I think it all started when my grandfather died because before then everyone got along. After he died, his sons all tried to take things for themselves and not share with their brothers. Then their wives got in the middle of it all and it became a big catfight. Now, 20 years have passed and the family doesn't talk to one another, much less get together. This is so destructive for our children who are cousins and don't even know one another.

What do you suggest? What can I do? Is there a spiritual solution to this? I am determined to get my family back together to reconcile before they die. I have received a spiritual message that this is my mission to accomplish in life.

CURANDERO'S RESPONSE:

I truly admire your mission, your spiritual sincerity and your determination to reconcile your family's differences. This is a case which will require profound faith and deep prayer to Saint Jude, the patron saint of impossible causes and especially to San Pascual Bailón. He will help you to make good family decisions and remember to honor him on May 17. Invoke Saint Jude and ask him to heal your family's spirit and soul and to have the differences simply melt away, pray to Saint Eugene de Mazenod, May 21, the patron of dysfunctional families and to San Nicolás of Flue the patron of large families, March 21. After all, they are insignificant compared to the importance of family.

Promise him that if your family receives this miracle you will not only organize a family reunion for the sake of your cousins, but that you will have a Catholic mass recited at the reunion. Plant the seeds of reconciliation and do it with the women of your family. If you can win them over, the men will agree. If your mother is still living, enlist her to heal her sons and daughters-in-law. But more than anything else, pray Psalm 28 to reconcile family issues.

COMMENTARY:

Here, the curandero reaches deep into the core of his faith. The Latino population deeply reveres Saint Jude, or San Judás Tadeo, and his ability to resolve their most impossible cases. The curandero senses the desperation in this person's voice, and that time is quickly elapsing for this family. Failure to resolve their issues will evolve into the next generation and literally destroy its spirit. Prayer is the answer which must be combined with a practical strategy to primarily resuscitate family communication, followed by unity and participation.

67. NERVOUS BREAKDOWN — *ATAQUE DE NERVIOS*

Hello, here I am again bothering you with my problem. Let me tell you, we carried out the procedure you ordered for nine days; passing the egg along my body in a sweeping motion and it looked like I was doing a little better, more or less, but yesterday a teacher came over to the house to give me a class and it happened again. I got really nervous and started crying and screaming. This is very frustrating for us; we don't know what to do. Please guide us and thank you so much. Do you think I have evil eye, *mal de ojo*? My girlfriend says that I am having a nervous breakdown, or what is called *ataque de nervios*, what is that?

CURANDERO'S RESPONSE:

Begin a spiritual cleansing of your home by burning incense such as *copal* and bathe with orange blossom water and Holy Water. Say a prayer to Saint Bartholomew who will protect you against a nervous breakdown. Bartholomew appreciates being honored on August 24 and to Saint Dymphna the patron of the emotionally disturbed, May 15. Do this three Fridays in a row and let me know if you improve and are less nervous. Pray the Psalms 11, 12 and 15 to resolve nervous issues.

The most traditional herb for calming the nerves is linden tea, or *té de tila*. There are many others including: wormseed or *epazote*; poppy or *amapola;* sweet basil or *albahaca*; coriander or *cilantro*; giant hyssop or *toronjil*; lemon balm or *abejera;* persimmon or *nispero*; violet or *violeta*; and white sapote or *zapote blanco*.

COMMENTARY:

It really sounds like this young man is asustado, that is to say that he has some level of fright sickness. At some point in the past, he must have suffered a scare or a startle which may have chased some segment of his spirit out of his body. His body is longing for its return. The missing part of the spirit can only be reunited with the body if the appropriate prayers and rituals are performed coaxing the spirit back into the boy's body to make him whole again.

Susto, or fright sickness, can also be a form of post-traumatic stress disorder (PTSD) which is directly traced to an experience or events that impacted the person years ago.

This can also happen during a pregnancy. The fetus is believed to experience the same emotions and trauma as the mother during pregnancy. Nervous breakdown or ataque de nervios is a very common occurrence and folk diagnosis or "culture-bound syndrome" in Latino populations. In reality, it's often a diagnosis of many conditions lumped into a singular concept referred to as "nervios." The most popular tranquilizer, or tranquilazador, for anxiety, or ansiedad, is té de tila, or linden tea, and marrubio, or horehound. Sedatives, or sedantes, and soporifics or soporíficos, and herbs for sleeplessness or insomnio, insomnia, such as the giant hyssop, or toronjil, and albahaca are used.

It is essential that you consult the Outline for Cultural Formulation and Glossary of Culture-Bound Syndromes (Appendix I) of the Diagnostic and Statistical Manual of Mental Disorders, DSM-IV, American Psychiatric

Association. The following are culture-bound syndromes identified in the DSM-IV and discussed extensively in this book: ataque de nervios; bilis and colera (not to be confused with cholera) or muinas; locura; mal de ojo; nervios; spell or trabajo; and susto.

68. DEATH OF A LOVED ONE — *UN PESAR*

My mother is near death and I am having a very hard time dealing with it. My mother and I are very close and she has terminal cancer. My whole family expects me to be the strong one and to lead them through what is about to happen, but I don't know if I can do it. We know that she will not live much longer and we are all trying to cope. I need to gather strength for everyone including my mother. Could you give us some spiritual advice on how to deal with the death of a loved one?

CURANDERO'S RESPONSE:

I am praying for you and for your mother. There are few things in life as painful as losing a loved one. Parents and children are at the top of the list. You must draw down deep into your faith and pray for strength. You must especially pray to La Virgen de Guadalupe and to Saint Joseph, the patron saint of the dead, dying and a happy death. His day is March 19. Ask them to give your entire family strength. Light their candles and keep them alongside your mother's bed in her hour of need. Sprinkle her room with Holy Water, keep fresh roses on hand and pray for a peaceful death. More importantly than anything else, be sure that your mother receives the last rites of the Catholic Church. In this way, she will approach death at peace and prepared to go and so will you.

COMMENTARY:

Most of our country's citizenry are culturally unprepared for the death of a loved one; which is never easy, especially with glaring cultural and emotional differences. Culture can lessen the blow when there is a remedial road map to prepare for death and to honor the passing of a loved one. Latino culture is by no means an exception for the unready, but the curandero does offer sage cultural and spiritual advice on what we can do to prepare.

69. LIFE IS A NIGHTMARE — *MI PESADILLA*

It's been three years since my divorce and since then, my life has become a nightmare, causing me deep emotional problems. I have lost everything: my health, my money, my house, and my job. I just can't seem to get ahead. I wish you could tell me if it's an evil spirit which has latched onto me or if it's simply life. Thank you.

CURANDERO'S RESPONSE:

Your situation reminds of the story of Job in the Old Testament. I don't know if you have ever read the book of Job. In life, these experiences are common. Life is worth living no matter what it brings, good or bad. Every day is a new day and every new day passes and becomes the old day. It's like the old sayings "there is no misfortune that doesn't come without good," and "there is no evil that will last more than 100 years or any person who can last that long."

Do you know what a scapular, or *escapulario,* is? I am sure that you have seen people who wear small colored wool pieces of cloth around their necks. They can be brown, or black, or red, or green and other colors depending on their intended purpose, saint or organization. It is a well-known fact that scapulars are miraculous and when the proper one is worn, the patron saint of the scapular will sometimes grant you an ordinarily unattainable goal. I recommend that you go to any Catholic store and purchase a green scapular dedicated to the Immaculate Heart of Mary. Pray for our Mother Mary to resolve your family problems and to restore your health and happiness.

Also pray that Santa Isabel will resolve your family problems and to Santa Clara so that you can see things clearly. Even life as a nightmare can be converted into a pleasant dream and everything you have lost can be regained. Another saying goes, "the last thing you lose is faith." And if you have lost your faith, you might want to recover that first. I'm talking about compassion and faith in God's mercy. If you have faith, Our Lord will help you come out ahead in your situation.

COMMENTARY:

Severe psychological and emotional problems often produce equally impactful physical symptoms. The concept of witchcraft is such an integral slice of Latino life and culture that it is almost always considered a cause before emotional problems surface. When people are facing difficult situations, emotional symptoms may be ruled out as reasons. Many of life's daily challenges are actually teaching tools which make us stronger and stimulate us to use our faith and common sense. Without life's ups and downs, many persons would become complacent and suffer a gradual loss of compassion.

In this most difficult and desperate case, the curandero recommends that the client wear a green scapular. Scapulars were worn by monks and other religious figures during the middle ages. They were popularized by lay or third orders to reflect devotion and affiliation to a confraternity, or cofradia. Scapulars are worn when individuals require special miracles and/or dedicate a novena to a saint for their personal intentions and needs.

70. BABY CRIES IN THE WOMB — *LLANTO DEL BEBÉ*

I remember as a child, hearing about the meaning of a baby crying in the mother's womb. I don't exactly recall what it means. I was born south of the border and I was raised in the old ways. I no longer have my grandma to ask about these practices.

I have a daughter who is pregnant and we have heard her baby cry from inside the womb. Can you tell me what this means? Could there be something wrong with the baby? We are afraid to say anything to the doctor again because when we mentioned it to her, she did not understand us. She did not even believe us and she looked at us as if we were crazy! Please help!

CURANDERO'S RESPONSE

I understand your concern. It can be very frustrating when one is in need of answers to very critical questions and issues in our everyday lives and one can't seem to find the answers or solutions anywhere. It is even worse when no one seems to understand, or much less, care.

In the traditional Latino culture, it has been my experience and belief than an unborn baby can cry in the mother's womb. While I have never heard it myself, many people have told me that it is true. In our culture, we are taught to believe that when a baby cries from within the mother's womb, that it is a sign that the child is going to be born with a gift from God. I hope and pray that this is of some consolation and comfort to you and to yours. I believe that your daughter is going to have a very special child. Pray to San Ignacio de Loyola to protect the baby and to bring the baby up in the spiritual life. Remember to honor San Nacho on July 31.

COMMENTARY:

Every world culture has unique, if not magical, beliefs about pregnancy and birth. They include the belief in what influences the fetus and what special qualities the fetus will display as an adult. Few parents have heard their fetus cry in the womb, but those who have, attribute special spiritual abilities to these unique children. The Latino culture uses the metaphor "gift from God" to describe these blessed children and fervently believe that they're destined to be clairvoyants and/or healers with a very special gift.

71. FRIGHTENED BEFORE BIRTH — *ASUSTADO EN EL VIENTRE*

I wanted to ask you if you think a baby can be *asustado/a* or frightened, while still in the mother's womb. My niece went through a traumatic event when she was about eight months pregnant. Could this have affected the baby in any way? We know that the baby shudders while she is sleeping.

Please let me know what you think. I also have a great-niece that I believe needs to be cured for *susto*. My grandmother used to do it for us and of course no one thought to write down the instructions to cure *susto* before she died. I know I need lime, called *cal* in Spanish, and mugwort, called *estafiate*, and that it is supposed to be done for three days. Are there special days when it is supposed to be done, and what about any prayers?

CURANDERO'S RESPONSE:

I am of the opinion that whatever affects the pregnant mother physically and psychologically also affects the unborn child to some degree physically or emotionally. The effects may be even greater where there has been a traumatic event, physical, emotional or psychological.

In some traditional folk beliefs, other concerns and symptoms might be present, such as cravings. It is believed that if the expectant mother does not satisfy her craving for a particular food, that the food will affect the unborn child. The fetus may develop hiccups in the womb and will be born with hiccups or will have an open mouth throughout its life. Sometimes these people drool and are called *babosos*.

Yes, I do believe a baby can be *asustado*, or frightened, while in the womb. It is the belief of some that if the expectant mother does not receive a treatment for the *susto*, the child will be slow to learn, to speak or will stutter throughout his or her life.

Shuddering is not considered a symptom or a result of *susto* and is more of a natural involuntary movement of the eyelids or muscles possibly due to dreaming. Another symptom of a person who is *asustado/a*, is that they will want to sleep all the time.

My mother used to have us jump over a hole in the ground filled with water. We would jump over it three times, making the sign of the cross each time and then drop on all fours to drink the water from the hole.

There are many variations on the cure for *susto*, so your grandmother had one and my mother had another. I bet both work.

To cure *susto*, I use fresh rue, rosemary and basil to sweep the frightened person. I recommend you look for a *piedra alumbre* or alum rock, at any *hierbería*, herb shop, and sweep the affected individual for nine straight days.

The frightened person should also drink a cup of spearmint tea in the morning during the same nine days and pray to the Archangel Gabriel.

COMMENTARY:

It should be noted here that the home remedies and advice from a curandero/a, should never serve as a replacement for suggested treatment by a medical doctor. The two treatments may complement each other, but always follow the advice of a physician. It is clear that the visits to the curandero provide grandma with comfort, but aren't meant as substitutes for medical attention.

It is widely believed that the developing fetus is influenced by both natural and supernatural forces. Therefore, the mother must always protect both herself and the fetus. Espanto is a severe form of fright caused by a ghost or spirit and pregnant women are always mindful not to be startled by them.

Pregnant women will wear a red ribbon around their waists, on their wrists or hang a key amulet pinned to undergarments. These are all designed to protect the baby from harm. The startle is believed to cause the fetus to be espantado or scared in the womb. Espanto might result in the baby being born with a scared looking or even twisted face, or unable to speak all together. The baby is also believed to be protected after birth by an ojo de venado seed or the deer's eye in the form of an amulet or talisman pinned to the diaper.

72. CANDLE DOESN'T SMOKE — *NO HAY MALDAD*

I was able to find everything you asked me to get. I still have to take the third bath, and that should be this Friday. I understood that when this candle finishes burning, I have to replace it with another and another after that, until my problems at work are resolved. I want to tell you this candle is not creating any smoke. The glass is clear. It makes me happy to see this happening. I think this is a good thing, right?

I would like to know how long it takes to travel to Espinazo, Nuevo León from the border. I made a promise to El Niño Fidencio that I would travel to his land and light some candles for him at his tomb. I'll wait for your response.

CURANDERO'S RESPONSE:

Complete the candle ritual I ordered and with time, your problems at work will be resolved.

It takes five hours to travel to Espinazo, Nuevo León, Mexico leaving from the lower Rio Grande Valley of Texas. It is very important for you to complete your promise and I hope that God grants you the wish to make the journey in order to complete your promise of lighting the candles at Niño Fidencio's tomb. That would be a life changing event for you.

May the shadow of San Pedro cover you and protect you on your journey, so that you may go and return to your home safely without accidents, happy and free of trouble.

COMMENTARY:

It is interesting to ponder that when a candle burns clean and without soot, it is deemed to be successfully bolstering the person's healing process and is in sync with the patient's prayers. Conversely, when it refuses to remain lit or is sooty, it's an indication that it is not functioning properly or that the healing requires a more detailed prognosis.

73. BAD AIR — *MAL DE AIRE*

My mother and my aunts have always said that if you venture quickly from a hot environment to a cold one without protection or vice versa, you will get sick. I don't understand this because my biology teacher says that viruses make people sick, not air temperature. Then, my anthropology professor was telling us about humoral theory. I know that many Mexican Americans still believe these things our grandparents taught us. Can you help me to understand?

CURANDERO'S RESPONSE:

Some people are more sensitive to a sudden or drastic change in temperature than others. That is, going from hot to cold or cold to hot. This sudden change of temperature could be caused by going from a cold air-conditioned room to the raging heat outside or vice versa during the winter. It can be a shock and very traumatic to the body by going from one extreme to the other. In *curanderismo*, this is referred to as *agarro* or *pesco un mal aire*, that is, to receive or "catch a bad air." The result from *mal aire* is usually a cerebral attack. It is believed that men are apt to be most susceptible to catching *mal aire* if they step out into the cold weather immediately after shaving. The result would be that the face or the mouth will pull to one side. Caution would be sufficient prevention in most cases. Massaging would be the therapeutic answer to this ailment. Headaches are another illness or sickness caused by going from hot to cold or cold to hot.

One cure for *mal aire* or bad air is to place a burning candle on a coin atop a person's back or stomach and then to place a drinking glass over the flame. As the flame burns out from lack of oxygen, the glass will press harder on the flesh, forming an airtight seal. When the glass is removed, it is pulled off gently and with its removal the *mal aire* or intrusive air is sucked out of the body.

COMMENTARY:

Latino folklore pronounces that a sudden change in the ambient temperature surrounding one's body triggers illness. For example, moving from an air-conditioned room to the warm or hot outdoors is believed to cause a cold, just as going from hot to cold is believed to do the same. Latinos will refer to bad air, or mal aire, as an invasive predicament affecting the body and the cause of illness. One ancient technique still practiced by today's curanderos/as is called la ventosa, or cupping. In order to remove the invasive air from the body of the patient, a coin or another type of metallic object is placed on the skin at the suspected site believed to be influenced by el aire, the air. A small candle is then placed on the coin and lighted; a glass or "cup" is then placed over the flame. As the flame flickers down, the skin is gently elevated, thus expelling unwanted air from the body.

The dichotomy of belief between hot and cold foods is also prevalent in curanderismo. In both food and in air, pre-Columbian cultures, as well as Europeans, believed influx retained a physical equilibrium for overall sound health. The slightest dip of this balance was thought to cause sickness. The Badianus Codex explains how an illness was precipitated by an imbalance in one's diet. Today, many of the curanderos/as' remedies are efforts to restore and maintain physical and spiritual balance.

74. EVIL EYE — *MAL DE OJO*

What can be wrong with my child? She was such a happy child but now she is irritable, can't sleep and cries a lot. This started after we attended a party where I know several women were looking at her. Do you think they might have given her the evil eye? Please pray for her. We have taken her to the doctors and they cannot find anything wrong with her. She is just one year old. She had never gotten sick before. We are scared and don't know what is wrong or what to do. I remember my grandmother talking about *mal de ojo* and I even remember being cured for it when I was little. We really don't know much about that stuff anymore, and they tell us at our church not to believe in it, but we do not know what to do. Can you and Niñito Fidencio please help us? Tell us what we need to do. Thank you.

CURANDERO'S RESPONSE:

You say the doctor has examined her and cannot find anything medically wrong with her, yet she is not doing well. I will try to help you. Let's check her out to see if she has evil eye, *mal de ojo*. Use a fertile chicken egg, one with a live yolk is best, to do a ritual sweeping, or *limpia*, cleansing on her by rubbing the egg over the child's body, especially her head and her eyes. Be sure to hold the egg in your right hand when you are sweeping her. Begin at her head and proceed down her entire body. Include her arms and legs. While you are doing the ritual sweeping or *barrida*, you must pray three Apostles' Creeds, or Credos. Another cure comes from an old Mexican belief that women's interior clothing may be used; especially if they are red.

Place yourself in a spiritual mood and pray to God and to the spirit of Niño Fidencio to remove all evil from her and to heal her. Crack the eggshell, dropping only the egg yolk but not the shell into a clear glass of water. Examine the egg yolk to see if you can spot what looks like an eye on the yolk or some other identifiable shape. If you can see what looks like an eye, that is a sign that negative energy of the evil eye has been absorbed by the egg from the child. Once this occurs, the afflicted child will settle down from what appears to be a frightening state of illness. People who practice witchcraft or who want to send the evil eye "back" to the person, who originally sent it will boil the egg and send the evil back to the one who sent it. Saint Lucy is the patron saint of everything having to do with the eye, including the evil eye, pray to her. Lucy's day is December 13.

If the child's condition does not improve immediately, the problem is not evil eye and the child should be taken to a physician for further examination.

A red string or a piece of red ribbon with an attached *ojo de venado*, or deer's eye, amulet may be tied around the child's wrist or attached to the child's clothing to ward off the evil eye. The evil eye may unknowingly emanate from seemingly harmless, yet powerful people. Negative energies can come from an unsuspecting person who admires the child, but without even touching the child on the head. We must always protect an innocent child from the transfer of a strong eye. Touching the child nullifies any energy transmitted by sight. Energies may be transmitted by people and even by animals such as owls, snake, and cats.

COMMENTARY:

In this question and response, it is clear that a multitude of variations exists in the cure of mal de ojo in the practice of curanderismo. One may not prove any better than the other and families maintain their own traditions. In the case of mal de ojo, it is important to always protect children from "powerful" glares or stares. This does not mean that people are evil; some may possess a "strong" eye that may befall a child by producing fever, restlessness, sleeplessness, and other similar symptoms. If possible, go to the hierbería and purchase an ojo de venado and pin it on your baby's interior clothing.

75. BABY SCARED IN SLEEP — *SUEÑO ASUSTADO*

My husband and I don't fight that much but we are loud. We both come from families that are very loud. Our baby boy is eight months old and very observant. Last week we had a yelling match and he watched it all. It seemed to worry him and that is when he began sleeping poorly and being very cranky with hurt feelings, or *sentimientos,* during the day.

My mother said that she noticed it and thought that he was scared in his sleep, or had *sueño asustado*. This behavior is very unlike him since he is a very good-natured baby. Please tell me how to cure him.

CURANDERO'S RESPONSE

I think your mother is correct and it is good that you are listening to her. A part of his spirit was scared out of him for some reason and must be coaxed back to make him whole again. Children who are very bright and alert begin to watch their parents at a very early age. If they see conflict between them, they become scared. I believe that is what has happened to your baby boy. I will tell you how to cure him with the help of San Marcos the patron saint of childhood illnesses. Be sure to celebrate him on April 25.

Let this be a lesson to you and your husband not to fight or yell in front of your child. In the long run, you can hurt him and warp his behavior. Their fears become part of their permanent personalities, their souls, spirits and their subconscious minds.

Here is what you need to do: Go to the *hierbería* and buy a large white candle called a *cirio*. Buy one that is not in a glass container. Also, buy three small alum rocks, or *piedras alumbre*. The store will probably have fresh basil, or *albahaca*, or can tell you where to buy it. You will also need rubbing alcohol, aspirin and tobacco. For three days in a row and, at precisely the same time every day, give your baby boy a ritual cleansing, first with the basil and then with the *piedra alumbre*. Be sure to cleanse him from head to toe while doing this. Hold all items used to cleanse in your right hand.

Light the white candle. The candle will let you know if the cure is working. If it burns without smoking, then the cure is working. As long as it smokes, more cleansing is required. Mix a small amount of the alcohol with one or two aspirins and use this mixture to make the cross on his hands, arms, legs and feet at the bending points; wrist, elbow and the back of the neck. While you make the sign of the cross on him, gently puff tobacco smoke around his head but <u>not</u> in his face. Be sure to recite three Our Fathers, Padre Nuestro, or three Apostles' Creeds, Credos. After the first day, you should begin to see an improvement in his behavior and he should sleep better as well. By the second day, if he really is *asustado,* the lighted candle should begin to crackle while you are cleansing him, letting you know that something is happening. By the third treatment, he should be a happy baby boy once again and totally cured. At the end of the three days, take the used alum rocks outside and carefully burn them in a small coffee or soup can. Always pray to the patron saint for preventing nightmares in children, Saint Raphael the Archangel whose day is September 29.

COMMENTARY:

Young children are most susceptible to a scare by their new or unknown experiences early in their lives. For example, newborns are sensitive to noise and motion, light and dark as well as hot and cold. All these aforementioned factors are equivalent to parents in their oblivious mode of incessant arguing and shouting, making their baby feel unsafe in the world. However, fright, or susto, is also known to occur during pregnancy and affect the developing fetus. The earliest medical texts available to us from the old and new worlds suggest many unpredictable situations during pregnancy which adversely affect the developing fetus. It is also commonly believed that factors which impact the pregnant mother or may scare her, could affect the fetus in a negative way.

If the fetus is believed to be scared while in the mother's womb, it is capable of violent shakes and can even cry in the womb. These are all ominous signs in the Latino world and indicate that something adverse is happening or could happen to the developing baby. The result could be something as benign as a birthmark or as serious as a birth defect.

76. WE ARE SUFFERING — *EL SUFRIMIENTO*

I suffer from schizophrenia and my wife also suffers from depression and extreme anxiety. Our financial condition is poor. We have had a lot of bad luck and I'm waiting to see if you can assist me with my disability application. We have a daughter and she is the only blessing we have. Many times I feel so desperate that I think about taking my own life, but I know that is a sin.

Please consult El Niño Fidencio on our behalf. We are honest and hard-working people but we never seem to get ahead. The only thing I know to do is pray the Holy Rosary and to burn candles to the Virgen de Guadalupe and to sprinkle Holy Water around our humble home. We don't want something for nothing; we just want our luck to reverse.

Will my attending Mass more often or praying the Rosary more often help us? Will these things take the salt off of us?

CURANDERO'S RESPONSE:

I always recommend that Catholics attend Mass regularly, participate in the sacraments and identify personal or patron saints. I will continue to pray for you and I invoke the assistance of San Leonardo who always helps the emotionally ill. Be sure to thank Leo on his saint's day of November 6. I feel for you so very much because I can feel your suffering. It must be so painful for you with your schizophrenia and with your wife with her anxiety. I know the only help you get to make it through the day is your spirituality, and your faith in God.

I will continue to pray for you, asking the healing spirit of Niñito Fidencio, and God to grant you and your wife a spiritual miracle. I will pray that God will grant you healing with many blessings and happiness. Make a special petition for luck or success in the home and place this written petition on your home altar.

Be sure to write all the names of the family members on parchment paper and place a green candle over it. Use specially-prepared sprays or perfumes for drawing luck and prosperity to the home. Be certain to ask your patron saint, like La Virgen de Guadalupe, for a special blessing for your daughter because she needs help to have a normal life. Many people in your situation ask for special blessings from San Ignacio de Loyola.

COMMENTARY:

This humble and sincere question deals with several very important concepts. The questioner begins with an admission of mental illness in the family and while it is revealing, that is not what the question is really about. Often the curandero must read between the lines, gathering as much information from the family as possible. In this case, the family is genuinely modest and the father believes that they truly have bad luck.

Luck, or suerte is something that the Latino population believes can be brought on the family and also altered and manipulated, and even removed. For example, an evil spell can be used to change luck from good to bad. While this is an issue that resides in the realm of curanderismo it is also related to the Catholic concept of prayer.

Prayer is believed to be a viable avenue to seek or petition a saint for his or her intercession with God for the purpose of reversing one's ill fortune. The curandero correctly says that he will continue to pray that the Niño Fidencio is able to intercede on their behalf for a positive outcome.

77. ABUSED GRANDCHILD — *NIETO VIOLADO*

I am a terribly distraught grandmother. I have custody of my four-year-old grandson since my underage daughter separated from the child's father. Now she is living with another man who is very abusive to my grandson. He even makes my grandson clean up the dog poop with his bare hands. He and my daughter do drugs and they all sleep together in the same bed. They have wild parties where they expose my grandson to all kinds of wickedness.

I don't know if my grandson has actually been molested or what has happened to him. He is not behaving normally.

I am his grandmother, yet he goes through the motions of trying to have sex with me. Where could he have learned these things, if not there with this man and his mother? I have explained to him that this is not proper behavior for a little boy and that we don't do things like that, but nothing seems to work. He has become very stubborn and I can't control him. I don't know what to do anymore. There are times he takes on an evil look as if it is not him anymore. What can I do? I can't afford professional help for him. Can you please help us?

CURANDERO'S RESPONSE:

Thank you for your e-mail. I understand that you are unable to afford professional help for your dear, troubled grandson. Please allow me to suggest other methods to help for your grandson. Never rule out the need to contact your state's children's protection agency, especially if the child admits to you that he has been sexually abused.

You understand that I am a traditional *curandero* so let's begin with spiritual healing baths with Holy Water and candle burning for a period of 40 consecutive days using plain white wax candles and prayers to Santa Agueda. Agueda is the patron saint of sexual abuse and her celebration is February 5 and to Saint Maria Goretti, July 6, to protect against sexual assault. Also, give him a *barrida,* or ritual sweeping, with fresh herbs once a week for seven straight weeks. Be sure to do this at the same time on the same day of the week. Be sure to let me know if you encounter any signs of unclean spirit possession when you do this. If you do, then we will have to cast out demons from his soul with an exorcism. Please keep me informed as you go along so that I can advise you. Also, I will place him in my special prayers.

COMMENTARY:

In today's world, more grandparents are legally responsible for their grandchildren than ever before. Never hesitate in contacting your state's agency for protecting children at the first sign of child abuse. Children are innocent and defenseless. As adults, we must be proactive or they will suffer horrible physical, sexual and psychological damage. When in doubt, call the proper authorities.

78. MOONBEAMS HURT MY BABY — *ECLIPSE DE LUNA*

My baby was delivered by a certified midwife, or *partera*. I went to this special birthing center because they specialize in Latino cultural beliefs. They explained to me that they were going to teach me the "old ways" and I would just love it. For the first time in my life, I felt connected to something, even though I didn't always understand what they were telling me. And, in fact, they don't really know or understand the origins for a lot of the things they taught me.

Can you help me to understand the influence of the moon on development and why we believe that moonbeams and eclipses of the moon can hurt the baby before it is born?

CURANDERO'S RESPONSE:

The moon is associated with both the natural and the supernatural influences and phenomena of prenatal development. Some believe that the moon is a heavenly body with magical or spiritual qualities. Others hold it to be virtuous and full of mystical powers.

Latinos believe that if an expectant mother does not protect the developing fetus from moonlight, when the moon is full there could be serious consequences to the child's well-being and the child runs the risk of being born deformed. People say that the moon will eat, or *comer*, the baby while in the womb if the moonbeams fall on the pregnant mother.

This is especially true during a lunar eclipse when pregnant women should protect themselves by not going outside or standing in front of windows where the moon is fully visible. To protect the baby and prevent the moon from eating away at an unborn baby, the expectant mother should attach a safety pin or a key to her clothes directly over her stomach. The mother-to-be should also wear red undergarments or tie a red ribbon around her body over her stomach to protect the unborn baby. Pray to the Holy Innocents, December 28, for the protection of the unborn.

COMMENTARY:

The belief that the stars and moon affect outcomes of conception and determine behavioral characteristics of the unborn can be traced back to the beginning of time. There are many ancient beliefs from all cultures about the harmful nature of moonbeams on the developing fetus. The belief that moonbeams "falling" upon the unprotected belly of a pregnant woman will deform a fetus is found in many ancient medical texts.

79. DEW HARMS BABY — *EL SERENO*

I am a young Latina and I have a newborn baby. I am trying to be a good mother, but I don't know how to do it. Everyone I speak to seems to have a better idea about how I should raise my baby, and what is good and what is bad. I don't know who to believe and I hope you can help me. On the issue of covering up the baby's head outdoors, I am told that the baby's head needs to be kept warm because it loses heat right away. Also, I am told never to let the evening dew fall on the baby's head because that will make him sick. Can you please help me to understand and what to believe or not to believe?

CURANDERO'S RESPONSE:

The condition known as *serenar* refers to illnesses influenced by evening dew, or *sereno*. This is a concern with many Latinos who have babies. The belief is that the baby should never be exposed to evening dew. If the baby must be taken out at night, the baby's head should always be covered because it is the most vulnerable place on the body. If the child is exposed to the *sereno*, the child may become susceptible to illness. The baby who becomes *serenado* may suffer chills, body pains and headaches, and the child's stool will be greenish in color. Additionally, it is believed that the child or baby may become ill if dressed with clothes left out overnight in the evening dew.

Chamomile tea is often boiled in milk and given to children as a remedy for this condition.

COMMENTARY:

All cultures swaddle newborn infants and know to keep them covered up. This is especially true of their heads. Curanderos, mother, and grandmothers will emphatically counsel their daughters to cover the heads of babies since they're believed to be conduits of illnesses. Most cultures once believed in the need for balance in the bodily systems and that a lack of balance actually triggers sickness. A balance of hot and cold along with wet and dry should be strictly observed and maintained. Anything that upsets the balance of these four factors will cause a dreaded illness. Latino folk beliefs include this established knowledge with advice on how to protect the fetus.

80. LOST VALUABLES — *AYÚDAME SAN ANTONIO*

I am writing to you because I have lost my mother's cross that was on a necklace given to me by my father. It was passed on to me by my mother while she lay on her death bed. I am so scared I've lost it that if I can have it returned to me, I will never take it off again. I am so worried that I won't find it again. Can you please help me to find my necklace? Use the spirit world and the saints to help bring it back to me.

CURANDERO'S RESPONSE:

I do not know where your necklace is, but Saint Anthony does and he can help you find it. Try lighting a Saint Anthony candle and pray Psalm 16 the first thing in the morning for three days in a row. Make a promise to Saint Anthony that if he finds it and brings it back to you, you will do something for him like visit his shrine or offer a novena to him for the redemption of lost souls. Be sure that you honor him on June 13.

Once you promise, he will most likely place it in your path where you will find it. Let me know when this happens as I know that it will.

COMMENTARY:

Latino curanderismo is inextricably intertwined with Roman Catholicism and its saints, beliefs and rituals. Saint Anthony is the patron saint of lost and misplaced items and as in Catholicism, curanderismo recommends that prayer to Saint Anthony will be rewarded by the return of the lost item.

81. CLEANSE GRANDMOTHER'S HOUSE — *EL DESPOJO*

I'm sending you this e-mail because my grandmother would like to know if you can come to her house to cleanse it of evil forces and spirits. I know that you have a ritual for completely cleaning up a home from bad spirits and evil influences.

She wanted to visit you this week, but she's still having pain in her legs. Yesterday, she did so well that it seemed like the pain was going to go away for good. She had even slept a lot better than most nights. She was so happy that she put the bedspreads on her beds and washed clothes like before she got this pain nearly four weeks ago. But, then, last night a little after midnight, she started complaining about the pain again and she didn't get relief until early this morning. She says that sometimes she gets relief after she cries.

Today she started drinking the *zacate de limón* tea with *cenizo*. I looked it up on the Internet and saw that *cenizo* is called sage and that *salvia* is also called sage. Are we preparing her tea the right way?

I am certain that her house needs a good *despojo*. Please let me know how to do it.

CURANDERO'S RESPONSE:

Thank grandma for her faith and trust in my prayers. There are many deserving needs and requests for my efforts and services. I am honored she and you would have me cleanse her house. However, I am unable to oblige her request since I have too much to do here and have very heavy obligations and responsibilities with my healing mission. I am unable to leave my house.

Another reason I am unable to cleanse her home is that I need permission from my spirit guide, El Niño Fidencio. Ask her to prepare a tea made from lemon grass, *zacate de limón*, and *salvia*, not *cenizo*, for the pain.

Pray a special prayer to San Cristóbal to cleanse your home and to keep it free of evil influences. Every Friday, burn incenses to the four winds and ask that the winds carry far away any and all negative forces that have attached themselves to your home during the week. Pray Psalms 61 and 62 to keep your grandmother's house always clean of bad influences. My prayers are for her good health.

COMMENTARY:

The petitioner is able, with directions from the curandero, to cleanse grandmother's home herself. It is not difficult and only requires a few items.

He also cautions that medicinal plants are sometimes confused and called by inappropriate names. Sometimes plants have duplicate names and there are variations of plants with similar names. One must always take care to have the proper plant because the wrong plant may produce undesirable effects.

Be sure to get real salvia and not sage. Salvia is the universal name for all sages in that particular plant family, but many varieties of sage are toxic to humans. The correct salvia will be sold by any credible *hierbería*, *botánica*, herbalist, or Mexican products store.

82. OUR FAMILY CURSE — *MALDICIÓN FAMILIAR*

Talking with El Niño is difficult because I do not speak Spanish. The last time I spoke to you it was a positive experience for me because I received the blessing I was expecting. I did some awesome praise and worshipping the day before, but I still have some questions.

The first time I made this request, Niño asked me to get two candles: a just judge, *justo juez* and Saint Gabriel, or seven Archangels' candle, for my happiness. The just judge candle would not stay lit. Each time I took out wax to find the wick, but it barely lit. I could only find the Saint Gabriel candle, which stays lit all the time. Last week, Niño told me to throw the candle away and get a new one. I did, but this one keeps doing the same thing. It has the dimmest light and does not seem to want to stay lit. I know that is not good. I am bathing in Holy Water and placing incense on the altar, as I was told for seven consecutive Fridays. The two new candles I got, San Ignacio de Loyola and San Alejo always stay lit so I feel I'm on the right path now.

There is this guy that I really like, but he does not seem to care about me. Is something wrong with me? Some say that we have a family curse. Will you pray about it? El Niño said that I was being tormented but I'm not sure how. I feel like this guy is playing with my emotions. He can be nice and then one minute later, he is heartless. He told me that he loved me, but now he acts as if he can't stand me. I don't understand. Does he really like me or should I just forget about him altogether? These are the things that I have been praying about.

CURANDERO'S RESPONSE:

It is difficult when you do not speak Spanish, but Fidencio will speak to your heart in his spiritual language and for that, you need no earthly language. Being in a spiritual trance helps us to communicate the union of the anointing and the giving and receiving of blessings. Niño understood through the translator that you are looking for happiness and for someone to love you.

The spirit of El Niño advised you to burn the just judge, or *justo juez*, and the Saint Gabriel or the Seven Archangels' candles whenever possible. Don't forget to honor the Archangels on September 29. With your faith and prayer petitions, the doors to finding true love and true happiness shall be flung open for you. If this man is not your true soulmate, you will find someone who will truly love you for who you are. I am picking up that he has deep emotional problems and a history of doing to other women what he is doing to you. Beware!

There is nothing wrong with you. It seems to me there is something wrong with him! Do not give up and you will soon find your true love. El Niño advised you to light the just judge candle for your petition so that the spirit could intercede and be your lawyer before God and plead on your behalf. In addition, you were instructed to light the Saint Gabriel candle as an offering to the archangel, who is the highest ranking authority of God's celestial spiritual beings. You want to seek the happiness of the petitions you have made for true love in the form of an earthly companion in life.

The bathing with Holy Water and burning incense is for cleansing the person of negative energies, forces and/or influences. There is a big difference between liking somebody and being in love with someone. You know he is not in love with you so I feel it is time to let him go. We believe that if he was meant to be with you he will return to you.

COMMENTARY:

Curses are routine in curanderismo. Curses result from spells which have been cast by witches or brujos/as on people on behalf of other people. In Spanish, spells cast by witchcraft are called works, or trabajos. Curanderos/as and brujos/as are known to conduct ongoing spell-casting and spell-

breaking in a continual spiritual tug of war. These mystical battles can last for decades and their *manda*, or cargo, can even be passed on to the next generation. Many times the children and grandchildren continue a war of the witches and warlocks that they had nothing to do with.

83. HELP ME SELL MY HOME — *AYÚDAME SAN JOSÉ*

I asked you for advice on whether or not I should sell my home and you advised me to sell it. Would you be able to find me a serious buyer for my home? I had a buyer but he didn't follow through. Right now, my son and I are living with my mother. I found a home that I like and put $500 down, but the owner of the house only gave me 30 days to close. Since I don't think I can get the money together that quickly, I will probably lose the house and my earnest money will also be lost if I back out for any reason. Would you be able to help me with this problem?

CURANDERO'S RESPONSE:

I will say a special prayer for you and I will ask Saint Joseph to help you to sell your home. If you say a prayer to San Onofre, who is celebrated June 12, he also helps people who are looking for a home. You should work it from both ends in order to be successful.

Sprinkle a pound of rice, a pound of wheat seed and a small packet of mustard seed in the yard of the house you want to sell. Pray to the Lord for your petition to come true. Check back with me in two weeks and let's see where we are.

I will try to help you. Write a special petition for the sale of your house and light a candle to the Virgen de Guadalupe and I will do the same for you here on my altar.

COMMENTARY:

Curanderos are consulted for a plethora of problems. The curandero may not be able to help this person sell the home, but the process of this magic is not any different than any other. More and more people believe that a statue and prayer to Saint Joseph is often helpful in selling a house. The mixture of rice, wheat and mustard seed is a time-tested remedy for cleansing a home of evil spirits which may be preventing the home from being sold.

Within the Latino population, the Virgen de Guadalupe is the most frequently petitioned saint. Since she is the Mother of the Americas, we ask for her help in all sorts of mundane issues.

84. CLEANSING AND SWEEPINGS — *LIMPIAS Y BARRIDAS*

I just wanted to give you an update and then ask for some help with the ingredients for my remedy. I came with my family to meet you about three weeks ago. We all received *limpias*, spiritual cleansings, and you also told my mom about what she needs to buy to help sell her house. You asked her to get *sándalo, sal y polvo sangre de dragón*, dragon's blood powder.

Well, I got the ingredients for my mom and as she spread them on the yard and began to clearly hear Indian chanting, but there were no Indians around. She also noticed that as she tossed the powder, it would just blow away in the wind without reaching the ground. Well, the curious thing was that there was no wind that day. The powder was simply being moved away from our yard as if something did not want the yard cured. But we didn't give up and continued to spread the powder until it hit the ground. It took some time but we finally prevailed.

Well, three weeks have passed and my father who was selling my grandma's house got about 25 calls after seeing you. Now he is about to close the deal. The same buyer might also be interested in my mom's house. So the *limpia* combined with the powders finally worked for us and the house was sold and another was purchased.

CURANDERO'S RESPONSE:

Thank you for the wonderful news. I am pleased you are receiving the positive results your family was looking in the selling of the house; especially after you had such difficulty selling it before you received assistance from Saint Joseph, and the spiritual world. Please, if I may be of any further spiritual assistance, do not hesitate to ask for help.

COMMENTARY:

Like most individuals, *curanderos* revel in testimonies of their successes. In this case, the ancient remedy of sandalwood, salt and dragon's blood powder sprinkled around the home is believed to have eradicated the evil spirits from the house allowing it to be sold.

The fact that the powder blew away without touching the ground is believed to be an indication that a powerful spirit stifled the remedy. Once the spirit was coaxed away or removed spiritually, the obstacle preventing the sale of the house was cleared.

85. HEALING PSALMS — *LOS SALMOS SANAN*

I hear a lot about the power of the Psalms. I am a Catholic and we pray the Psalms, but not as much as the Protestants. My mother is a born-again Christian and they really pray the Psalms. In my limited experience with *curanderos/as*, I have noticed that they almost always use the Psalms in their healing rituals. Do you use the Psalms and are they important? Should I be reading and praying the Psalms for my situations in life?

CURANDERO'S RESPONSE:

I am a healer and considered by some to possess *el don,* the spiritual gift of healing. My efforts are mainly concentrated to accompany those with health issues and in comforting and consoling them when I am asked to do so. I am a firm believer in the magical ability of the Psalms as handed down by King Solomon and Kind David, which is, El Rey Salomón and El Rey Davíd. In my altar room I have both the Holy Bible and the little book called the Secrets of the Psalms. I use them constantly. I read them during healings and you should do the same.

For example, in *curanderismo,* a lot of our work is reversing bad luck and attracting good luck, but this is not a guarantee when it comes to wealth, money or winning the lottery. Divine Providence is always in the hands of God.

Many people try cleansings with heads of garlic and many other items to remove evil forces, spells, curses and bad luck, while others try spiritual healing baths to remove negative energies. Any method can work for you. It's all up to God.

Any one of Psalms 4, 8, 41, 43, 57, 61 and 63 may be used to return good luck or fortune to the household or to your business. If you need better luck or help with prosperity, then prepare an amulet bag of green flannel and place in the amulet black and yellow mustard seeds, a male garlic head, a copper coin, red and white coral, buckeye seed, juniper berry, and a whole spice and clove. Add a hot pepper, three coriander seeds and Irish moss leaves, two rose petals and horehound root. Mexican marketplaces sell these items as well as printed prayers for good luck, money drawing and items believed useful for winning the lottery.

Personally, my favorite spell is to use essence of basil and seven male billy goats' lotion, *loción siete machos*, for money-drawing purposes. Good luck and I hope you are granted all your wishes.

COMMENTARY:

Most curanderos perform simple white magic rites as spiritual trappings in their repertoires. Curanderismo is not just about healing, it also encompasses magic; this is why churches are mainly opposed to it. However, if curanderos/as had actually discovered how to win all the lotteries, there would be no curanderos. They'd all retire as millionaires.

Traditional curanderismo is not self serving. It is about helping the needy both materially and spiritually. Curanderos habitually use spells to reverse a straying husband's ways, but spells used for personal gain are believed to lead to negative consequences. As curandero Don Perfecto used to say, not only will you lose your spiritual power, but the spells you cast on others will come back on you. It's not worth it.

The Book of Psalms in the Old Testament, is believed to be handed down to us by King Solomon and David, and is critically important in curanderismo. The pamphlet entitled "Secrets of the Psalms" by Godfrey Selig is readily available in hierberías and is considered an essential part of the curanderos/a's tool kit. This little book addresses all nuances of life issues like court cases, escaping danger, how to receive holy blessings and many more.

Antonio Zavaleta and Alberto Salinas Jr.

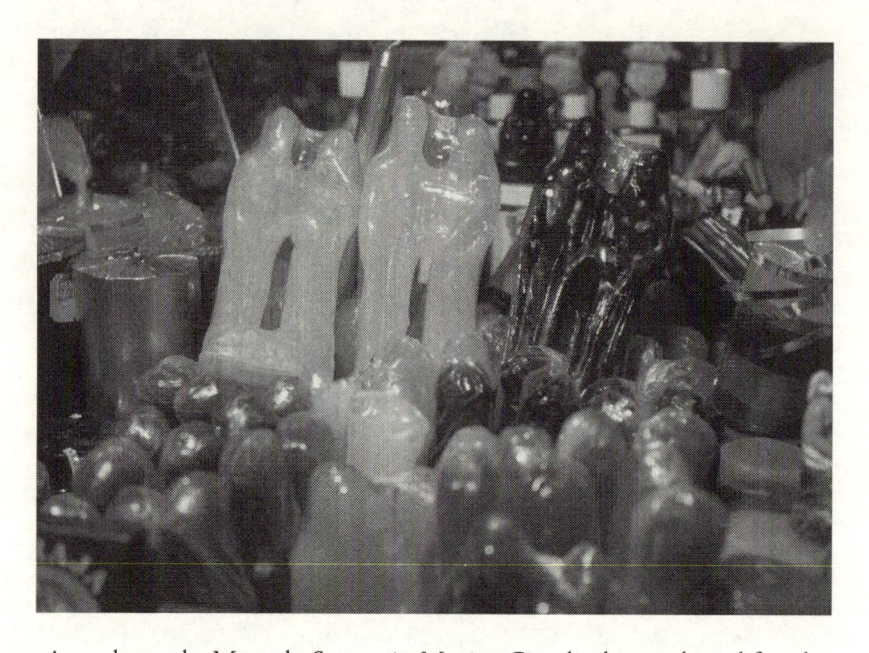

A vendor at the Mercado Sonora in Mexico City displays male and female candles intended for love attraction or breaking spells.
(Photo by José M. Duarte)

PART SIX

Healing the Heart: Cheating Husbands and the Other Woman

"Both men and women come to me for help. They are all worried that their husbands and wives are having affairs. They come to me to save both their marriages and their families and they are always desperate. It is wrong to think that only men have affairs. There are just as many cheating wives as cheating husbands."

– María Tamayo, *curandera*

86. MY HUSBAND LEFT ME — *LA ABANDONADA*

I spoke to you briefly about buying candles. My situation is that my husband has left home. He left for work a month ago and never returned. We know that he is living with another woman at her parents' home. What kind of people are they to allow their daughter to live with a married man?

When he first left, he would talk to me by phone, but if I mentioned the woman's name, he would just hang up on me. Now he has cut off all contact with me and our daughter. He left all his clothes here at home. Everything he owns is here at home. He refuses to come back for his belongings.

He will not answer my phone calls or calls from anyone we know. He has stopped communicating with everyone that we know, including his family. He told me that he can't step a foot back or on our property. He runs from me if I try to make contact with him at his job. He shouts and yells for me to stay away from him. I found out that the woman he is living with keeps a close watch over who he sees and talks to. He never goes anywhere by himself except to work.

We have been married for many years. He has never acted this way to me or our daughter. He will not let us get close to him, touch him, and now he will not talk to us. His childhood was an abusive one because he was a foster child. He always felt rejected. I don't think he understands or knows how to love. But I do love him and I want him back home with his family. Our daughter is suffering and it hurts.

These people have taken control of his mind. He thinks that I am a witch but in reality, they are the ones who have placed spells on him. Please help me if you can. Please tell me what I need to do.

CURANDERO'S RESPONSE:

Purchase these four candles: San Ignacio de Loyola, San Alejo, a San Cipriano and a plain white candle for San Eduardo, the patron of good marriages and for Saint Gummarus, who is acknowledged on October 11, and is the patron of the unhappy marriage. All are seven-day candles. Once you have all four candles, or four plain white wax, seven-day candles, place them in a triangle. Position one on the east side where the sun rises and the other two on the west side where the sun sets. Place his picture in the center of the three candles. Place the fourth candle in the center along with a clear glass of water over his photo. Light the candles and make your petition to the Lord asking to have your husband return home. Once you light the candles, do not extinguish them. This candle-burning ritual is to clear him of all the witchcraft influences that have been placed on him by the other woman or by anyone else. This should work within about seven to nine days.

Once the goal is achieved, it will be necessary to do another "work" to get him to return to you, his rightful family. God bless you.

COMMENTARY:

It is ordinary in Latino culture to use magical spells performed by practitioners known as brujos/as or witches to draw people into sexual relationships or to break up relationships. More than likely, this is what the other woman has perpetrated on the husband. While it may sound very strange or foreign to those who have not heard of this, it is actually one of the most routine requests made of healers and witches, curanderos and brujas. The witch is asked to destroy a marriage and the curandero is asked to return the husband to his rightful wife. The curandero intimates to the wife that this is why her husband is afraid of her and stays away from his daughter, family and friends. This strange behavior can only be understood within the context of witchcraft. This is supported by his inability to go anywhere alone except to work.

87. DESTROYED MARRIAGE — *BRUJERÍA DESTRUYE*

Hello. I have been going through some very troubling times. My husband has been seeing another woman, but recently and with your help, my husband has broken off with the woman that he thought was the love of his life. This illicit relationship was destroying my marriage and my children at the same time.

I have been feeling awkward the last couple of years and have found myself spiritually weakened at times. I went to see a psychic and this lady gave me a reading that was completely accurate. She also told me that someone went to an evil witch, or *bruja,* and asked this witch to cast a spell upon me and my marriage using the devil, pure evil. This bad witch was paid a lot of money and agreed to cast the spell, *trabajo.* Together, my husband's girlfriend and the witch have brought misery, pain and suffering upon every aspect of my life.

I hired a psychic to perform a ritual to reverse the spell. I think I wasted my time and my money. I was really very nervous about it because she asked me to bring $1,800 and I wasn't sure what it was being used for. She said that the money was needed to use against the warlock, or *brujo*, who laid out the curse on my marriage. She said she spent it all to destroy the spell against us. I don't know if this is true or not. This has been going on for a couple of years now.

The psychic also rubbed an egg on my body to pull out of me anything that was evil. During this ritual we broke the egg and I saw something in it that really scared me. I was in total disbelief. I saw the mark of a hand with a claw with blood and it looked like the devil's hand. That's what my psychic said it was also.

My husband and I are caught in the devil's hand and the devil is squeezing the life out of our marriage. This is really evil stuff.

The psychic then cut the $1,800 I gave her in half because she said the people that did this to me used the mark of the beast or 666 on me because they thought that I would not be able to raise this amount of money to reverse the spell. They used that same number to break the curse. The psychic said that we had to cut up the money and mix it in with the egg. The psychic says that the evil is attempting to destroy my marriage so my husband will be under the eternal spell of his girlfriend.

What kind of woman would do this to a marriage with children? I was told that the number of the beast, 666, adds up to the number 18. So the psychic has told me that $600 times 3 makes $1,800 which is the amount I would need to reverse the devil's number. The psychic says she has to complete the ritual and has asked that I call her back later to learn the results.

I now know that my husband's girlfriend also spent a lot of money to purchase the evil necessary to cover my eyes and take my husband away from me. I keep asking the psychic for the name of the person who has cursed me but she says that it is too dangerous to tell me the name right now until the spell is reversed. But I think I know who it is. I just want her to say her name out loud so I can be satisfied I know. I know it was my husband's girlfriend because they told me at work it was. Her girlfriends are also terrified that she will take their men away.

Since I contacted you and you put me on the righteous path I know that there is a spiritual battle taking place right now between me and my husband's girlfriend. The witch she is using is one of the most powerful in this area. People have even seen her transform into an owl, or *lechuza*. Flying witches are the worst.

The psychic told me that she would go to church and complete the ritual in order to reverse or break this spell. She said that she had to burn my money and the egg and bury them in the church yard and then it would be finished. But I don't believe her. I think she just ripped me off. I threw my hard earned money away. I ask for your continued guidance and for your intercession with El Niño Fidencio and Pedrito Jaramillo, with our Lord and for all your prayers to help me win in this matter. I don't want this evil on me. I want to walk the path of light, and I want my marriage put back together. So with this, I ask you to give me the strength and will to live a good and healthy life. I ask you to show me the light and the right way to live. Show me how to love and restore my husband and to help my kids and most importantly, help my husband not to want to see his girlfriend again. I wish to know the truth. I thank you for reading this and look forward to hearing from you.

I am very confused, and my mother and aunt asked me to consult you for guidance because you have helped them in the past. I do believe I need your help, this evil spell is too strong to defeat by myself.

CURANDERO'S RESPONSE:

I am saddened to learn of all your troubles. First of all, you made a huge mistake giving the psychic $1,800. Your problem will be solved with faith and prayer and the workers in the light; not with dirty money.

Secondly, I believe I can guide and help you in your situation. I will pray over you for your spiritual deliverance and healing. To begin your spiritual cleansing and healing, light three Niño Fidencio candles forming a triangle with the three candles, one on the east side and two to the west side, placing a picture of yourself in the center and a clear glass of water over your picture. You need to call out Niño Fidencio's name three times and make your petition to him. Niño Fidencio's spirit will come to you and will begin to help you. Also, buy a green candle and dedicate it to San Cipriano who will also protect you from any kind of witchcraft that is affecting your marriage and a candle for Saint Columba to protect against witchcraft, her day is May 20. Also pray to Saint Margaret on December 22, the patron saint of single mothers.

COMMENTARY:

We are very proud of this wonderful story which is the basis of the original artwork gracing this book's cover. It was skillfully and painstakingly painted by Professor Carlos Gómez of the University of Texas at Brownsville and Texas Southmost College. Carlos was inspired by this story. Study the painting carefully. It will definitely speak to you. Every story in this book will "talk" to you or reflect upon some particular aspect of your life or perhaps someone you know.

88. ARGUING GRANDPARENTS—*ABUELOS PELEONEROS*

I just wanted to let you know about the way my grandmother is acting toward my grandfather. Just before I left my grandmother's house tonight, she told me that he had said that tomorrow he was going to ask you who the person was that had put the white powder by the living room door. And also, who made the cross that looked like drops of blood on the sidewalk in front of the steps that go to the kitchen?

From the way things look, my grandmother is not too happy about him asking those questions. My grandfather is very jealous and thinks that my grandmother has a lover. My grandmother even told me tonight that she wished that my grandfather would have had a daughter that could come take care of him. She said that she was already tired of him crying at night because his back hurts and that nothing seemed to take the pain away. She said that she wished that they could send another provider to take care of him at night because she has to be awake all night watching over him.

My grandmother was never like this before. It was just not in her nature to act the way she is acting toward her husband of 50 years. I believe that someone is working them. Do you think it is possible that my grandmother could have a lover?

CURANDERO'S RESPONSE:

It seems to me like your grandfather might have some legitimate concerns regarding the mysterious white powder and the cross and drops of blood. What is going on? Why does grandma not want grandpa to look into this? I will talk to them, and I will do all I can to help them. You may be correct that someone has placed a spell on your grandfather.

You must pray to Santa Inés who protects marriages against infidelity and pray Psalms 45, 46 and 140 for making peace between spouses. Her feast day is January 21. Pray to Saints Anne and Joachim on July 26 to protect our grandparents. Many people are now using the power of La Santísima Muerte to protect their marriages which is what she was originally petitioned for by people in Mexico City. Either way, we will find out and reverse it.

COMMENTARY:

More than likely the grandmother is an innocent player in this real-life melodrama. The grandfather is very elderly and must be monitored to avoid seeing visions. Belief in witchcraft is very prevalent within the Latino population and its practice is part of life. Because of this, witchcraft or spells may be the initial thoughts when there are negative or painful familial occurrences. However, in this case, it seems like the white powder and unusual markings by the kitchen door are mysterious.

89. HE DOESN'T LOVE ME — *YA NO ME QUIERE*

My husband has abandoned me and the kids. I don't know what to do or what's going on with him. Do you "see" another woman in his life? He has not given me any reason to think so. I have been taking my garlic baths but so far I don't think they are working. The kids miss him a lot and I don't know what to tell them. I don't have the money to move. I thought we had a happy marriage. Can you see if there is something else that is bothering him? Help me to save my marriage?

CURANDERO'S RESPONSE:

The garlic baths are for spiritual cleansing and the ridding of evil curses, witchcraft spells, hexes and bad luck. Place a pinch of cinnamon powder inside your shoes every morning when you get up then say a prayer. Cleanse yourself with a lemon while praying the Lord's Prayer, El Padre Nuestro, and pray to San Joaquín to protect your marriage. Honor him on your home altar July 26. Pray Psalm 139 to preserve love between married couples. Do this for seven consecutive Fridays.

Another thing you can do is purchase three yellow candles, and beginning on a Thursday, place his photo and your photo facing one another in front of one candle. Tie the photos together with yellow string always circling clockwise never counterclockwise. Place the photos and the candle on a yellow cloth and sweeten the item by either sprinkling a little sugar on it or dripping a little honey over it. Get a yellow rose and pull off the petals and place them around the candle and photos. Repeat the procedure for three weeks, always on Thursdays and always starting during the early morning hours. Start each week with a new candle, the same photos, but with a new yellow rose. At the end of three weeks, dispose of all the materials you used in water in which the water current is running in the direction of your home. This ritual will also serve to bring your husband home to his family.

COMMENTARY:

One of the most popular reasons people seek advice from a curandero/a is for marital or relationship issues. Not able to resolve personal problems themselves, these suffering individuals seek aid from the curandero or resort to witchcraft to influence an errant loved one, morally guide a wayward spouse home or to extinguish the other woman's hold.

90. IT'S DEFINITELY OVER — *HASTA AQUÍ*

I want you to know that it is definitely over between me and my spouse. I am also aware of the message that El Niño sent me through you. Just know that my wife and I have grown apart throughout these past years, and if you recall when I created a small shrine to El Niño, she tossed everything out. She never really cared or respected any of my spiritual values. Of course, I myself am not without sin and I carry a very big burden on my soul and in my heart. I expect that the next few months will be very difficult for us as we split up. I will try calling you one of these days, and I hope that I have not let you down because I know how much you value the family unit. Take care and God bless you now and always.

CURANDERO'S RESPONSE:

I am sorry to learn of your problems, my friend. I can only say that my prayers to Saint Ann the patron saint of marriage and family are with you. Saint Ann, El Niño Fidencio, and the Lord will grant you strength, valor and peace. I am here for you, in your hour of need as you have been there for me in my hour of need. May the good Lord bless you.

COMMENTARY:

A Roman Catholic priest once counseled "do everything you can to save the marriage, but if it cannot be saved, save yourself." Very often and over many years of knowing a person, curanderos/as forge very strong bonds and caring relationships with their clients. People seek out curanderos in the same way they do a priest or counselor. The curandero tried over the years to save this marriage, but ultimately, was unsuccessful. Unfortunately, one of the reasons was that the wife had a different faith and could not accept her husband's spirituality and rebelled against her husband for consulting the curandero/a.

91. DRUNK AND USING —*VICIOSO*

My husband is ruining our marriage. He simply will not stop drinking and doing drugs. Is it true that sometimes destructive behavior in people who are loved is due to other spiritual forces that are controlling them? I know many people who have beaten alcohol and drug addiction, but there always seem to be a few who need more than the typical 12-step program. Could you explain how I can help him?

Antonio Zavaleta and Alberto Salinas Jr.

CURANDERO'S RESPONSE:

A woman and a man came to my altar room, or *consultorio*, for the first time. The Latino male was about 40 years old and she was a Latina about the same age. They brought with them another Latino about 50 years old and they said they had all been living together for about a year. They seemed to care very deeply for each other and they wanted to know if there was a fee for a consultation. I told them there wasn't, but that I welcomed donations.

With that, they said they would be back, but then they began to bicker. The woman wanted a ritual cleansing for the older man, but he said that he did not believe in these things and refused. I said they could come back any time. She pleaded with him to get the cleansing and he agreed that she could get one if she wanted. He said he was an alcoholic and that the only reason he came was to please the woman.

I cut some fresh branches from the lavender shrub to use for the cleansing ritual, and the three of us went back to the altar room to perform the healing ritual. While we were there I asked him if he believed in God and he said that he did. I explained that during the cleansing ritual he could ask for a healing from God. I told him that I was there just to help him along. He looked into my eyes and he acknowledged once again he did believe in God. So I asked him to pray to San Benito, to Santa Bibiana, Saint Matthias whose day is May 14, also pray to San Cipriano and San Ignacio de Loyola for strength. I lifted my hand to touch his forehead with the herbs, and as the herbs touched his forehead, he began to jerk frantically backward and forward. His legs were unable to support his weight, and as she tried to keep him from falling, he fell into a chair.

The ritual instantaneously brought about a terrible resistance in him and the prayers brought about an even greater torment from within the subject. Luckily, for me I was able to control him with her help. With a simple touch, something changed in him and he was no longer the same person. There seemed to be the appearance of another being in him.

I immediately could see that this other being was very angry and could possibly turn violent at any moment. As the violence built up, I was fearful and wanted to get away, but I had a job to do. I began the healing ritual and it became an exorcism. He calmed down and appeared to become himself once again and acknowledged that he was an alcoholic, and that he used cocaine and marijuana on a regular basis. He said he would return for further healing. In the old days, there was another way in which women would control their husbands' drinking. In the *hierbería* you can find *habas de San Ignacio,* a sort of round flat bean from a tree in Mexico. Women grind them up and mix them in their spouses' meals in small amounts to induce vomiting when they drink. Thus, it is believed that they would not want to drink. Any women with drunkards for husbands should pray Psalm 37 to combat drunkenness. Saint Bibiana protects husbands from hangovers preventing them from going to work or any other productive work. Celebrate her on December 2.

COMMENTARY:

Extensive research has been conducted on gender and cultural factors which influence drug and alcohol addiction as well as rehabilitation. There are many cultural methods which mimic current medical treatments for addiction. For example, the habas de San Ignacio bean mentioned by the curandero should be treated very carefully because it has been proven to induce vomiting. The same type of therapy that induces nausea is used in some medications and produces similar results. The person who is feeling nauseous does not feel like drinking. Control of substance abuse must always be sustained by a combination of behavior modification with physician-prescribed medication. Families with alcoholic relatives will often give them tea made from estafiate, or mugwort. Antihepatotoxins are medicinal plants believed to fortify the liver. An antidote, or antídoto, is the action of a plant used to reverse an action from another plant.

92. NOBODY UNDERSTANDS — *NADIE ME ENTIENDE*

Thank you so much for listening to my plea for a special prayer. I just wanted you to know that even though I am back with my family, I am really not happy despite the concessions that my wife is willing to make. For me, most importantly, I want to set the record straight with my children and get my finances back in order, giving our marriage another try. All I can tell you, and strictly speaking on a spiritual level, is that I am madly in love with another woman. We have each done a lot of crying over this, and she and I agree that our souls are united. We communicate with each other in our dreams and this love we have for each other is beyond this world. We have said that they can put us in cages, but we will still see each other in our dreams. One thing you should know is that absolutely no one will ever understand this strong love that we have for each other. We don't even understand it. Maybe we were together in a past life time. At the same time, it seems as if no one wants us to be together, and I know that our relationship is not clean. However, I have repeatedly told her that we are two old, ancient souls that are meant to be with each other but our love is crossed. We must have really sinned in the last life.

I am already seeing a psychiatrist, which I spoke to you about. But, anyway, please let me know what you think of my situation and give me some of your spiritual insight on what I should do.

CURANDERO'S RESPONSE:

I am trying to understand what you are going through and your feelings for the other woman. But you must understand that your wife and children also have feelings. Our prayers are with all of you. I am sure you are on the right track in trying to make your marriage work and to get your family back together again. Pray to Saint Daniel. He is the patron saint of putting families back together. Honor him on July 21.

It is the right thing for many reasons. It will take some time and quite an effort on everyone's part for you to be successful. I am sure with your spirit guide and protector, you will succeed. You have too much to lose to fail.

For awhile, you had been listening to the voices of unclean spirits that have been misleading you. You must separate yourself from the other woman because it is not fair to her either. Once you do that, you will prevail. You must pray for the path to marital love to be shown to you. Pray that the road be opened, or *abre camino*, between you and your wife and for you to erase the memory of the other woman from your thoughts.

Pick any Friday at midnight when there is moonlight. Stand in the moonlight and visualize your wife, pray that Venus and the moon reunite your love.

COMMENTARY:

Because curanderos/as steadfastly follow a moral and spiritual compass, they almost always support the institution of marriage; advising the client to end the illicit affair and work out the marital problems for the sake of the children, their families and cultural/religious beliefs. In traditional Latino culture, marital partners will stay together for the benefit of their children. As time passes and technology advances, this tradition, sadly, has deteriorated.

93. MENDING FENCES — *CONFORMÁNDOSE*

Please send me some information on a special prayer. As you know, I'm trying to mend fences with my family and there is extensive damage in my relationship with my husband and my children. I ended my relationship with the other man. I'm asking for a special prayer so that there will be true and genuine peace for everyone involved in this situation.

CURANDERO'S RESPONSE:

Create your own very special prayer for a husband and wife and a happy life together. Pray together before retiring for the day. If the other is absent, pray alone, but for the intentions of the couple. Pray something like this:

"Santa Ana, we pray to you to continue to bless us, help us to appreciate you for what we have. We are united by the sacrament of matrimony. Grant that we will truly be one in heart and mind, and that we respect each other's person. Grant that we love one another, remembering it was you who gave us our love because we should be parents to your children. Help us to give one another completely and be less egotistical and trust one another. Help us to trust our difficulties in you and to always count on the promise that you gave us in the sacrament of matrimony. Help us to be good parents to our family. Be it your will to grant us health and the strength for our duties in the happiness that supports us in our love. Grant that we not forget that we have been given a blessing from heaven by the grace of our Lord and Savior. God give us strength, valor and blessing so that it may go well through our journey. Amen."

Also, it is a good idea to maintain a specially-prepared candle for Saint Ann, lighted at noon every day for 21 straight days. Be sure to write both of your names in red ink on a piece of paper and place the candle over it while it is burning.

Some spells for repairing broken marriages or relationships use the root and the seed of High John the Conqueror. Then write the name of the man on the root and the name of the woman on the seed, sprinkle them with perfume and place them in a small red cloth bag. The bag is then carried on your person, either in a pocket or pinned to inner clothing.

COMMENTARY:

The curandero composed a very special spiritual prayer in this case. The petitioner asked for and received the specially-requested prayer to save her marriage. She also received a vital healing regimen which included her husband's participation. Praying together can show the spouse a form of rededication to God and the marriage.

94. HE DOESN'T HELP US — *NO NOS AYUDA*

I need some help. I am having trouble with my children, but most of all with my husband. Everyone is fighting and not helping with the house and they are never home, and my husband and I are always fighting. He is never happy and everything bothers him.

I have been trying to get a divorce for years, but he won't let me go. I have received housing assistance, but I need to find a four-bedroom home that will qualify and once I do, I want to leave him and get a divorce. I have lost my job due to a funding cutback and right now I am very dependent on my husband. I can't take the fact that he is so very cold and mean to me. To make matters worse, he seems to hate our kids.

My son is in trouble again, facing charges and he'll be going to court soon. I am so scared that he is going to go to prison for a long time. Maybe that is what he needs, I just don't know. I know my son's actions were wrong, but he is very stubborn and never listens to anyone. I know that he needs to straighten up, but he is my son and I love him and will do anything for him even though at times he is very mean to me. He is just a teenager, but I really need guidance and help with him and with all of my problems.

I pray to El Niño Fidencio and I even drive almost an hour to purchase his candles. I try not to run out of them and I also pray to my *Diosito* to help me, but I feel so weak and very tired at times. I am always sad and my diabetes is out of control. I know it is all of the stress. I really need your prayers and counseling. Thank you for listening.

CURANDERO'S RESPONSE:

I know you are going through a lot and my prayers are with you. Do a cleansing/healing with a lemon for nine consecutive days. Don't throw the lemons away. Say a prayer to the Virgen that unties knots, her name is Santa María de Desatanudos, and make your petition while doing the cleansing. Saint Helen the patron of divorcing couples is celebrated on August 18. At the end of the nine *limpias*, make a fire and burn the nine lemons you used for the nine days of cleansings. Let me know how you are doing.

COMMENTARY:

Here the curandero does not address the reason that the husband has emotionally abandoned his family. In all likelihood, he has his own problems and is not able to provide support for his family, especially his son. There could be another woman or another family involved here, we simply don't know. He may also be ashamed of his son and blames his wife for the son's problems, refusing to be accountable for his own parental role and responsibilities. Often, the personal issues of husbands and wives are interwoven, further complicating familial issues.

95. DAUGHTER'S BABY'S FATHER — *ENREDADO*

I have a couple of problems. I will tackle the most pressing and the most important one first. My daughter, who is 18, has a baby girl who is one year old. Right now my daughter is living with me, but she is trying to decide if she should go back to the baby's father or not. She is not married to the baby's father and he does not treat her well. She admits this to me.

Then there is this other guy she says she is in love with, but because of her entanglement with the baby's father, she cannot bring herself to leave him. She says that she loves them both, but that she is drawn to this other guy. She loves the other man so much that she cries for him. I know that this other guy would be good to her.

The short time she was separated from the baby's father and with the other man, he treated her and the baby very well. They seemed to be a happy family. My daughter told me that going back to the baby's father would be the biggest mistake of her life, but she is still considering it. I don't understand that attraction, do you? I don't know what to do or how to make her come to her senses. Is this her fate or destiny?

The baby's father has told her that if she would come back, he would change, so she is seriously considering it. She tells me that he has been treating her well, but how long is this going to last? Her one true love is still calling her and begging her to get back with him.

What can I do? I don't want her to hurt anymore.

I can't stay out of her life because this is the same thing that happened to me when I was young and I made the wrong decision staying with her father and had a miserable life. Now my youth is gone and I have not been able to find anyone to truly love me. They just want to sleep with me. I don't want this same life for my daughter.

It is like there is a curse on us that is passing from one generation to the next. I guess I would like to know if I should leave things alone and let time take care of things. Please advise me on what to do and let me know if you need any material or information on them so that you can "work" them for me.

CURANDERO'S RESPONSE:

Hello. I can see you talking to your daughter, providing her with advice, but you need to keep your life out of it or she won't listen to you. After all, she knows your histories as well as you do. She will think that you are trying to meddle in her life and you are. If you can, try to get her and the baby's father to professional counseling maybe from your parish priest. She is confused and being pulled in different directions. She does not know which way to go. She needs to see what would be best for her happiness and most importantly, for her baby's welfare. She needs you to be there helping her find a solution, but don't be overpowering.

You should advise your daughter not to make hasty decisions. She should not rush into any relationship with either one of these men. I don't "see" a future with either one of them. Her whimsical behavior is what got her into serious problems in the first place. You and your daughter should place your daughter's child's welfare first and foremost before making any decisions around that issue.

Whatever you do, do not use her father as a bad example you throw at her. That will surely backfire and turn your daughter against you.

I am sure you are keeping her in your prayers. Please, light a Niño Fidencio candle, a Santa Irene candle or a Saint Michael the Archangel candle for your daughter. Place a glass of water by the candles and say a prayer to Saint Irene. She will help the true couple that is meant to be together. Saint Eustace is the saint of difficult choices, his day is September 20. You may need to pray to him in order for her to make the right choice. Make your petition for your daughter. Please keep me posted.

COMMENTARY:

The close-knit nature of the Latino family produces situations where everyone is very connected in each other's lives and decisions, both good and bad. In this case, it is quite obvious that the mother is too mettlesome in her daughter's life. The mother's life is possibly not much better than her daughter's. The mother has committed so many mistakes that she's now living vicariously through her daughter's situation. The generational differences between the mother and daughter further exacerbate their problems.

This projection of the same fate is both unhealthy and inappropriate behavior. The only thing that counts here is the welfare of the child. What the daughter and the mother want are not as important. The mother must set aside her life and experiences so that the daughter and granddaughter can prosper.

96. HE DOESN'T KNOW HIS SON — *DESOBLIGADO*

I want to get my teenage son out of trouble and get him some emotional help. I have already sent my younger daughter to live with my ex-spouse in order to save my son. His father is no help and takes no interest in the fate of his son. It is a very sad and tragic fact and the reason my son has now joined a gang. Not long ago, my life was getting better and all of the kids were doing well, but my world has turned upside down. My son has been in and out of juvenile detention and his next step is county jail with older and more hardcore boys. My son is running with a bad gang and I am afraid for his safety and his future.

My son is being influenced by older boys. He doesn't know any better. All this time he has been holding inside of him this horrible situation and has refused to talk to me about it. We have also learned that his stepfather, my ex-husband, sexually molested him. I'm afraid to tell his father what happened to him because he will kill my ex-husband and emotionally abuse his son. Our lives are in shambles.

I do not want my son to spend his life in jail and that is where he is headed, or worse. He wants to come home. He misses his school, and his friends and his music. He is a troubled and confused boy. We do not know what is going to happen to him.

Please help us and pray for our family. It seems like everyone in our family has had a terrible secret and now they are being revealed and they are tearing us apart. Everybody is against us each other and blames everyone else. This situation is ripping our once-happy family apart. What can we do? Please help us before we go to court this next time.

CURANDERO'S RESPONSE:

I have kept you in my prayers for the last two days. I hope and pray things will get better for you and your family. Please let me know how things develop so that I know what further instructions to give you. If you ask Him, God will give you strength to cope with all your anguish and pain and he will resolve your problems. Ask God to grant you a miracle.

Not only was your world turned upside down, but also your son's, as well as the whole family. He is a very confused teenager. It is going to be very hard to hear all the ugly truths of his actions, and your case will require constant prayer and ongoing professional counseling for him for many years. Pray Psalm 126 for the return of wayward children to the fold. The patron saint of caregivers is Aloysius Gonzaga celebrated on June 21. Aloysius should help grant you the miracle you seek.

COMMENTARY:

This is a classic situation in which the spiritual assistance of the curandero must be reinforced by state law enforcement agencies. That is, the family must be assisted by an attorney, a social worker and child protective services. The young boy is a victim, as are all youth which are pulled into gangs. All too often, Latino families find themselves in this desperate situation and prefer to hush it up and/or never discuss it. This is a mistake. Cases like this can lead to a lifetime of loss and damage. Always be sure that children who are drawn into gangs or cults have someone to confide in. Don't become biased toward one side or the other. Provide the child with good advice and support.

97. LIFE'S TROUBLES — *DILEMAS*

I am having problems and troubles in my life. I have been very sad lately, and emotional. I have three children that depend on me. I also have a stepchild who is living with us and who is involved with drugs. Worse, he is now stealing money from me to buy his drugs. I know from experience with my own brothers that it is going to get worse from here if he doesn't get help.

I have tried not to tell his father because his father will think I am just picking on him. But now, the situation is out of control. His behavior is interfering with my marriage.

I constantly talk to my husband about his child by another woman, but he does nothing because he feels guilty about the divorce. Even though the child's mother was a whore, my husband defends her against me. He says he feels sorry for his son because he does not have his mother.

My husband is not willing to see that I can act as his mother, as well. My husband is not willing to take the necessary action to get him off drugs and he won't allow me to be his mother or correct him in any way. Anytime I talk to my husband, we argue about this. We are even talking about separating because of it. I find myself questioning why my life has taken this horrible direction. Can you help me find a way through this for my family and me?

I ask that you pray for me and help guide me to peace. I find no happiness or peace in my home. I work very hard every day and I do not enjoy coming home at the end of the day anymore. I fear it. I am constantly frustrated and feel like I am going crazy. I have no appetite, so I do not eat. I am afraid that my family will have to be broken up to keep my sanity. I do not want that to happen.

My stepchild's behavior is also having a negative effect on my children. They fight when they see us fighting. They become very aggressive with each other. Please help me be the mother and wife that I used to be. Help my husband to open his eyes and see the truth. Help me relieve all the pain and hurt that I have inside me. Please bring me out of this darkness that I am constantly in.

CURANDERO'S RESPONSE:

I understand what you are telling me. Light a Sagrado Corazón, Sacred Heart of Jesus, and candle for peace. Cleanse everyone in the household with a San Alejo and a San Ignacio de Loyola candle. Use the same ones for all the family. Put a pinch of cinnamon powder, a pinch of sugar, a few mustard seeds and a few rosemary leaves inside the candles. Place a clear glass of water over the pictures of everyone in the family next to the candles. Light the candles and make your petitions to the Holy Spirit. Boil rosemary in the evenings and make your petition to God and El Niño Fidencio for light, understanding, love, happiness and peace. Do this for nine consecutive nights. Let me know how it works and if you see any change.

COMMENTARY:

Blended Latino families have emotionally-thorny issues to resolve and always represent a significant share of the curandero's caseload. The victims are always children who have allegiances and love the absent parent. The stepparents can never fill the void of a missing parent. Sometimes, the stepparent is even blamed for having broken up the original marriage although this may actually be far from the truth.

98. LIFE IS TERRIBLE — *ERRORES*

During these past 10 years my life has been terrible and I was hoping that you could send some kind of spiritual light or hope into my heart. I was also just wondering what the garlic bath is for. I will, of course, do as you say.

I am so tired of suffering and not being loved by my husband. I wish I could just pack up and go, but without money and with two young kids, it is impossible.

CURANDERO'S RESPONSE:

The garlic baths are for spiritual cleansing from evil, curses, witchcraft spells, hexes and bad luck. Place a pinch of cinnamon powder inside your shoes every morning when you get up to start your day and pray to San Eduardo, saying "Follow in my footsteps and answer my prayers this day, oh, San Eduardo. Favor me before the eyes of my fellow man, oh, San Eduardo." Cleanse yourself with a lemon and pray the Lord's Prayer. And pray to San Casimiro or Casimir the patron saint of bachelors to bring your husband back to you. His day is March 4.

Purchase a magnet stone, or *piedra imán*, from the nearest *hierbería*, along with nine white candles and oil for peace and calm as well as *conquistador*, or conqueror oil. Place three white candles in a triangle with the *piedra imán*, magnet stone, in the middle for three weeks always beginning Thursday. Be sure that you drip or spray the two essences of peace oil and conquistador oil over the area. Write your name and your husband's name on parchment paper and also place this in the middle of the three candles. You will see your husband begin to change his attitude toward you.

COMMENTARY:

Many Latinas find themselves in despairing situations. They are trapped in marriages without love, but with children who depend upon them. They are culturally bound to stay in their marriages despite being miserable. This causes behavioral health issues that need an outlet. Persons in great need of an emotional safety valve often find solace in curanderismo.

The informal networks of friends they encounter at the curandero's spiritual healing sessions are similar to a 12-step program. While waiting to be seen by the curandero, much is discussed and learned by and from the people awaiting their turns.

99. SOMEONE FOR ME — *ALGUIEN PARA MÍ*

I am going to be a bit selfish and ask for some help for myself. I have a very special person in my life. We are in love, but our timing is way off. Every time we plan to spend time together, something gets in the way. Is there something we can do to "clear paths," *abre camino*, so we can spend some quality time together? I hate feeling so helpless in this situation. Hope you have some helpful advice for me.

CURANDERO'S RESPONSE:

This is for my special friends who are in love, but never seem to spend time together. The person, who finds love, peace and happiness in himself, has these same qualities to share with others. To remove these barriers and clear the way, or *abre camino*, the spirit indicates you may place seven *pencas de nopal*, or cactus leaves, in a bucket of water and set the bucket out in the daylight for seven consecutive hours. Most importantly, call upon San Antonio to protect the lovers in this case. Once you have done this, use the bucket of water to bathe in, while calling on the spirit of the Niño Fidencio out loud three straight times.

Then petition that the obstacles to your love be removed from your path. Pray Psalm 138 to produce and nurture love. Always remember to pray to Saint Dorothy the patron saint of women without men. Her day is February 6. Also, pray to Saint Andrew the patron saint to find a husband. His day is November 30.

To remove obstacles from her way she should place seven *tunas*, or prickly pear fruit, in a pail of water left in daylight for seven hours, and thereafter bathe with the water while calling aloud El Niño Fidencio's name three times and then state her petition. The leaves and the fruit of the cactus are the male and female elements of the common Mexican cactus, or *nopal*.

It is also possible to bind up love with a red ribbon saturated with special love potions or perfumes. Write your loved one's name on the red ribbon at high noon on a Friday, then, apply the perfume. While you do this, always concentrate on the name of the person and visualize their face. Pin the ribbon inside your underwear for 21 consecutive days.

COMMENTARY:

The curandero offers a classic love-attraction ritual intended to draw the lovers together. Incantations designed to attract or inspire the affection of another were practiced within European as well as in Mesoamerican magical rites. Over the centuries, methodology has evolved, but always retained the intent of using magical means to transform outcomes of romantic attractions. In the world of today's curanderos/as, the practice uses all of the modern paraphernalia found in the hierbería for this purpose. This includes sprays, wax figures, powders, oils, soaps, perfumes and much more. There are many ways to do this and there is no single or absolute method.

The curandero uses an element of sympathetic magic in the male-and-female aspects of the same cactus plant in a ritual to consummate the relationship.

One of the most frequently consulted books in the hierbería is the book of San Cipriano. This little grimorio, or book of magic, claims to have been compiled in the year 1001, by Jonas Sufurino a monk who studied mysticism and magic. Today, San Cipriano is considered the patron saint of magicians and is believed to protect them against spells, demons and overall evil. The book contains many commonly-used spells, or *sortilegios*, regarding marriage, relationships and love affairs. For example: How to fall in love; how to discover if a woman is seeing another man; how to know if a husband is faithful, and many other romantic spells are contained in this mystical tome. Sex, love, and relationships are among the most requested categories that curanderos deal with on a daily basis.

100. THE OTHER WOMAN — *LA OTRA*

You are a very busy person helping people in the spiritual realm. That is your gift. All I want to do is talk to you because today was a very strange day. My wife is always complaining about how she hates her job and how she wants me to get a good job, but it is really not so easy for me to find a good job at my age.

Yesterday, I stopped over at the home of this woman I know from Spain. She is Basque. I told her she looks Irish and she told me the Basque people have a lot of Celtic heritage. I tell you, my friend, if I wasn't married, I would definitely want to be "hooked up" with this woman and I'm certain she knows it.

After I visited her, I felt so attracted to her. I felt that my marriage was ready to break up because of the differences in our relationship. Who knows, maybe I'm going through a midlife crisis. I can't land a good job, my marriage isn't the greatest and I have an infatuation with another woman. I am all screwed up.

CURANDERO'S RESPONSE:

Hang in there my friend. Something is about to break loose for you. I am going to pray over this for you for the next three days. I understand you are frustrated and need someone to talk to. I appreciate the trust you have in me as a friend and as a spiritual advisor.

Tie a pink ribbon and a blue ribbon together and write your names on the ribbons. Sprinkle a little patchouli on the ribbons. Do you feel you have tried your best to get a job or make your marriage work? Have both of you talked about seeing a marriage counselor? You would do well by doing so. Be sure that you pray to San Eduardo to save your marriage. Pray Psalm 56 to release oneself from false passion. Don't go back to see the other woman. It will only cause you temptation and more problems. I feel that the devil is placing temptation in front of you and you must see it for what it is. Love your wife and be faithful to her.

COMMENTARY:

In this particular case, the curandero failed. He needed to clearly state to the man, who happens to be his friend, that as a married man, he should not be visiting single women. Visiting a single woman who lives by herself can only lead to trouble. The subconscious mind is titillating his sexual desires.

101. GUY PROBLEMS — *EL TONTO*

I had trouble with a guy and I'm still having trouble with him. I met him and fell in love with him. Then, all of a sudden, he stopped calling and e-mailing me. Now I have no contact with him at all. I am writing to you again because I don't know what is going on. I find myself constantly thinking about this man. It is like a feeling you get when someone is talking about you, a very strong feeling. I tried forgetting about him, but it didn't work. I still like him and that is not all.

There's another guy I know and I don't understand why I think about him all the time, too. He comes and goes out of my mind and I don't know what's going on. I don't understand why I have all these desires. He seems like a nice guy and I like him a lot, but I haven't seen him since we were teenagers. But back then we were never given an opportunity to have a relationship. Please help me out and let me know what's going on in my head and in my heart. I would like to get married and have children someday. I'm still single and am lonely. Has someone put a spell on me so I can't fall in love and have a normal relationship?

CURANDERO'S RESPONSE:

If the guy is not meant to be the love of your life you should try to forget him and move on. I am sure there is someone out there that will fall madly in love with you and you with him. Please try my spiritual healing advice. You shall see what I am talking about.

Light a candle to Saint Gabriel the Archangel and make your petition for happiness in life. If you do not find that candle, look for the seven archangels' candle and boil *gobernadora, alhucema,* cinnamon sticks, four, cut apples and rose petals with a cup of honey and bathe in this water at noon on Friday while saying a prayer to Saint Gabriel Archangel and to Saint Dorothy and make your petition for attracting love.

COMMENTARY:

Single Latinas are under a constant psychological cultural barrage from their own families and friends to enter into a relationship leading to marriage and a family. As more years pass, those still not engaged begin to feel a gradual buildup of familial pressure and a sense of personal failure. This tía, or aunt, syndrome requires them to take on the role of the surrogate mother to their nephews and nieces. But they go unfilled as wives and mothers in life.

102. VANQUISH THE OTHER — *LÍBRAME*

I was writing to tell you that this weekend went okay. But my ex-boyfriend has missed two days of work due to a woman he is messing around with. He told me yesterday that he is probably going to have to move back with my son and me because this woman refuses to leave his apartment. Now she is threatening that she will go to his probation officer to tell him he's been doing drugs if he leaves her. She is telling him that she has pictures of them doing drugs which she plans to e-mail to his probation officer. This evil woman is holding him hostage from his past. I guess the hold that she has on him is sex and drugs.

I always thought that he wanted to live a decent family life, but I'm no longer certain. I am still praying the prayers you sent me and I have lit some candles. I do not understand why this woman is being so difficult and will not leave. I trust and have faith that pretty soon with Niño Fidencio's help she will go and leave us in peace.

CURANDERO'S RESPONSE:

I don't believe that the two of you are compatible. Why can't you see that he is no good? Your relationship may never improve. You are having problems admitting that you are not right for each other. It may be time for you to do the right thing for yourself and accept change. Move on with your life. Expect powerful and positive changes for yourself.

Go to a *hierbería* and purchase a San Alejo and a San Ignacio de Loyola seven-day candle. When you do this, call me and I will explain how you will use them to rid your life of all the problems that this woman has created for you.

Also, bathe in a bath prepared with rosemary, mint, anise, star anise, basil and myrrh and add High John the Conqueror seed. Pray to Saint Adelaide on December 16, she is the patron saint of second marriages and second attempts at the first marriage.

One way women may control their men is through the use of jimson weed, or *toloache*. If she is truly evil, this is what she is using. Jimson weed is a powerful herb and, in small amounts, it's used to control men and women and to settle them down to stay home and not fool around. Usually they don't know that they are being given the substance, which keeps them docile, or *mansitos*. Pray Psalm 14 which should free you from slander.

COMMENTARY:

In this case we simply do not know what has transpired between the woman and the curandero. It seems like the curandero has not offered hope, only an easy exit. The ex-boyfriend is vain and maybe he just wants to come home and feel loved. The curandero psychically "sees" the truth and sometimes there is no hope for the relationship to survive. The curandero tells the woman about jimson weed, also known as toloache. This is a datura, and Mexican populations have used it for centuries to control straying husbands. It has a very powerful effect and should not be used by someone who is not fully versed in how to properly prepare and dispense it.

103. THE DIVORCE — *EL DIVORCIO*

My wife has asked me for a divorce and we have a seven-month-old baby boy. I really love my son and I will do anything for him. I am very confused about why my wife is doing this to our family.

My wife and I just had an apartment so we split up and I moved to my sister's house and my wife moved to her friend's house. She told me yesterday that after living with her friend, she realized that her mom was the real reason she was mad at me all the time because her mom would tell her how to be a good wife to me and she would get upset and, in turn, get mad at me. This has been going on since she got pregnant and finally she decided that she had enough and wanted a divorce. After causing all of this confusion in our lives, now she tells me that she would like to try and work things out. She would like to get an apartment and live away from her mom instead of living in our house, which is being built next to her mom's. She says she would like for us to live on our own so she can have a chance to grow up without being in her mom's shadow.

I told her that I would also like try and work things out and that we could get the apartment and sell the house. I told her that she and her mom had to get counseling to deal with their problems. She is very quiet and never wants to talk about her problems, and avoids confrontation and holds everything in until she finally blows up. She agreed to get some help and also take her mom to get some help.

I am willing to try and make our marriage work so we can be a united family and my child can grow up in a complete family instead of a broken home. Can you ask Niño Fidencio if moving in with her and working things out is the right thing to do, or if she is just setting me up? My brother is going to see you tomorrow and I will try to see you soon. Please let me know if this is the right thing to do as soon as you can.

CURANDERO'S RESPONSE:

I have been keeping you in my prayers for some time now. Regarding your situation now is not the time to rush into anything. Take your time about getting back together until you are sure she is not setting you up for anything nor has a hidden motive. When she is sure she is ready to settle down and be a responsible mother to your child and a wife, you will know it. When she is convinced that she is ready and can convince you of it, then it will be time to make the marriage work, not before. Pray to San Isidro Labrador to protect your rightful family and to Saint Helen the patron saint of the divorced and divorcing. Her day is August 18.

COMMENTARY:

Divorce can truly be one of the most traumatic and bitter events individuals experience in their lives. Persons should not have to go through a divorce without a support network. In the Latino culture, curanderos/as play major roles in the familial support network. If you decide to consult a curandero/a for delicate issues like this one, you must find a reputable person to assist you. Expect the consultation's results to impel you to reach a long-term, as well as a life-altering decision.

104. MY RIVAL — *MI RIVAL*

I am writing you in regards to my mother. She wants your prayers and any advice you can give her. The woman that my father had an affair with is making it as hard as she possibly can for my mother. First of all, this woman filed a restraining order against my mother, but my mother is the one that is severely hurt in all this mess. Then, this woman keeps trying to get a hold of my father by calling our home, knowing all along that my mother is bound by the terms of the restraining order she placed against her. There is not much she can do.

To make matters worse, my father refuses to answer my mother's calls and now my mother has been fired from her job. My mother worked at the same place with this other woman, but my mother is the one that got fired. This other woman has been trying to get my mom in trouble for any little thing she can. If my mother goes anywhere, she has to be looking over her shoulder because if the other woman sees her, she calls the police. The woman tells the police that my mother is following her, but of course this is not true.

My mother and aunt were out recently and were walking out of a store and they saw the woman and her mother. My father's girlfriend's mom pointed out my mom and my aunt, and the woman created a huge scandal by yelling at my mom that she was going to call the cops. She got on her cell phone and called. My mom left before she could finish the call, but the cops showed up at my mom's home and told her that the next time, they will take my mom to jail. The officers told my mom that there is a stack of complaint forms at the police station against her.

Then, as if that was not bad enough, my mom has received a letter with a court date accusing her of violating the restraining order. She spoke to a lawyer today to represent her. It will cost her over a $1,000 to defend herself and the lawyer said if anyone should have a restraining order against anyone it should be my mom against the other woman, and I agree. My mother never asked for any of this. She is very worried about her court date.

Please pray for her so that she will have a just judge. My mom wishes that the woman would just leave this town forever. I wish she would just leave my mother and my father alone. Why can't she find her own man, why does she have to have my father? I hope that in court the other woman can feel the shame and embarrassment my mom has been feeling. Can you help us?

CURANDERO'S RESPONSE:

I am praying to San Cipriano for all your family. I am burning some candles for your mom's safety, protection and well-being. Tell your mom to call me and, if your mom could, have her go to a *hierbería* and purchase a San Alejo and a San Ignacio de Loyola seven-day candle. When she does that, she can call me and I will explain how she will use them to get rid her of all the problems this woman has created for her.

COMMENTARY:

Some persons know how to manipulate the system, but they are definitely on the other side of the righteousness fence. Frequently, they use the police and courts for selfish and harmful gains. The wife needs an authority figure to serve as her advocate. There must be someone who knows the reputation of the other woman or her work situation who can help or testify against her. It appears this other woman has done this before. The mother should enlist her personal network of family and friends to resolve this troublesome issue. Notice that this is a perfect example of a case that could include the use of witchcraft to manipulate the situation, but it wasn't mentioned by the petitioner or by the curandero.

105. BRING HIM BACK — *VEN A MÍ*

I followed your instructions and the candles are now burning. They should burn out in seven days. What do I do next to get my husband to return to me? I have been praying and believing in God for his return. Please let me know what I need to do next.

CURANDERO'S RESPONSE:

Pray to Saint Gabriel the Archangel and to San Daniel, then, make your petition. Place a clear glass of water on your kitchen table or on your home altar. Call out the name of the archangel aloud three times and repeat the prayer. Do this for nine consecutive days. Light a just judge, or *justo juez*, candle, and another plain white candle. Get romance and attracting perfumes or sprays named, come to me, or *ven a mí*, from the *hierbería*. Place them or spray them on your left hand and place your left hand over your heart. Pray for your man to return. Pray Psalm 32, that the other woman will be sent away or that she will find another lover. Never wish someone harm because it will be returned to you.

COMMENTARY:

Candle-burning rituals are universal in the practice of magic around the world. The Catholic priests introduced candle burning to Latin American populations in the 16th century. The dark side of witchcraft is thought to reverse Catholic rituals. Therefore, candle burning is common in the practice of both white and black magic. Black magic is used to darken good which is opposite of the original intent of illuminating our prayers with candles.

106. MY HUSBAND'S AFFAIR — *EL ENGAÑO*

I have been married for years and now my husband has left me. We have grown children. He went to truck-driving school, and soon after went out on the road. Not long after that, he met a woman who is also a truck driver and they started a relationship. Now they are driving a truck together. In the last six months, he has gone from being a loving family man to no longer caring about neither being home nor seeing his family. Can you please tell me if you can help me to get my husband back? Is it possible?

CURANDERO'S RESPONSE:

Thank you for your inquiry. You have a serious dilemma if your husband abandoned his family for another woman. If he is unfaithful to you this time, how can you be sure that you would have a good marriage if he were to return to you? What is to keep him from doing the same thing again and again? If you ask me, I would suggest that you start anew. If you want him back, you will have to pray to El Niño Fidencio and to Santa Ana for his return. Do not ask someone to do witchcraft to get him back. Also, pray Psalm 136 to rid him of his willful sins. My prayers are with you but be careful what you pray for, as you might receive it.

COMMENTARY:

Curanderos use multiple time-tested means to work with wayward spouses and their lovers. First, illnesses that are attributed to all three of those involved, are believed to have natural origins. God and the saints find the situation morally repugnant and mete out punishment through sicknesses. At one time, curanderos/as would recommend the herb toloache, or datura for wayward husbands to keep them docile, or toloachado. This dangerous herb would literally render them physically unable to leave their homes, or keep them mansos.

You may have noticed from this series of spousal relationships, that partners stray when the relationship becomes mundane and new persons enter the lives of one or both of the marital partners. This is why it is always important for couples to maintain communication and be open with each other. Like a beautiful garden, marriages also need constant tending for successful growth. This care could manifest via a date night without the kids, a weekend getaway, and notes of affection or even romantic poems for emotional sustenance.

107. MOTHER ACUSED FATHER — *EL ACUSADO*

As for my mother, there is surprising news. Though it is not pleasant for me to mention it, I have to wonder about my father's conduct with the new widow neighbor in his neighborhood. Supposedly, this new neighbor is building a home funded by the housing authority.

There was a large tree that was in the way of the building project. She promised to pay my father if he would cut it down and he did, but my father has not mentioned if she has paid him or not. The tree was large and I know that my family helped remove and clean it out. The neighbor also needed to use our electricity for the carpenters to continue construction of the house.

This neighbor is avoiding my mother and giving her the cold shoulder. Even worse, my father is now acting distant toward my mother. Mom told me that dad called city hall concerned this woman's house would be damaged if it rained, and since housing is in charge, he also called to complain to the housing authority. My mother and I don't understand what his interest is in this woman's house. It is not any of his business. The whole family thinks that he has taken too much interest in this widow woman.

To make matters worse, this woman has a lover that comes in every now and then. My dad doesn't seem to care about that because now all he does is flirt with her all the time. We have found that my father is drinking a tea of *damiana* and everyone knows that is for sexual power. I know that my mom is worried about the situation and wants answers fast. The situation gets more complicated every day.

CURANDERO'S RESPONSE:

Call out the Holy names of the archangels to come to your aid and make your petition for justice. Please, don't play innocent! I don't mean to insult you but if you have doubts about your father having an affair with his widowed neighbor, just approach him with the family's concerns before it gets completely out of control. It is disturbing that your father is taking an aphrodisiac. If your father is already having sex with the widow, then it is too late. Follow the signs and check it out. This sounds like a special case for La Virgen de Guadalupe. Make your petition and promise to her to bring your father home. Also pray to Blessed Angela to protect against sexual temptation. Her day is January 4. The situation is even more difficult since this widow woman will be living right next door to your father and mother. Sometimes tall fences makes good neighbors.

COMMENTARY:

It seems like the daughter has enough worries within her own family without involving herself in her father's life. Where is her mother or her own spouse? Sometimes, persons who visit curanderos/as do so because it feeds or nurtures their intrusions in situations where they do not belong. The daughter is a meddler which is a red flag; indicating she needs to undertake constructive and dignity-building activities in her own life. The fact that the father has started taking a tea made from damiana is a clear sign that something is up. Why else would he take an aphrodisiac or afrodisiaco?

108. THE OTHER MAN — *DESÁTAME*

I want to ask you about the candles you asked me to buy to get rid of all negative forces and bring my girlfriend back to me. I found out this man she is seeing has my picture buried inside a glass jar somewhere in my yard. A family member told me about this, and that I need to be careful because the man is trying to steal my woman away from me and maybe even kill me. I have talked to my former girlfriend and she feels that some force is keeping her in the other man's house and won't let her leave. When she tries to come to my house, something pulls her back. She told me she wants to leave him and that if she has to, she will move out. But when she mentions this to him, he flies into a rage and says that his *bruja,* or witch, will kill her if she leaves him. So, she is afraid to leave him. This is a clear sign of witchcraft. Please let me know what to do.

CURANDERO'S RESPONSE:

My prayers are with you, and you are not alone. The spirit of San Valentín is with you. I am attaching some prayers to El Niño Fidencio for you as well. He is a healing spirit of light, a spirit guide, a spirit protector, a spirit doctor, a spirit lawyer, a spirit counselor. His spirit will help you. Drink a clear glass of water daily and call out the name of El Niño Fidencio Constantino three straight times aloud and then drink the water. His spirit will place medicine in your body, mind and soul. This spiritual medicine will give you strength, valor, and the will to overcome any witchcraft that has been placed on you.

Make yourself a red stone amulet bag. Obtain a small red felt bag or make one and place a red stone signifying the heart inside the bag. Sometimes, you can find small red hearts which would be perfect. Apply love and attraction perfumes on the stone then carry it with you.

COMMENTARY:

Since the practice of witchcraft is so widespread, it is understandable that persons who do not partake in witchcraft encounter mystical items without even realizing what they are. Never touch these items with your bare hands! When in doubt, always contact a competent person who is experienced in destroying these objects in the proper manner, which is usually by fire.

109. LET HIM GO — *DÉJALO IR*

I am so very sorry I haven't written sooner. So much has happened and I have been trying to cope with my depression. Just last week I wanted to take my life, but I asked God for strength. My heart is heavy because of that woman who lives in my ex-husband's home. He threw her out once and we started to work things out and planned to move back together. Things were going great until she started writing to him again and then he took her back.

Last week he was so ugly to my son and me. Someone sent the police to my job, and claimed that I broke into his house. That is a lie! Someone broke into my home and took a lot of things from me. I have a chance to file charges against them, but I am torn because I love him. My son is also deeply disturbed. He loves his dad very much and does not want him to go to jail. Do you see any chance for our relationship? Do you see him in my picture anymore or is he gone for good? I really need your advice now as I have no one to turn to.

Everything in my life had started to change for the good and suddenly things have turned ugly again. Please tell me if there is anything good coming my way in the future or are things just going to get worse?

Is my ex-husband going to be a part of my son's life even if we are not together? He has been the only father my son has known since he was three years old and he is now 17. Please reply as soon as possible and let me know what to do! I would greatly appreciate it.

CURANDERO'S RESPONSE:

You may need to let him go for your welfare and your son's. Your son is old enough now to understand. He received the benefit of a father for all those years. You had a man, but if he cheated one time, he will do it again. I don't think he will change back to the man you once knew. It may be time for you to turn the page and start a new life. You might be asking God for something that is not good for you in which case He will not grant it. Ask Santa María Desatanudos to "untie the knots" that bind you and to give you strength to go on with your son and your life. Also ask Saint Gudule the patron of unmarried women to help you. Her day is January 8. If your life and your intentions are pure, love will come to you again when you least expect it.

COMMENTARY:

False accusations, accompanied by robbery and lying to the police, are obvious and very disturbing warning signs.

Suppressed rage and domestic problems always lead to violence. Try, at all costs, to avoid situations that may lead to domestic violence before a family problem escalates into serious legal problems.

110. COUPLE PROBLEMS — *ENTRE DOS*

Today, more than ever before, I need your help and advice. I am living in a situation where my partner and I keep bumping heads. This woman that I'm with also has her sons and mother living with us. I can't stand it and it's making me desperate. They only use me and take advantage of my generosity and hospitality, and I have had it with them.

I'm so distressed I do not know what to do. I miss my own children and wish to be with them and not another man's children.

And to top things off, my job has been terminated. I am working at the hospital in my town, but now I can't even meet my grocery budget. Enlighten me, Fidencio. Can you help to soften my employer's hearts so I can get my job back so I can support my own children? I live permanently in communication with you, Niño Fidencio.

I pray with faith and devotion and I can feel Fidencio's presence in my heart. I know El Niño is with me. I implore Fidencio to send me the miracle light, his infinite light and give me his strength. I'm living in a terrible economic and emotional crisis.

Even though I attend a self-help group, I can't seem to understand how to make good decisions. Please help me.

First, I need a job, and secondly, may the people who live in my home have a change of heart and help me financially and emotionally. I need the strength to make the decision to leave these people who are leeching off me.

CURANDERO'S RESPONSE:

It will all be okay. I'll share my faith, my help and my advice with you. I'm sorry to hear that you are not happy with your partner. My prayers are for your happiness and also for hers. God is going to help you because you are good and charitable.

Be patient and you will be able to see how God will help you more than if you are not patient. Go immediately and reconnect with your natural children. They are also in need of your love and support. Help your relationship by carrying a small aluminum triangle on your person, and write their names on it in red ink. Place it in a red felt bag and carry it over your heart. Concerning your job loss, maybe it is as the saying goes "one door closes and another opens."

It will be good if you can make a pilgrimage to Fidencio. Get close to him and he will enlighten your path and give you warmth. If it is true that you feel El Niño Fidencio's presence, you wouldn't say that you were living in the worst crisis economically and emotionally. If you really and truthfully wanted the help, strength, courage, light, peace, love and understanding, El Niño Fidencio would hand it to you. You have always preferred a different road and not El Niño Fidencio's. Isn't that true? My advice is that if you truly seek his assistance get close to God and El Niño Fidencio. You need to find humility and put your vanity and pride aside, ask Saint Rose of Lima to help you through to see through the mess you are in. Her day is August 28.

COMMENTARY:

It is significant to observe that the curandero has worked with this individual for some time and is acutely aware of the client's fragile emotional and psychological well-being. The overwhelming majority of Latinos in the United States simply do not have access to mental health professionals. These needs are exponentially greater in Mexico and all other Latin American countries. When we encounter a person who obviously needs help, it is crucial to help him/her access any and all available support systems. This is especially relevant when the person is contemplating taking his/her life.

111. CANDLE MAGIC — *LA VELA MÁGICA*

My mom is at the store right now and she will be so happy to hear that I have spoken to you when she gets home. She'll be purchasing the candles and calling you soon, I'm sure. Thank you for your prayers. As I've told you before, I have been in the same unhappy, abusive relationship for nearly four and a half years. For some reason, I've let this man keep hold of me and control my mind. This past weekend he let me know that he doesn't want to be with me anymore. He now says that he has been as unhappy as long as I have and that he is ready for us to go our separate ways.

Even while he tells me this, he says that I can continue to live in our house. Do you see how controlling he is? Why should I move out? Why doesn't he move out? He has told me and several other people who live with us in our home that he is happy to sleep on the couch. And to make matters worse, he tells them that he is hoping that we can all remain friends.

I was so caught off guard by all of this. I have been physically and emotionally abused by him and I have been mostly unhappy during the years that we have been together, but for some reason that I don't understand, I don't want to let him go. I think I still love him. Maybe it's obsession. I never really thought of being with anyone else. I just want for us to try and make it work or to let it go.

I know that I am not a very easy person to get along with. I always want to be right and I like to talk rather than listen. But now I am ready to change all of that.

My bad qualities have gotten me in trouble with others as well. I tend to lie, also. I don't mean to, but I have such a need to be right all the time that I find myself lying. Even when I doubt myself, I want others to think I am right. So I'll change things or add things to gratify myself. Either way, I know I need to change this. Please help and pray for me.

The thing I want to know is what would be the wisest thing for me to do? As far as I'm concerned, I love him a lot and I believe that I would be faithful to him until the end of time. I always thought he felt the same. It feels like he is just really mad at me and is saying things to hurt me but he doesn't really mean them. If that's the case, I just want us to try to stop fighting. But if he's serious about it being over, it is going to be so hard to move on. I want to be strong and I have a lot of work ahead of me either way.

What can I do to stay focused on what I need to do? What can I do to help him see that I still love him and want to always be with him? He is being so mean to me right now that I can't see how this is happening without a real reason.

CURANDERO'S RESPONSE:

Please light a yellow wax candle and keep one lit for three straight months. Boil rosemary on Fridays so the aroma fills the house for cleansing and peace in your relationship and the household. Do this for seven Fridays in a row. Boil *verbena* and bathe in this water, and pray to the spirits for peace. Do this for nine Mondays in a row.

You are both trapped by what you think is love. What happened to that wonderful love you felt so deeply for each other? What was it that made it fade away as time passed by? Apparently he is listening to someone else's questionable advice. On the other hand, you admit you have been confused and at fault about many things. I have to believe from your story that you are not telling me everything. There must have been an event or series of events that sent him over the edge in his decision to break up with you. Tell me the truth especially since you admit that you are a liar. The positive is that you are ready and willing to do something about it and improve yourself and your relationship.

COMMENTARY:

Persons ensconced in an abusive relationship seek some type of support network. Almost every community and/or phone book lists help-lines that can point them in a rehabilitative direction provided by support groups. Also, seek support groups in your area via the Internet.

112. SPITEFUL STEP-FATHER — *MALICIOSO*

It seems whenever there is a break for us and things look better, something goes very wrong and we're in another financial mess. My husband needed to pass a test to keep his job. If he does not pass, then he is going to be laid off again.

Well, my husband passed his test and it seemed as if we were going to be financially stable again. But now he is acting strange. He is mean to me and my children. Four of them aren't his, and he says he is tired of feeding and taking care of four children that are not his. He says that they are not his responsibility. He knew that when we got married. Now he complains that our house is never clean enough, and that my kids get on his nerves.

He curses and says the ugliest, meanest things and calls me every name in the book. He makes my kids cry all the time, puts them down and swears at them.

I want to leave him, but he gets really mad when I bring this up and he scares me. Does he want out of our marriage?

I now believe that would be best for all of us. I am confused, financially unstable and scared. I have family that say I should get away from him and move back to where they are because there are many more opportunities for single moms there. But my kids do not want to leave their schools and their friends. I just need some advice on what to do. Please help. I am all alone and have no one to talk to me that I can trust to give me good advice, except you. I am very tired of living this way.

CURANDERO'S RESPONSE:

Have you considered seeing a counselor? I think both of you should. Both of you could talk with your parish priest or pastor and ask for guidance. I will keep you in my prayers. How are the children coping with all of these problems between you and your husband? What do they say about him? Do they get along with him? You and your husband must pray Psalm 132 so he can settle down now that he has passed the test. He is acting like he is under some kind of pressure. Do you know what is bothering him? It's not you and the kids; it's outside of the home.

Do the children get child support from their own father? If you are having financial problems and you need assistance, have you tried applying for food stamps or government assistance, or from church organizations that have assistance programs? You and your children have already gone through the hardship of a divorce. How do you think another one will affect them? Can you seek professional counseling for the children? This may be much more serious than you think!

Begin your prayers to San Cayetano, the patron saint of work and for the blessing of the home and to Saint Flora to protect you from betrayal. Her celebration day is January 26.

COMMENTARY:

This case is extremely serious and the curandero senses it. Curanderos usually act as a one-stop referral agency. It is evident that the husband feels trapped in his situation. There are clearly many more underlying facts that we don't know. But if this woman feels that the relationship is over and that her family is willing to accept and assist her, then the curandero will guide her toward that scenario.

It is also the moral responsibility of the curandero to contact child protective services at the first sign of abuse or physical violence in the home. The wife has already admitted that she fears him.

113. REMOVE THIS WOMAN — *QUÍTAMELA*

Help me get rid of the woman that lives with me. This woman, together with her mother and her children, does me much more harm than good. I'm so depressed about all of the many dreadful things they do to me. I don't know why I put up with it, force of habit I guess. They are not happy and don't appreciate that I'm providing housing, education, and supporting them, despite them not being my children.

They pay me back by making fun of me, screaming and humiliating me. They do not value anything I do for them. She drinks a lot and gets home late. I don't know where she has been and I put up with it because I don't want to live by myself again. I am afraid to be alone and that is why I put up with this.

If Niño Fidencio was still alive and standing in front of me, I'm sure that without a doubt he would give me a helping hand, he would be my voice, my sight, and my ears. I know you have your own problems and that you receive tons of e-mails and telephone calls to help other Fidencista brothers. But who do I appeal to if not another Fidencista to plea for us? How else do I find comfort and support? Please help me and don't lecture me that I don't have faith. I do. Don't be mean to me, and please don't abandon my needs.

CURANDERO'S RESPONSE:

Yes, of course I will help you. But you must want to help yourself first! Yes, I will help you, first God, and then El Niño Fidencio. Beforehand, prepare a crystal glass with water and keep it in the middle of your kitchen table. Every time the woman leaves the house, without her knowing what you are doing, throw the water from the glass toward her back on the floor or outside just after she walks out.

Also, have a regular household broom and position the bottom side up and behind the front door of the house. At every opportunity, when she leaves the house, sweep behind her and out the door. Whatever you do, don't let her see what you are doing. This is in order to avoid her becoming angry; because then the one who'll be running out is you. Do all this with caution and everything will work out. Most importantly, pray to Saint Martha the patron saint of unwanted guests. Her day is July 29.

COMMENTARY:

The majority of the healing missions of El Niño Fidencio are located in northeastern and north-central Mexico. While help from the Niño Fidencio may not be found everywhere, there are always curanderos, who work with different saints and spiritual beings, or seres espirituales, that can be found around the United States and in Mexico, or, wherever Latinos reside. Inquire where these visionaries are located, at any hierbería or botánica. After learning their names, ask for the following: authenticity, reputation, and effectiveness as related by persons who possess personal knowledge of their work.

114. MANIPULATIVE WOMAN — *CONTROLADORA*

At my mother's request, I'm sending you my brother's picture. He lives with a manipulative woman in a common-law marriage. She tells him all kinds of gossip to get him further away from our family. He has asked her to leave, but she refuses and everything he does comes out wrong. She has him with no money because she keeps everything that he earns as if she owned everything. What can I do to help my brother to get rid of this woman?

CURANDERO'S RESPONSE:

My regards and respect to you and your mother. Either you or your mother should read Psalm 119; it's made up of 22 verses. Read one verse at a time for 22 consecutive days; making your petition on behalf of your brother at morning's first light, in order to free your loved one of all bad things happening. After the 22 days, you will witness a miracle that the Lord has granted. While in prayer to San Judás, the patron of desperate and difficult cases and El Niño Fidencio, ask for the Spirit of the love Our Lord has for us. Ask Saint Leopold to help get her out of your life. His saint's day is November 15.

COMMENTARY:

Sometimes family members become embroiled in situations where they shouldn't. This type of familial interference is unhealthy for everybody.

115. DIFFERENCE OF OPINION — *PUNTO DE VISTA*

I thank you very much. I gladly receive your good wishes. I hope you are in good health and I always have you in my prayers. I am continuing my spiritual development but it is difficult for my husband. I know that in order for me to become a trance medium I have to abstain from sexual relations while I am developing my spirituality, but my other half does not agree with the rule of no sexual relations for three months. He asked if it could be done differently and I am afraid he will wander.

What I think is that if he wants to see me accomplish this great challenge, he will have to accept the abstinence and support me. It's up to him now. I am not going to look back. I wish you could speak to him and perhaps explain to him in a better way so he can understand that this is good for both of us. I don't have a problem with the abstinence. I'll do what it takes to reach my goal.

CURANDERO'S RESPONSE:

I believe the three months will pass very quickly and that this is a very small sacrifice compared to the healing you will receive and give. El Niño Fidencio will help you sacrifice for the good of both of you. This, above all, needs to be done in good faith, hope and in agreement. Ask Our Lady of Good Counsel, on April 26, to enlighten you toward your spiritual growth.

COMMENTARY:

What is not crystallized in this dilemma is the fact that the curandero has been counseling the questioner on how to develop, desarrollar spiritually as a medium. This process usually requires abstinence. Problems with a spouse who is neither sympathetic nor in agreement instigating and forcing the decision to walk a righteous and spiritual path in turn require patience and tolerance.

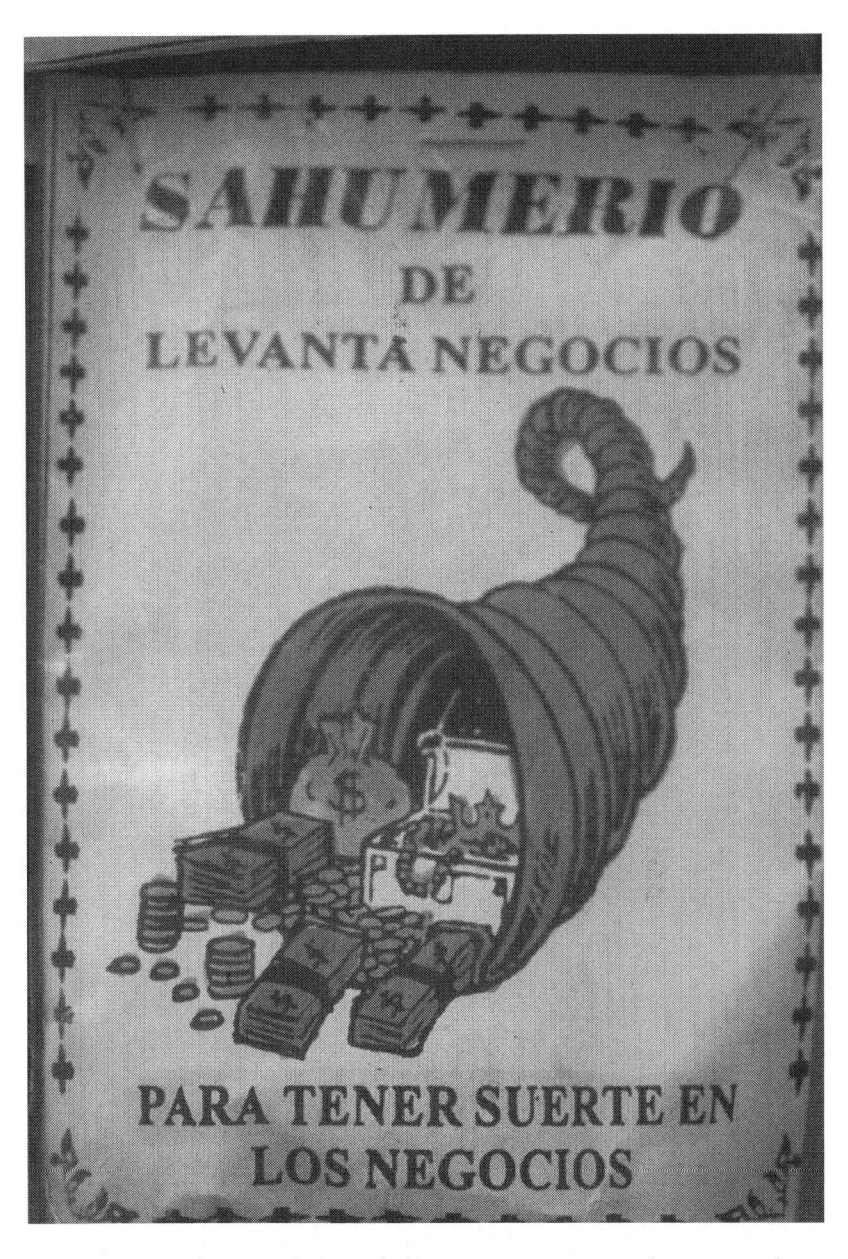

A pre-prepared incense is intended to promote success in business and is displayed for sale at the Mercado Sonora in Mexico City.
(Photo by José M. Duarte)

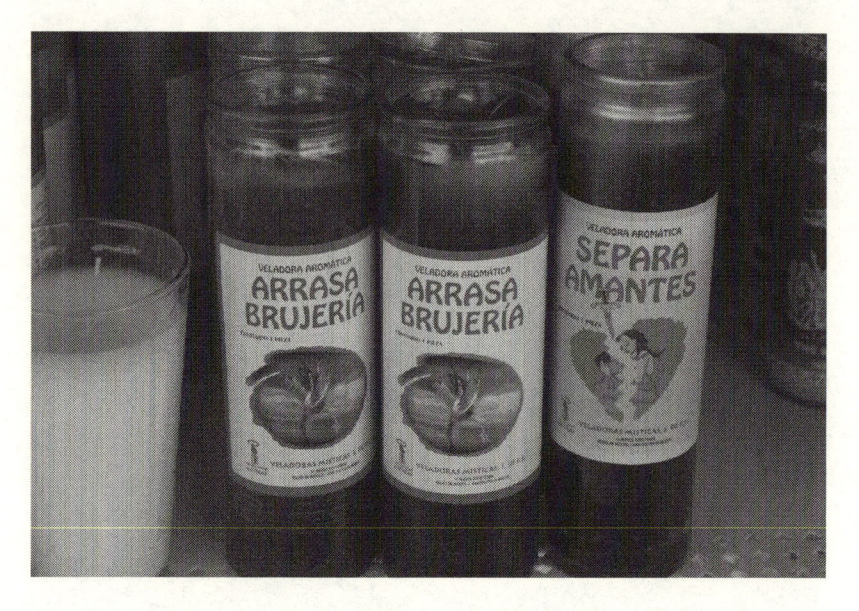

Votive Candles are used to reverse witchcraft spells and are also used to destroy relationships and love affairs. (Photo by Zavaleta)

PART SEVEN

Healing the Workplace: The Treacherous World Beyond the Home

"Latinos consider their home a place of safety from the dangers of the world. They view the world outside the protection of the home as hostile. Therefore, Latinos feel they must be ever vigilant of neighbors, co-workers and even relatives."

—Joseph Spielberg Benítez, anthropologist

116. BAD PEOPLE — *GENTE MALA*

Hoping you are well, please pray for my forgiveness. I write to you because my votive candle to the Virgen of Guadalupe has become smoky and this week I have been feeling ill at work. There are some persons at work that as soon as they get close to me, give me a headache and I have to go to the restroom to throw up. I am just a secretary so I don't understand why they don't like me. When this happens, I pray the Rosary and I feel better. Could you please help me to understand what is happening?

CURANDERO'S RESPONSE:

Your votive candle is smoky because it is working hard to clean the bad vibrations and the entire negative situation that surrounds you. Be sure to pray to San Isidro Labrador, the patron saint of work. He will help to rid you of negative influences at your workplace.

Thank you very much for the reliquary. The *estampa* or holy picture that you sent me is in vigil on my altar. Apart from you having an impious spirit, you are very sensitive to the currents of benevolent and malevolent spirits. This is why you react and feel ill when different persons come close to you. In order to combat this, you must wear around your neck a blessed talisman or amulet. Always be sure to keep your yard and home cleansed by using special waters prepared with ammonia, and for uncrossing, *descruce*, use perfume. Also, please pray Psalms 41, 43 and 44, which will help you to rid the workplace of bad people. There is no such thing as just a secretary. Secretaries rule the business world and that is why they don't like you. Pray to Saint Cassian the patron saint of secretaries to protect you at all times at work. His day of recognition is August 13.

COMMENTARY:

Witchcraft belief in the Latino community is pervasive and the workplace is one of the most frequent examples of where a person suspects co-workers of "working" them. One must always be protected with a personal talisman and must never show it to co-workers. Certainly never talk about your feelings or your protection with co-workers.

117. CHANGE MY LUCK — *ESTOY SALADA*

I hope you remember us. We used to live near you, but most of the time we were unable to go see you. My daughter e-mailed you the other day and you sent her some prayers. We wanted to see if you could help us out because my husband has been having some bad luck at work. This week he had two minor accidents. Now he is worried that he might lose his job because of them. We wanted to see if you and El Niñito could help us. We really do like it here and don't want to have to migrate to find work again. I hope you and El Niñito can help us.

We have had some questions answered through a *materia* near us, but she doesn't work all the time, so it is hard to reach her. Through the Internet, we know that we can reach you almost every day and that is a wonderful support network for us so far from home.

CURANDERO'S RESPONSE:

To cleanse your husband of bad luck at work due to *envidias,* or jealousies and negative energies due to witchcraft, your husband should have a *limpia* with a cluster of *verbena,* vervain, *yerba buena,* mint or *albahaca,* basil. He should be swept outdoors at 3 a.m. The spiritual cleansing should take place out in the open under the stars and with a full moon in the sky overhead. You may perform the ritual yourself on him. Pray to San Antonio that your husband be delivered from all curses and that he be blessed in abundance by the good spirits. Be sure to pray for his protection from evil. Saint Francis Xavier celebrated on November 13, protects migrating families.

Go to the *hierbería* and purchase a *piedra imán,* or lodestone. Be sure that they give you a female *imán*; you will also need the iron filings to feed it. Be sure to feed this stone every Friday morning and once it becomes fat, it will bring good luck to your husband and your entire household. You could also purchase a small statue of Buddha or an elephant with raised trunks to help change your luck.

Always pray Psalms 4, 57, 63, and 65 to rid your family of bad luck or salt. I shall keep you in my prayers. Boil three heads of garlic in a pail of water. You and your husband should bathe with the garlic water to ward off any curses, evil and other bad luck he is having. Also try using a good luck stone prepared with special essence and carried in your purse or pocket.

COMMENTARY:

The curandero/a is asked to use his powers and connections with the spirit world to intervene in the workplace and with the boss. We implore the spirits to help us with our own human frailties so that we may be shielded beforehand. The curandero/a is asked to reverse bad luck and aid us in sidestepping accidents which would take a loved one from us or because of serious injuries, depriving needed income and emotional-familial support.

Magical items reversing bad luck and attracting good luck are some of the most popular items found for sale at *hierberías*. In addition to lodestones, sprays, amulets and talismans, it is not unusual to find the desiccated hummingbird, *chuparosa*, or *colibri*, believed to attract good luck. Every traditional home and/or business will also feature items hung over the front and rear doorways of homes. Today, you will usually encounter a preprepared collage consisting of a horseshoe, a living aloe vera plant with red ribbon and other items thought to attract good luck. These arrangements are usually embellished with a holy picture, or *estampa* of the *Virgen de Guadalupe, San Martín Caballero, Pancho Villa* or other highly regarded patron saint.

118. SHE NEEDS HER JOB — *NECESITA SU TRABAJO*

I am still working on getting the pictures of my family you requested so that I can send them to you. My sister told me today that the new job she just started is beginning to go sour, just like all her previous jobs. I think she is *salada*, has bad luck. She only started a week ago and she loved it in the beginning and then it started to turn bad for her. Do you think it's her?

We think it is her behavior and not the job, but she refuses to see that and says we are against her. She feels differently now and said it seems as though her boss does not like her. I cannot tell her to put cinnamon in her shoes as you suggested because she will tell her husband and he is not a believer. I feel so bad for her because she cannot seem to hold a job. I plan to send their pictures to you as soon as possible. Is there anything you can do at your end to help her? At this point, she has to work because her husband cannot support them alone right now.

My mother has also been very moody lately and my daughter told me that she yells at the baby because he cries. For awhile, my mom is fine and the next moment she blows up. It hurts my husband and me to know that our children are being yelled at daily by their grandmother while we are at work, but at this point, we have no other options. We cannot afford to pay for daycare, so my mother has to watch them for us. I will keep you posted and I hope to hear from you soon.

CURANDERO'S RESPONSE:

I am trying to help you the best that I can. In the meantime, you should light the Divina Providencia, Divine Providence, and the Holy Trinity candles. Have your mother light a Sagrado Corazón, Sacred Heart candle, so that she may have peace in her heart and maybe she will not yell at the children so much. I continue to pray that you may be blessed and comforted. While this situation continues, you should give yourselves and your children three *limpias*, or cleansings, with fertile hen's eggs. Do the cleansings on Monday, Friday and Sunday of the same week. Don't miss days and always carry it out at the same hour and in the same place.

COMMENTARY:

Our loved ones can be subjected to jealousy in the workplace. Being busy, they may face real evil worked against them. Brujos and brujas, or witches, are utilized by jealous co-workers to cast spells to cause us harm and even death. We need spiritual protection through sweeping to ensure constant vigilance by the spirits of light. Verbena, vervain, is an herb used to remove evil influences from the body.

119. GOSSIPY WORKMATES — *CHISMOSOS*

Who are the people that will cause me the problems you wrote about? Last week my husband was fired as I predicted. I tried to help him out spiritually to no avail. We work for the same company and my husband told my supervisor that I told him to call and tell him about some bad things that are going on at work. Then, my supervisor called me to tell me what my husband had told him. He also asked me if it was true, but I denied it. I could not tell the truth. I had to deny it or I would have blown my cover, and I cannot let that happen because I am working undercover for the owners of the company on an internal investigation. Not even my husband knows what I am doing.

I felt that I had to help my husband because there is a lot of injustice and fraud at work involving lots of people. I am not getting paid for this undercover work. I am doing this for myself and for all of the workers I see being abused because I am tired of everything I see going on.

We all work hard while others don't work at all because they are relatives, friends or drinking buddies of the supervisors. They go to bars during working hours. They add extra names on the payroll and receive checks for people who do not exist.

I don't want you to think that I am a snitch. It's just that we all work our butts off while they party or don't even come to work. There is more to the story, but I am afraid to put it in an e-mail. I know that El Niño knows what I am talking about.

In your last letter to me, I was very surprised that the Niño was able to tell you the names of the people I am talking about because I never told you the names of the people at work. That just shows the power of El Niño Fidencio.

CURANDERO'S RESPONSE:

I feel good about your concern and believe that you are doing the right thing. You must be very careful. I still believe things will work out well for you and your husband. I know you are going through a terrible experience.

Please boil seven heads of garlic in a bucket of water, saying prayers and making your petition to the Creator and Lord while bathing in the water. Also, call upon the help of San Miguel Archangel, San Martín Caballero and San Martín de Porres to gather around you and to protect you at work and at home. Pray Psalm 7 to keep your enemies from plotting against you. They will always assist you to keep negativity away from you and your loved ones.

COMMENTARY:

In this case, the livelihoods of an entire family have been placed in jeopardy because she has been asked to work undercover and inform on co-workers; some of whom happen to be friends and family members. While wanting to comply with the request, they are very vulnerable and fearful of losing their jobs as a result of this work. The request has also created great anxiety and a frightful condition labeled as nervios, or chronic nervous anxiety. Having consulted with El Niño Fidencio on this issue in the past, the petitioner asked that the Niño be consulted for further advice. The husband has already lost his job, the supervisor is suspicious and the wife may be in way over her head, lose her job and throw her family into chaos.

120. TEACHER NEEDS A JOB — *ABRE CAMINO*

I have great news. I was called at work today and offered a job as a fifth-grade bilingual teacher. I am a qualified bilingual teacher while many teachers at this school are not. It is going to be a challenge since I have never taught this grade, much less a bilingual class of fifth graders. I don't know my exact assignment yet, though my former sister-in-law offered to help me by giving me a copy of a book on ideas once I know what subjects I have to teach. I hope she follows through with her promise.

Please pray for me because tomorrow is going to be my first day in the fifth-grade bilingual class at a new school. Please pray that I do well. My former principal said that I have to do well in the area I teach because it is a big responsibility and if the children do not learn, then it will look bad on me and the new principal will not renew my contract. I need to work and cannot lose my contract. I don't want that to happen and I pray that I will have a successful year. I need all the help and prayers I can get.

I just wanted to let you all know of the good news and my apprehensions, and thank you, Niño Fidencio, and especially the Lord for all the Divine spiritual assistance. I would not have made it without their kindness and mercy. I am truly grateful. Now the challenges lie ahead.

CURANDERO'S RESPONSE:

It is always so good to receive good news. You don't know how happy I am for you. The Lord has blessed you. The Lord has answered our prayers. I know you will do fine but you must have confidence in yourself and your abilities. It sounds to me that you have very low self-esteem and are not thinking of all the skills you learned in college. What's the matter with you? You were a good student and you will be a good teacher, and the children will love you. Thanks to our Lord and the Niño Fidencio. Your job is a miracle. By the way, don't wait for your former sister-in-law to help you. Help yourself. If she helps you, that will be good, but there are many resource materials available to you online to help you with fifth-grade bilingual kids. Help yourself for a life filled with success and stand on your own two feet.

Ask Pope Saint Gregory the Great, the teacher of teachers, to bless you by maximizing the use of your educational accomplishments so that you will serve as an example to all of your friends, family, and especially to your employer. Pray Psalm 132 to keep your job and avoid future problems. You may also pray to another well known patron saint of teachers and students, Saint John Salle. His day is April 7. Most importantly, believe in yourself.

COMMENTARY:

In this case the curandero has established a relationship with the client. While this woman is educated, she is a single parent and in great need of constant moral support. The curandero has provided her with support through her divorce, her college education, and now with her job. Yet she lacks confidence and self-esteem and will need many years of support before she will be able to fly on her own. She maintains a home altar with her patron saints and visits the curandero at his home whenever she can.

121. SHE BURNED ME — *ME QUEMÓ*

I hope you remember me. I am just going to write a few lines. First of all, my health has been good and so far, my pregnancy is going well thanks to God and El Niño.

I do have problems at work. Maybe you can help me with them. The problem is a co-worker who's also a relative and works with us. I feel she is trying to cause problems for me with my supervisors. I don't want to lose my job. I am good at what I do and with the children I care for. I know that she talks about me with the co-workers behind my back because they have made comments to me about her. For example, they say "if she is your cousin, why does she say these things about you?"

I know she likes to gossip because that is the way she is with the rest of the family as well. I don't understand why she has it in for me. I know I have never done anything bad to her. I hope you can help me so she will leave me alone.

CURANDERO'S RESPONSE:

Niño Fidencio asked you to light a just judge, *justo juez,* candle as well as a Saint Michael the Archangel and a seven-archangel candle, and to pray for happiness. Remember that San Judás Tadeo is the patron saint of difficult cases, and this surely sounds like one to me. I will check with you again. You should also bathe with Holy Water, or *agua bendita*, for seven straight Fridays. Pray and make your petition to the Lord while bathing.

Burn three kings incense, *copal* and myrrh. Burn this incense mixture for seven Fridays in a row to cleanse yourself and your house of any negative energies, evil forces and evil spells. Also, sprinkle a mixture of rice, wheat and black mustard seed around the house on the first day of each month for protection from evil. This should help to *amarrar*, or tie up, your cousin's tongue.

COMMENTARY:

Situations at the workplace can be particularly stressful and problematic. When a relative is involved and the principal troublemaker is a family member, the situational stress levels escalate in both the workplace and within the family. How is one to handle this delicate problem? The curandero asks that the petitioner purchase a just judge, or justo juez candle as well as a Saint Michael the Archangel. An elaborate ritual is prescribed to be conducted on seven consecutive Fridays for protection and to silence the gossipers, tapa boca, cover the mouth of her cousin who is causing all the problems.

122. THE BUREAUCRACY — *ENREDADO EN LA POLÍTICA*

I am e-mailing you because my electricity was cut off this week and I couldn't get in contact with you. However, I want to inform you of what is happening to me regarding college and the program I am in at the university and at my work.

I was called into the school district office where I work and told by a human resources employee that the university program that I'm enrolled in does not cover the grade level that I am currently teaching. This personnel lady is the same one that pushed to help me get a job at the school in the first place. She has been very kind to me. She called another program that helps people get into teaching and they told her about a new law that verified what she told me about not qualifying.

It seems that the people at the university are not keeping up with the changes in the state laws, or they just didn't tell me or don't care. I have already signed up to take the state teaching exam to be certified to teach, but now, unfortunately, it is for the wrong grade level. If I can't get a transfer to another grade, I will lose my job.

I talked to an administrator at the university and she told me that they were not aware of this new change in the law. How is that possible?

So, after work I headed to the district office not knowing why they had wanted to talk to me. When I arrived, they broke the news. I had the choice of staying employed with the district or changing programs at the university.

In the university office I encountered several other high-positioned people who were called in to listen to my case on a conference call. A higher university administrator said that he would try to have the class fees waived and that he would release me from the program without academic penalty. The only thing is that I invested so much money in it. The district knows this as well.

Now, the school district is telling me that all of the classes I took at the university will not help me retain the teaching position I am currently in and I want to stay there. Perhaps there was a reason for all this. As you can see, things are changing rapidly and I can only ask you to pray for me. Please let Niñito know what is happening. I feel like I am getting the runaround and that I am in a box with no way out. I have worked so hard for my education and now my job just to have it all go up in smoke. I need the Niño's help, and fast. Please pray for me.

CURANDERO'S RESPONSE:

I understand you are having major problems with your finances, with your university, with your teaching job, with your family, with your children, with your transportation, with your mom's health, and so on. It will be quite a challenge to help you, but I will try my best. The fact that you are a single parent of three makes your situation even more difficult.

I recommend that you take a spiritual healing bath with boiled California pepper tree, *pirul*, leaves. Do this for any nine consecutive Saturdays at noon. Or, when school is out for summer, take the baths on nine consecutive days. Say a special prayer to Saint Scholastica, the sister of Saint Benedict, and ask her for her special assistance in your case. Saint Thomas Aquinas is also an expert on university issues, so pray to him as well. Also pray to Saint John Salle and to Saint Brigid to ensure that your students will like you and will learn. Saint Brigid's day is February 1. Pray Psalm 134, which is meant to assist you to succeed in school. Sweep yourself with three lemons, holding them in your right hand while standing in front a mirror, and praying, and making your petitions to the spirit. Do this right after your bath. Please contact me for further instructions when you have done this. I am here for you.

COMMENTARY:

This single mother has the weight of the world on her shoulders. Because the university cannot get its act together, her job is now in jeopardy. Additionally, she worries about her kids, her mother, and her car. The curandero prescribes a specialized spiritual bath consisting of leaves from the California pepper tree, or the sacred pirul tree of El Niño Fidencio in Espinazo. Also note from this case that visiting a curandero is a cultural event and has little to do with educational status. While more low-income people seem to visit curanderos than the middle class, this is probably more due to socioeconomic status than it is due to cultural tenets.

123. SUCCESS — *ÉXITO*

I am e-mailing you to inform you that yesterday after school I interviewed for a second-grade bilingual position with the principal and her staff. I think that they were a little hesitant of me because they are not bilingual certified and I am. Also, they have a new second-grade bilingual teacher who is not certified either. She is being trained by someone on another campus. While I am a certified bilingual teacher, I don't want them to be threatened by me. I just want them to give me a chance. I hope that they will consider me and help me get the training from another campus as well.

I have another interview for a fifth-grade position in bilingual teaching this afternoon. I have to travel through many winding roads to get to a distant country school where I will teach if I get the fifth-grade job.

If I get this provisional job, I will have to change my degree plan again. I have already changed it twice and this is the reason that I have to take a state bilingual teacher exam again for a different grade level.

This time it will be for a kindergarten bilingual teacher. If I pass, I will now be qualified to teach in three different grades and I pray that some school district will want me. I had always planned to be a first-grade teacher and I don't know if I have the confidence to teach the older kids. I know that is my problem. Please pray for me to have strength and confidence in myself. I have come from the migrant fields to become a certified teacher, but I still lack confidence, I am afraid and I don't trust people.

CURANDERO'S RESPONSE:

If you can, come by for some spiritual cleansing, or *limpia*. You will need to bring some fresh rue, rosemary and basil cut in heavy bunches for the *limpia* ritual to rid you of the negative forces that keep you from progressing and to build your confidence.

You should consider having a *limpia* at least once a week for at least seven weeks. You may also light a Holy Trinity and a Divine Providence candle on your home altar for a period of 40 straight days. Also, recite Psalm 8 so you will be successful and state your petition aloud on a daily basis. May God bless you.

COMMENTARY:

Continuous spiritual baths are the most common prescription for a situation like this one. The curandero will usually ask the petitioner to come by his consultorio or the location where he/she spiritually consults for spiritual sweepings if they are able. If they cannot visit, he will instruct the person exactly how to carry them out. The intention of the remedy, or remedio, is to keep envy, envidia, and evil forces at bay and to reinforce confidence.

People who work hard and climb the career ladder out of poverty often find it difficult to rid themselves of low self-esteem. Many psychological studies have proven that success greater than three levels of social status can cause failure through self-sabotage. The traditional solution to the problem can be attained through constant prayer and spiritual sweepings.

124. FATHER'S CREDIT — *EL BUEN NOMBRE*

My brother and I wrote to you on a Friday, three and a half weeks ago. Do you remember? I find myself still in desperate need of your help. You see, I have not found a job yet, and to make matters worse they stopped sending me unemployment checks on this very day. I am very worried that if I don't find a job soon, I won't be able to make the payments on my car. I don't want to lose it and I don't want to ruin my father's good credit because I got my car on his credit. What do I do?

I feel so helpless, like everything is falling apart before my eyes. No one at all has called me for a job interview, much less an actual job. I can honestly say that I have just about given up. I find myself not caring anymore or wanting to be in this world anymore. I am tired of everyone else getting what they want and I can't even get a job to pay for my car! I feel very angry inside and I feel cheated. Please help me! I'm begging for your help.

CURANDERO'S RESPONSE:

My prayers are with you. Saint Rita is the patron saint of good deals, pray to her. Her feast day is May 22. You should boil *ruda*, rue, *romero*, rosemary, and *albahaca*, basil, in a bucket of water and then remove the herbs from the water. Add one half bottle of green rubbing alcohol to the water. Add one tablespoon of salt to the water. Add one half cup of honey to the water. Bathe with the water. Pray one *Padre Nuestro*, Our Father, and make your petition to the Lord. Light a *Santísima Trinidad*, Holy Trinity candle and a *Divina Providencia*, Divine Providence, candle on either side of your picture with a glass of water setting over your picture. Do this with faith whenever you can. This should help you out of this problem, God willing.

COMMENTARY:

Spiritual baths comprised of rue, rosemary, and basil with alcohol, salt and sometimes honey are the usual remedies used for ongoing spiritual cleansings. In order to ensure success, special candles are burned on the home altar with one's photograph between them. You may notice here and in the following curandero's response that the spiritual remedies are very similar and repetitious. Just as in a doctor's office, ensuing patients receive a similar prescription if they have the same symptoms. No difference here.

The petitioner should also be encouraged to continue applying for jobs and keeping busy doing odd jobs around his father's home to show his intent to help his father, as his father's credit has helped him.

125. A SPIRITUAL TEST — *UNA PRUEBA ESPIRITUAL*

I am writing to you because I have failed you and let you down one more time. I was terminated today from the job that the Niño Fidencio just helped me get. They had me working out in the hot sun and in a hot warehouse all day until I went home. They kept giving me responsibility after responsibility and I could never catch up with the work that needed to be done. It was like they wanted me to fail. I am not lazy.

Then today, they wanted me to help these other guys that were installing an air conditioning unit. That's not my job to do, so I told the assistant manager and he told me to go home, which I did. I called him about an hour later to see if I was fired or not and he told me that my manager would have my termination papers ready tomorrow. So now I am fired. I mean, I feel bad about losing my job, but I also feel I did what was right to stand up for myself.

They would not help me. No one would find me a helper to help me with all the work they gave me. If this was a spiritual test, I failed it. I'm really sorry. I feel that I have failed you and disrespected you as well. I am begging for your help again. Please let the manager give me another chance or help me to find another job that is not so stressful. I feel so terrible for letting you down. I don't know what to do anymore. I need you to guide me, please.

CURANDERO'S RESPONSE:

If you are given another chance, you have to work harder and not complain. If you do your best you will always win. They probably just wanted to see what you were made of and you failed. Try to apply for another job with another company or at a different place. As I told you, I will pray for you. Light a Holy Trinity candle and a Divine Providence candle and place them near a glass of water. Boil *ruda*, rue, *romero*, rosemary, and *albahaca,* basil, in a pail of water. Then, take the *hierbas*, herbs, out of the pail of water, leaving the water and adding one half a cup of honey, half a bottle of rubbing alcohol and a tablespoon of salt, and bathe with the water. Say the Our Father and make your petition to the Lord that you be given another chance at work. Please keep me posted. Pray that the Holy Infant of Prague grant you prosperity. Celebrate Him the third Sunday in May each year.

COMMENTARY:

The Holy Trinity and the Divine Providence candles are the most referenced in curanderismo for this sort of candle magic but others may be substituted for specialized issues. For example, in this case, the petitioner feels that he has been unjustly fired and he may replace or add a Changó or Santa Bárbara candle from Santería for added force and aggressive protection, or he may pray to San Isidro Labrador to work more diligently. Any person should be grateful for having a job. Simultaneously, employers should not ask workers to work in dangerous conditions without support and protection from the elements and their subsequent effects.

126. I NEED WORK — *NECESITO TRABAJO*

I'm just writing to you to let you know that I have submitted four applications today. Three of them are hiring right now; the other is not looking for anyone at this time. But I do have the experience that they are looking for. Plus, it's only five minutes away from my house, and that is why I would love to work for this company. They have two people checking in shipments and stocking parts. Please help me with either of these jobs. Also, I have done what you asked me to do with the herbal bath and the candles you told me to light to be sure that I do not have a witchcraft spell on me. I have a lot of faith in you and that you will help me. Thank you very much.

CURANDERO'S RESPONSE:

Please boil three heads of garlic in a bucket of plain water. Then, bathe with this water reciting one Our Father and make your petition to the Father, the Son and the Holy Spirit to cleanse you spiritually from this witchcraft spell that I believe has been cast upon you. Then, you should buy a Holy Trinity or a Divine Providence seven-day candle and light it. Once again, make your petition to the Lord for a spiritual cleansing from witchcraft plus ask for a blessing from the Lord for employment.

COMMENTARY:

Note in this remedy the curandero is drawing from Roman Catholic prayers and rituals. Reciting the Our Father and sometimes the entire Holy Rosary in difficult cases is not unusual. The petition to the Father, the Son, and the Holy Spirit is a Catholic tradition. Research has shown that most persons who seek out curanderos for help are also practicing Catholics.

127. LONELY — *LA SOLEDAD*

I have been doing alright, but I could always be better. As you suggested, I have been trying to make new friends and do new things. But I'm still having a lot of trouble finding a job. I am also very lonely. I had a lead on an office job that looked promising, but at the last minute the company was sold and they started laying people off. I am a very good computer operator with good people skills. I would love to have another opportunity like the last one you got me. I will continue to try harder. Please pray for me.

As far as my loneliness is concerned, my two girlfriends that I share an apartment with easily attract a lot of male companions. Almost every night they are out with new guys or the same old ones that they bring home from work. Well, I could do that, too, but I have not and I won't. I do not want to be that easy and develop that kind of reputation. I don't want to be like them. They have very bad reputations with all of the men at work.

I just want one man to start a new relationship with and maybe, if he's the one, I would like to marry someday. I don't want to date or sleep around.

I have a special friend at work that I like a lot. He is so nice, down to earth, and he works very hard every day at a good job. He seems like he likes me, too, but he is surrounded by these friends that will never leave us alone together.

They just want him to party. I think we've only been able to sit down and talk together alone twice for maybe 15 minutes and, boom, someone knocks on the door. I'm trying to get to know him and it seems like he is trying to know me, too. I think he sees that I am a decent woman. They say that he has never really had a steady girlfriend, although many from work have tried to catch him. I really, really like him. What should I do?

I'm so confused, lonely and tired. I just want to cry. I have lost my confidence. I miss having real friends that care about me and love me. I think that is why I want to find my soulmate. To me, your soulmate should also be your best friend. I desperately need a best friend, someone who will just sit and talk to me and one the Lord would approve of. Please help me. I'm scared and feeling all alone.

CURANDERO'S RESPONSE:

You are very lonely right now and I understand your feelings from your e-mail. You also want a meaningful relationship, and not just a passing relationship. You want a permanent, lasting and loving relationship. For that, you know you need to be patient, and even then you never really know when it will come your way. Anyway, as you already know, there are no guarantees in life.

Yes, you must maintain faith and hope and I shall continue to pray for you to have patience, too.

Light a Holy Trinity or a Divine Providence candle for finding a new job. Pray to Saint Gabriel the Archangel for finding your soulmate and happiness. I am praying for you. You must know that you are not alone, even though you feel this deep loneliness. I hope that you won't be alone for long. Be patient and you shall be blessed, believe me.

COMMENTARY:

This petition points out the pitfalls of the workplace as well as why and how they can prove to be so treacherous. At times, the workplace presents openings for romance between persons who are already married, but not to each other. This decent woman wants a viable relationship with God. The guy she likes is drawn away from her by his partying buddies. She asks the curandero to pray for her and to point out a method for a steady relationship without her resorting to promiscuity. Never compromise your values. It only takes one minor slip and your reputation is ruined forever.

128. NEED GUIDANCE — *ORIÉNTEME*

I've been doing really well, but lately I've been in need of your prayer and the guidance of the Holy Spirit. I got hurt a couple of months ago on my new job. They sent me home until I was completely well. I now have a permanent physical disability and my doctor has released me saying there is nothing else they can do for me. I was receiving workman's compensation checks as income, but now they have stopped because the doctor released me.

My employer does not want me back and has fired me because I have restrictions that they cannot accommodate. I'm not sure that is legal and I need your prayers and help. I am going to go to the unemployment office as soon as I get my last check. I have to wait for a check because I have no money for gas.

I have also been trying to find a lawyer to fight for me because this does not feel right. I do not think that what they are doing is just and fair and I think it might even be illegal.

Well, as you know, I was in legal trouble over drugs, but I have been doing great. I am completely clean. I am involved with my church and I drive the church van. I love to work with the kids, and I recently got married. My husband and I live with my parents and help with their bills. Ever since I got hurt, the worker's compensation company had me running around close to 100 miles a day, all week long; going to doctors and to physical therapy. It was all really stressful and then the company decided to cut off my benefits and fire me.

I have sort of gone off the deep end and I'm ashamed that I did some drugs this past weekend. I regret it and beg for forgiveness. I have faith that I will be forgiven.

CURANDERO'S RESPONSE:

Yes, of course I will help you. Search for three candles: St. Michael the Archangel, San Alejo and Saint Ignacio Loyola. Write the names of the people who you feel have denied you your benefits or are keeping you from being successful. Write their names on dirty underwear with a red pen and throw them away. Also write their names on a piece of parchment paper and place the paper in a private place where you will also place the three candles in the shape of a triangle around the names. Place a glass of water over the parchment paper with the names in the center of the three candles. Light the candles and pray to the spirit, make your petition that actions against you be reversed.

COMMENTARY:

This example is from the workplace and deals with an average person who is simply trying to get through life and feels that she has been wrongly treated at her job. Now, she finds herself up against a powerful system and the influence of corporate attorneys. She feels desperate and terrified. The curandero asks her to purchase candles for a special ritual to rid her of evil.

129. ANGUISH — *LA ANGUSTIA*

I gladly greet you; I know you have given yourself, body and soul, to the Fidencista order. Without your prayers, many of us would despair and be lost to Satan. I continue with my prayers and spiritual baths, but I remain sad and desperate because I am at the point of losing my job and the anguish is killing me. I have already lost my family and I am in an immense loneliness. I live far from my parents, brothers and sisters, and I am now separated from my wife and children as well, and it feels terrible. I know that being a Fidencista means to tolerate the pain; to be a Fidencista is to have hope and kindness; to be Fidencista is to have patience and faith in God and in the Niño.

I continue to request that you speak with Niño Fidencio and request that I can count on a job with dignity; that he shine his light and strength of spirit so that I develop and continue to support my children, and that he clear my path of evil and illness and place in my path good health. Ask him to distance my debts and continue to look for happiness for me in all of its aspects. I request a job, stability with emotions and family and an end to my debts. Help me. Do not abandon me to oblivion. What do I do? For the love of God, tell me what to do.

CURANDERO'S RESPONSE:

I will not abandon you, but God helps he who helps himself. I feel you are looking for an easy way out and that won't work. If you are ready to help yourself then, boil *ruda*, rue, *romero*, rosemary, and *albahaca*, basil. Let the water sit for one night and bathe in the water the next Friday, while praying and making your petition to God and to the Niño. Ask the Virgin Mary to intercede for you. Invoke the sacred name of the Holy Spirit three straight times asking to be favored before the eyes of man according to the will of God the Father, Jesus the Son and God the Holy Spirit. Ask for protection of Saint Michael the Archangel, and health of body, soul, and spirit of Saint Rafael and happiness of Saint Gabriel. These are the three archangels. Take the baths for seven Fridays in a row without missing at the same time of day or night.

I know it is awful to be alone. Loneliness is a very difficult and sad situation. The Niño Fidencio will walk with you and accompany you if you have true faith. He will comfort and console you in your hour of need. You will see how quickly your luck will change and God will grant you a good job. You will have your good health, money and blessings in abundance in your home, love and happiness. It is up to you to change your attitude and behavior.

COMMENTARY:

The faith that many people have in the Niño Fidencio is no less supportive or significant than one's faith in God. For those who believe, the Niño Fidencio is a saint who sits at the right hand of God and seeks his intercession on behalf of those who petition assistance.

130. HOMELESS — *SIN TECHO*

I am desperately trying to find a place to live. My husband has gotten to be really bad and I want to leave him. I have been offered a very good paying job and I am wondering if it's a sign to take it so I can leave my husband and live alone with my kids. I called the housing authority and they said my application is really close to the top and that I will probably be picked in the next group to be called for a house. So I am going to try to stick it out until I can find a place to live. I will stick it out as long as he is not abusive to my son.

CURANDERO'S RESPONSE:

Please say the prayer to Saint Edwin and to the El Niño Fidencio for nine consecutive days. Fast in the morning during these nine days of prayer. After you pray, open your Holy Bible to Psalm 119. There are a total of 22 verses, so recite three verses per day. One in the morning, one at noon, and one before you go to bed. Pray to Saint Benedict Labre on April 16, to protect you from homelessness.

The first thing every morning make your petition and ask for what you want to happen in your life. If you fast and pray in the morning, you can expect that God will grant you a miracle and open the road for you, *abre camino*.

COMMENTARY:

Prayer and curanderismo go hand-in-hand. In fact, you can say it's a symbiotic relationship of spirituality; encompassing all remedies and situations. This woman is approaching desperation, wants to leave her husband and is afraid of his abusive behavior to their son.

The curandero suggests she offer a novena, nine days of prayer and fasting in his hope that she will receive a miracle; allowing her to escape from this desperate situation.

131. BAD LUCK — *LA MALA SUERTE*

We have two children, 10 and six years old. I'm writing to tell you that my husband and I are desperate. First of all, he was fired from a very good job and we have no idea why. They are now giving him very bad references and it is hurting his ability to get another job. He has applied with several good firms and so far he has not found a permanent job. This year, lots of things have happened to us. We had an accident, but luckily our children were not with us and it was something minor. I've been hospitalized several times, one for the accident, the other for gastritis, and the other for an endoscopy. My blood pressure went up while they were checking for ulcers. Test results came back showing I was in good health. But I feel a burning sensation like hot peppers that starts in my stomach, goes to my chest, and then to my arms.

Do you have any idea what I have and can you help my husband get a job?

CURANDERO'S RESPONSE:

My regards to you and your husband, I understand that you find yourselves in a desperate situation. Let's continue to fight the battle. I hope that you are able to boil some aromatic herbs so that you and your husband can bathe with them, and get rid of this bad spell that was cast on you both.

The herbs you will be using for those baths are pepper tree, rue, rosemary, common basil and *chaparral*. You should do these seven days straight at about noon and then cleanse yourselves with a wooden crucifix while reciting the Our Father and asking the Lord to help you with your needs. Also, cleanse yourselves with incense such as white *copal*, the sacred resin incense of the Aztecs and Mayans. Add a mixture of storax, hibiscus, mixed with ground coffee and brown sugar. Add bay leaves and dry rosemary. This should take care of your bad luck and may God bless you.

Let's plead with our Lord for your petition so that your husband and you will soon recuperate totally and be able to find a good job. Did they let him go from work for a motive or reason? It looks like someone continues to give out bad recommendations. How much longer can you continue to take this bad deed that keeps happening? I hope the Lord answers your prayers very soon. Our God will have mercy toward your needs.

COMMENTARY:

Securing and retaining a job is crucial in the Latino culture. Traditionally, Latinos possess an exceptionally strong work ethic. Latinos face many challenges and often, many have not even completed high school. This is compounded by inadequate transportation and/or proper child-care options.

In this case, the curandero is treating the patient for the ill fortune and job loss, but he does not address the gastrointestinal symptoms. It is always important that both the physician and curandero ask the patient to consult each one in a complementary way. Many medical doctors might best be approached by the patient and mention that the curandero is used for the patient's spiritual well-being during the physical healing process.

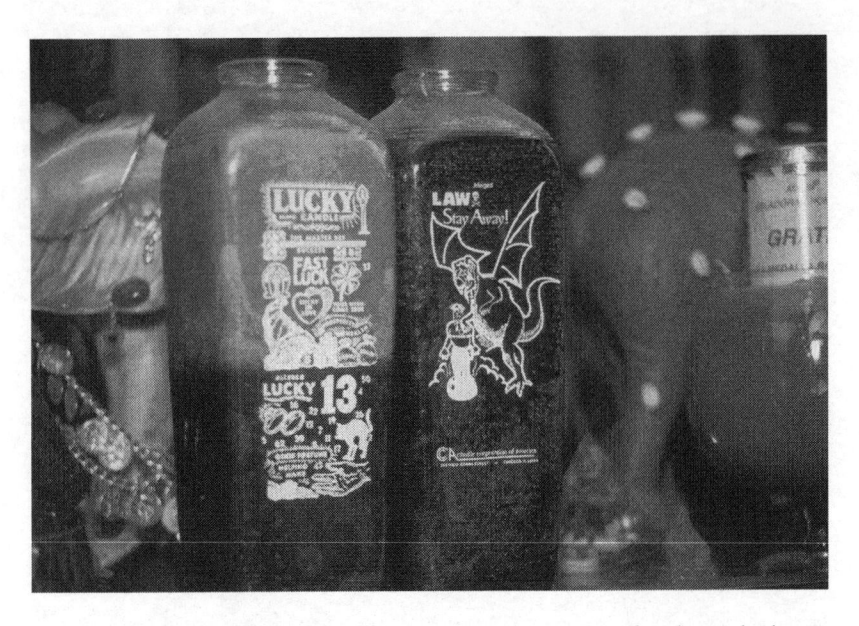

Pre-prepared votive candles intended to attract luck and to keep the law away are displayed here. (Photo by José M. Duarte)

PART EIGHT

Healing Injustice: In and Out of Jail

"I served as a partera for more than 40 years delivering thousands of babies. Now they are all grown up and they live all over the country. They always come back to see me when they are in need of special help or are in trouble. They don't have faith in the system but they have faith in me and especially in God."

— †Josefa Contreras, partera and curandera

132. DARK SECRET — *SECRETO OBSCURO*

I am sorry to have asked for something, and I am writing you from work. My home computer went out. My ugly, dark secret is out and it has totally broken my heart. We now know that there is widespread multi-generational sexual abuse and incest going on in our family. I can now bring myself to talk to you about it because it gives me peace of mind. I hope that you, with your connection to divine intervention, can help us recover peace of mind in our families. I thank you for all your prayers.

All was going well with all the older kids when we got a visit from my oldest son. I spoke to you before about my youngest son having emotional issues. Everything was going well with his therapy, but some days are better than others. I noticed that he is depressed a lot. I asked his therapist to get him into a home where he could get more help than just going once a week. She said that only in severe cases would they accept him into a facility.

Sometimes I feel so hopeless because I cannot help him enough. It was in that situation when my daughter called and told me what had happened. I tried to understand what she was saying. When we got out of the therapy session, my son broke down in tears and told me that he had sexually molested his younger sister. He was so sorry and crying. That is when I learned that he had also been sexually abused by his other sister. One sister molested him, and he in turn, molested his younger sister.

During our visit, the therapist called a hotline and was told that the police were coming to interview him. That is when he was picked up and taken into custody. I spoke to a public defender and she said it was going to be a difficult case. We have tried to provide mental health records for them to review, but for some reason the defender keeps putting my son's case off and our court dates have been continuously postponed. Why do they keep putting it off?

I asked my friend who worked for an attorney if they could help me. She spoke to her friend, the attorney who said that he might be able to help us.

In the meantime, so many things have happened to him in custody. The place that he is in is very dangerous. They took his glasses from him and broke them. The other kids tried to make him fight for them. I saw him after his last court appearance and he looked very scared. They tried getting a therapist to visit him, but I am not sure they did.

I have been praying the Rosary and have placed a glass of water to the spirit on my home altar. I have also asked my son to pray. Please help us. It is very painful for the whole family. I cannot see any of my daughters because they have been removed from the home. They cannot come over to my house, which is a very depressed and lonely place. Please help this mother who is scared for her son and daughters.

I want him to get intense therapy. I don't want him in that place anymore. Please help us.

CURANDERO'S RESPONSE:

Your explanation will help me better understand where I can be of assistance to you and your family. Check the *hierberías* and New Age stores for a Saint Eduviges candle or prayer card. The prayer to her is stamped on the back of the candle or card. Say the prayer to her spirit, which will help you with your son's mental and emotional state and condition. Also pray to Santa Agueda the patron of sexual abuse and to Saint Louise on March 15, that the social workers you encounter will be compassionate. Please continue to inform me how matters develop.

I pray your house, your family and your heart will once again be filled with happiness and joy. Your faith has given you strength. The Holy Spirit will not abandon you and your family. Things are very bad now, but your hope and prayers will be answered. The Holy Spirit will bless you, and your family will become better for it. Since your children have been taken by the State and are currently parentless, you should pray to Saint Jerome for them to be returned to you and to their home. His saint's day is February 8. I shall walk with you in spirit and shall help you all. The Lord will allow me to do this for your needs.

COMMENTARY:

The family in this tragic story has been torn apart. Only by intensive and constant counseling along with the curandero's support can it be healed. Families of faith must combine counseling with faith in God. The curandero serves as the intermediary between God and the reality of this world.

Saint Eduviges is not very well known in the Latino world of curanderismo. She spent her lifetime pushing back against the trials and tribulations of life and knew that sacrifice and good works are the way to God. She is the patron saint of incarcerated persons as well as needy and suffering women.

133. ARRESTED FOR DRUGS — *ARRESTADA*

My mom was arrested an hour ago. She has a warrant for dealing drugs. Please help her! I am so worried. She is basically a good person, but has made some bad mistakes in her life. She helps many other people who are less fortunate and has a ton of faith. But now her mistakes have caught up with her. Please pray and tell me what I need to do to help my mom.

My aunt said she is going to call you later this evening and hopefully you will e-mail me back soon. Please help us.

I have two younger sisters and they are very scared and my dad is trying to figure out a way to get the money to get my mom out of jail. She has a cash bond and it is going to be very hard to get her out. No bondsmen are allowed, just cash. Please help us!

CURANDERO'S RESPONSE:

Your mom is in the criminal justice system now and it will be very hard for me to do much for her, but I will pray for her. I will pray to Saint Maximilian Kolbe, the patron saint of drug addiction. I know he will help her beat this terrible addiction. His day is August 14. Pray to Saint Faustina Kowalska on October 5 for your mother to have mercy.

First of all, she will need a good attorney. May our prayers give her strength, and I pray that if she comes out of this, she will refrain from ever doing anything like selling drugs again. That is putting her children and the welfare of others at risk. But I am afraid the Holy Spirit is telling me that this time your mother is going to do some hard time.

COMMENTARY:

The competent and successful curandero knows when to refer a client to medical care or legal help. Ongoing counseling is important, but in today's world, one must know how to work with and against the system. The curandero has worked with this family for years but this time he seems to be resigned to the fact that the mother is going to jail. The curandero's support will have to shift to the children left at home without a mother, and how to help guide them along the right path.

134. HARD TIME — *ENCARCELADO*

I have been very reluctant to ask for your guidance because I don't know if I would be able to handle any bad news you may have for me. I have been married for over three years, and my husband has been in prison for almost seven and a half years for drug trafficking. He is to be released in about two years. So, he has now been moved out of maximum security to a potential release location.

I have doubted his feelings for me because I found a letter from a so-called pen pal he has, who he says has fallen in love with him. To me, this is infidelity. When I questioned him about it, he simply said he was sorry, but that he did it because he wanted to see if he could get money out of her and he wanted someone else to write to. I guess I have some fault in this because I don't write to him as often as I should. Recently, he said that he does not feel that I love him. He told me that he didn't care if I was with another man. I know this is the end of our marriage.

I was very hurt by this, and he doesn't seem to understand the extent that it hurt me. It makes me wonder if he will be faithful when he comes home. Sometimes I think we should just get a divorce and get it over with. But that is not what I want. I do love him and I miss him and I feel that he is my soul mate and he is the person I want to spend my life with. He's been in prison for so many years and that has really made me struggle with the thought of our being together again after so many years. It will be like sleeping with someone you don't know.

His first wife is no help at all. She told me this weekend that my husband has asked her to get a divorce packet from the courthouse and mail it to him, and for her to pick up his things from my house. She also said he wants to get back together with her when he gets out.

It upsets me that my husband would talk to his ex-wife about our personal matters other than about the children they share. My *comadre*, (a ritual kinship term used by those who co-participate in a baptism as a godparent) said not to pay any mind to what she said; that she just wants to upset me and she's jealous. My *comadre* was going to write to my husband to let him know what she'd said. I don't want to divorce my husband, but I don't want to question his feelings either. I think he and I deserve to be happy, and to give our marriage the chance to strengthen when he finally is able to come home. I don't want to give up on him. I want to be able to speak to him face to face, not just by mail, especially about something as important as divorce. I want to know if he really does want a divorce. He does tell me to let him be a father to my daughter if we split up, and that he will always love me no matter what. He has been great with my daughter and he is the only father she knows. I don't know what to do.

He called me to wish me a happy Mother's Day, and it was the greatest feeling to hear his voice again. My daughter was just as happy to hear from him. I really can't afford to visit him, but I am going to try to go some weekend soon. It is a 20-hour drive, so it is very hard. My step-kids also said he was going to be released this year or next year. I wish they'd just bring him back so he would be closer and I could visit him at least every other weekend like I used to. Please let me know what you feel is in our future. Thank you so much.

CURANDERO'S RESPONSE:

I see very serious troubles for all of you. From what you tell me, I can tell you have been holding up well on your own so far. Your *comadre* is right. Do not listen to his ex-wife. Listen to your heart and try to feel what is in his heart and begin each day anew. I feel that it is critical that you speak to him face to face no matter how difficult that may be. You must have some advanced notice of what to expect and prepare now before he is released. I wish you both much happiness and the best in life, but it will probably not be as a couple. I will light a candle to Santos Inés and Daniel for you and I will keep you in my prayers. Santa Inés protects against infidelity and Santo Daniel protects spouses who are away from the family. And finally, the Santo Niño de Atocha protects prisoners while they are away from home. He is celebrated on December 15. Pray Psalm 19 for those who are in prison or going to prison.

COMMENTARY:

Sadly, this case reflects situations all too familiar in Latino culture. Within the Latino population at large, there's an inordinate number of Latinos in our nation's prisons; placing extreme hardship on their families, friends and loved ones. It is critical that those on the outside be provided with ongoing counseling during the time a family member is in prison. Prison life is definitely not normal, and raises all sorts of unforeseen problems for the family at home. Additionally, there are many unseen and unspoken pressures the inmate faces which those on the outside cannot even begin to comprehend.

135. WINNING IN COURT — *JUSTO JUEZ*

Is there a certain candle that is used to influence the outcome of court cases? I know that there is and that it is blue. What I don't understand is does the glass have to be blue, the wax or both? Also, if I want to win my divorce case, I was told to put my husband's picture under the candle and to have a plain glass of water next to the candle. Is this correct?

CURANDERO'S RESPONSE:

Yes, there is a specially-made candle for petitions for legal matters and court cases and it comes in a blue wax. You may use a plain, blue wax candle if you do not find the original. You may also elect to use a Saint Jude candle, the patron saint for impossible causes and a *justo juez*, or just judge, candle. Saint Joan of Arc may always be invoked to protect the powerless against the powerful. Her day of celebration is on May 30. Either one will work. Pray Psalms 38 and 39 to protect those who are being punished by the law. Importantly, the correct candle for a court case is always in blue wax. Yes, place the glass of water over your husband's picture next to the candle you have lit.

COMMENTARY:

The use of justo juez and law-stay-away candles has become increasingly popular in the Latino community. Additionally, powders, oils, sprays and other items are believed to be spiritually effective in legal cases. As an unfortunate side note, La Santísima Muerte, Malverde, Pancho Villa and other entities are commonly used to influence the law and legal cases. They are not bad, in and of themselves, but are frequently used by people who commit evil deeds. Attempting to influence outcomes of court cases has become a common exercise among law-abiding citizens as well as scofflaws.

136. DRUGS KILL — *DROGAS DESTRUYEN*

I wrote to you before and am writing again in regards to my out-of-control life! I have been smoking marijuana for a long time and I have used other kinds of drugs as well. I was in a yearlong abusive relationship and have been in jail 10 times or more and I am finally ready to go straight. I prayed last night for the first time in a long time. I left my boyfriend and all my friends to free myself from the pressure to do drugs. I do not want to be close to them. I am scared because I am still in trouble with the cops, the court and probation. I am ready to clean up my life and serve God, for once and all. I want to confess all of my sins and start over.

I regret and hate the things I have done in my life. I am a very smart girl who the Lord has blessed with many talents. I do not want to go to jail again. I no longer want any drugs in my body. I am ready to start over without my old boyfriend coming around.

I do not want to be weak and give into the pressure of drugs. I want a new life and I want to be finally out of trouble! Please, is there anything I can do to get my body clean of these drugs, other than giving it time? Are there any prayers you can send me to help me? Most of all, please pray for me!

CURANDERO'S RESPONSE:

The Holy Spirit turns away from those who disobey Him. It is good that you have repented from evil and your wicked ways. It is good that you want to turn your back on disobedience and turn to the Lord's ways.

Pray to Saint Maximilian Kolbe that you abandon a life of drugs and I pray that the Lord will answer your prayers and bestow His blessings in abundance upon you. Are you ready to take the high road in your life? Allow your spirit to be your guide. You have reached a critical fork in the road of your life. It has become clear to you which path to take. The journey through life can be what you are willing to make it. The best in life will not come easy. It will take hard work to get you to where you want to be. If you live your convictions, it will help you live a happy and full life. The spirit of Fidencio will help you through hard times. If you truly are ready to confess you must do it out loud and pray to Saint Pio the patron of confession to hear your confession and to absolve you of your sins. His day is September 23.

COMMENTARY:

As in all populations, many Latinos suffer from a combination of physical and emotional issues; exacerbated by social and cultural nuances. Often, these individuals are unable to access professional counseling, so they turn to culturally-based systems like curanderismo. Additionally, they feel more at ease talking to someone from their own culture.

137. THE BIG LAW FIRM — *GANANDO LA CAUSA*

I'm writing to you for my mother. She wants me to ask you to pray for her upcoming court date. A while back, she was injured on the job. Her back has been hurt very badly since then. She is trying to get restitution due to her for her loss of wages. The corporate lawyers are going against her in a big way in this case. It is a pretty big law firm. She is worried because some things they ask her about she cannot remember. She is worried that her bad memory will be held against her. The lawyers are not very nice either and she is intimidated by them. She thinks her own lawyers will sell her out to the corporate lawyers. You know how it works. Please pray for her. She has so many doctor bills and debts, it's outrageous. She worries constantly about this, and she just prays it will work out in her favor.

CURANDERO'S RESPONSE:

I pray your mother is feeling better. Have her use essence of basil for money-drawing purposes. Spiritual-healing baths with *loción de siete machos*, seven male goats' lotion, added to her bath water should help. She should make a small green pouch out of cloth and place *cáscara sagrada*, holy bark, three *ojos de María*, Mary's eyes beans, three *lágrimas de San Pedro*, Saint Peter's tears beans, *semillas de mostaza negra*, black mustard seed, and three *colorines*, red beans, inside the pouch. She should bless it with Holy Water and carry it with her for money drawing and protection. Finally, pray Psalm 5 for the outcome of court cases. She can find all the items I have requested at any *hierbería*. Let me know how it goes with her.

Finally you are going to need spiritual assistance and you should light a candle on your home altar for Saint Peter of Verona and to Saint Ivo who will send you a powerful lawyer. Saint Peter's days are April 6 and 29 while Saint Ivo's day is May 19.

COMMENTARY:

Curanderos are often consulted for court and legal cases that seem insurmountable to the petitioner. As in this case, the woman who has been injured is facing a formidable corporate law firm. Since she is not likely to find adequate help on the physical plane of life, she must enlist support from the spirit world to win. The curandero recommends that she create a spell for attracting money and for spiritual cleansing. Bathing with spiritual water is an often prescribed remedy. Loción siete machos, is a widely-used scented water or florid water used in spiritual healing and rituals. It is one of the most popular spiritual waters. It may be found at any hierbería. The green amulet pouch containing the cáscara sagrada herb, sacred husk, three lágrimas de María seeds, tears-of-Mary seeds, three lágrimas de San Pedro, Saint Peter seeds, black mustard, and three colorín seeds are highly recommended for attracting money. Colorín, lágrimas de María and San Pedro are seeds found at most hierberías or botánicas.

138. GOING CRAZY —*VOLVIÉNDOME LOCA*

I just wanted to tell you that I do not know what is wrong with my head. I feel like I'm going crazy. I feel almost insane. My mind says bad words on its own and it feels satanic, like there is a demon making me say these words. I do not know what to do when my mind comes up with the weirdest evil thoughts. I am afraid that when I get like this I will hurt someone or myself. I do not want to go back to jail, but I need help. I am also afraid that I will never get out of purgatory when I die.

I think that I picked up an evil spirit in prison and, when I got out, the evil spirit left prison with me. I had to go to Mexico to find someone to remove this demon from me. I felt God's mighty power and I felt the Niño's power work through this man in Mexico, who healed me.

My grandpa used to work with El Niño, also, but he died 11 years ago. He used to work with the spirit of San Miguel Arcángel and channel him through his body. My grandfather understood these things, but my father does not.

I don't get along with my dad and he does not understand what I am going through. He is a man of faith in God and he knows that evil is out there, but he doesn't believe that witchcraft works and that it can be used to kill someone.

I have so many psychological problems. I do not know if I am crazy or not, but I do know I cannot handle it anymore. I seek guidance from the Niño and I just want to live in peace. God bless you and all who have this blessed power.

A *curandera* told me that my 10-year-old brother has the gift of healing, but he does not have faith in his power and does not try to use it. I hope that someday he can know that God has blessed him as you are blessed.

I feel paranoid and have many worries. I do not know what to think, but I do know that I really need the Niño's help. I am praying for help and it seems to be working, but I really would like to talk to you in person. I am also worried that I may still be possessed by spirits that I cannot control. They control me. I would like to be blessed by you. I worry so much about my little brother who is also traveling the dark path. His mouth is full of fire from the lies he tells.

CURANDERO'S RESPONSE:

What you have related to me is very sad. You are suffering so much. If only your father could bring you to me for healing. In the past, I have conducted spiritual-healing rituals for others who were in the same state and condition that you describe you are in and suffering through. I know that in the past you have informed me your father is not willing to bring you here. Why don't you try cleansing yourself?

Go to a Catholic Church with a small vial and fill it with Holy Water from the back of the church. If someone asks you what you want it for, tell them it's for your home altar, which is true but don't tell them you are seeing a *curandero*. Go straight home after you get the water and bathe in it. If you have a violent reaction from the Holy Water then you are surely possessed by an evil spirit. Ask your father to take you to a priest or go yourself right away.

Pray your father will change his mind and bring you to me or find some way to get here on your own. And don't be afraid of purgatory. Pray to the *ánimas solas,* or souls, in purgatory and to Saint Odilo the patron of getting souls out of purgatory. His day is January 1. Only then, may God grant me the ability to help you.

COMMENTARY:

In this case the young man is suffering from many emotional problems worsened by his time spent in prison. He was treated for demonic possession and was raised in a family with a grandfather who channeled spirits. He was drawn to the spiritual lifestyle, but upon the death of his grandfather, a void transformed his life. He had no way of summoning the spirits after his grandfather died since his father is not a believer. He lacks a support base in his belief in the spirit world. His father, who is a Catholic, rejects his son's beliefs and provides no emotional support for his son. The curandero senses this, and wisely recommends that a Catholic priest become involved for counseling and/or an exorcism. This must be supported by the father for sorely-needed family harmony.

139. MOLESTING STEPFATHER — *ABUSADA*

Oh my goodness, where do I begin? Last night my daughter told me and my other kids that my husband, her stepfather, has been molesting her for years. I was so shocked I got a restraining order against him, and the older kids were placed with their biological dad just to make sure that I am taking the right measures to put him away. Now, child protective services are involved and it has been so awful. My children are out of my home, even though they are just five minutes away. The silence in the house is deafening and it is killing me. I cried all night, the first night, and all day today. I miss my children so much.

I am so scared for my little girl. How could I not have seen this? Am I so blind? Looking back now, I see it clearly. I blame myself. I should have left him and gotten my children away from him a long time ago. Please help me get my kids back. I am so scared for them and myself as well. How could he have done this to his stepdaughter? Please help us.

CURANDERO'S RESPONSE:

May the Spirit of the Lord give you strength to see you through this entire terrible ordeal. You must ask the Virgen de Guadalupe to assist you. The good news is that she had the courage to tell you about it and you did not let her down; otherwise, it could have gone on for many more years. Prayer and meditation will, with time, make very clear what really happened and what did not.

I will pray for you and your children, and for you to be protected by the Spirit of God. Please keep me informed and let me know if I can be of help in any way.

COMMENTARY:

This is another terribly desperate case requiring the curandero to engage the shattered family in prayer. In all likelihood, once the legal ramifications of this case play out, everyone involved will need years of support and counseling by professionals, as well as a permanent support network with curanderos.

140. PLEA AGREEMENT — *UN ACUERDO*

We have been offered a plea agreement in a case that my husband is charged in and we are not sure what to do. It wouldn't be much jail time, but we were wondering if we accept it, would we still have a chance of getting back together and adopting children together in the future. I was just wondering if there is anything that I can do to make this go smoothly and have my husband back home with me and not have to spend much more time in jail. I was told that he should not plead guilty to anything, especially to things we know that are not true and that he is not guilty of. I will keep the candles burning until this is resolved and I will keep the faith. I was also told that all he needs to do is have faith and it will work out.

Once before, we took a plea on something he was not guilty of and it backfired on us. I do not want him to do it again. Would it be wrong to accept the plea? On the other hand, if we do not take the plea, will everything work out for us? My biggest worry is that it will turn around on us again. You know you can't beat the system. We go to court today to have verbal arguments on inconsistencies in the case and the prosecuting attorney is trying to combine two different cases against him into one case. The system has already started stacking things up against him. If we take a plea agreement, we can put this behind us and hopefully move on, but I don't trust them. Can you see if we will have any chance of adopting down the road?

CURANDERO'S RESPONSE:

Your husband should not plead guilty if he is not guilty, but I know it's not that easy. If your husband pleads guilty, he will most likely not be allowed to adopt children in the future. What is his lawyer doing for him? Did the adoption agency say you could not adopt?

A plea agreement is not an admission of guilt. He has not yet been found guilty of any crime. You have other children you should be thinking of now, and not of adoption at this time. Our prayers are with you, please pray to Saint Nicolás of Myra, who is the patron saint of lost law cases. We know you care very much for each other. May the good Lord grant you all the miracles that you need so desperately. Pray Psalm 26 for those who are in danger of imprisonment and to Saint Blandina on June 2 for those who have been falsely accused.

COMMENTARY:

Other than family members, the curandero may be the only person who has followed certain cases over time and who is in a position to offer wise advice. Issues and judgment in legal cases can become murky. Due to his experience in this case, the curandero wisely advises the family not to accept a plea bargain.

141. CAN'T BE GOOD — *MALO MALOSO*

I am so sorry for the way I have gone back to my old ways. I really do want to be a better person. I don't want to do things to get me put in jail again, but they just seem to happen to me. I think my life is *salada*, or someone is doing witchcraft on me. Up to now, I have kept myself from calling my drug dealer and I will continue to be strong. I so badly just want things to get better. I am so lonely and scared.

I am so sorry for backsliding while everyone is praying and looking out for me. I have been home from jail for nearly five days and I feel better about that, but I just feel so empty. The drugs make me forget my loneliness. I guarantee you, if you could please just help me just once more, I will make sure to keep trying and doing good. I will try my best not to backslide into drugs as I have done repeatedly before. For the first time, I feel like this is a real new start.

CURANDERO'S RESPONSE:

You are not alone. The Holy Spirit and the spirit of El Niño Fidencio are with you. Together, we will give you strength, valor, spiritual guidance and protection. You may light a candle to the *Sagrado Corazón*, Sacred Heart of Jesus. Place a clear glass of water next to the candle. Say your daily prayer where your candle and the glass of water are located and the spirits of light will answer you.

COMMENTARY:

A curandero who has received a true calling, a gift from God, is not judgmental. In life, people have ups and downs and then lapse into destructive patterns of behavior again. They are always welcomed back into the world of the Holy Spirit and of God. The understanding and compassionate nature of healers is usually the same as that of El Niño Fidencio when he lived. Everyone is capable of change and can heal if the desire exists.

142. TEMPTATION —*TENTACIÓN*

Thank you so much for your advice. It has helped me out a lot. I lighted my candle and have been praying and have been going to church the past two Sundays. But I am still having some trouble letting go of drugs. Please keep praying for me. I am struggling with a few things, namely temptation to do drugs and depression. I get tempted to do the things that I know would keep my mind off my problems for the moment. I know that if I do that, I will get caught and go back to jail.

I am depressed because I seem to hear about my ex-husband every day from different people. Everyone wants to tell me about his new job and I've been told that he is now dating an old friend of mine. I keep thinking about how unfair it is. I was the one that was always there for him, and he hit me and talked to me so badly. He showed me absolutely no respect. And to make matters worse, he is the one that got me hooked on drugs.

CURANDERO'S RESPONSE:

Thanks to God, you are free from the chains of drugs and the abusive relationship you were in. Your old girlfriend will find out soon enough what kind of man he is. You are the lucky and the blessed one, not your girlfriend. He is unclean and he wishes he could be free like you, but he does not have the desire or the strength like you do. You are more powerful than he is. You are moving in the right direction. Keep going. I will continue to help you. You are not alone. He is empty inside. Pray to Saint John the Evangelist to help keep you away and out of the influence of bad friends. Pray for him on December 27 in order to know God. Be strong and keep me posted.

COMMENTARY:

It is not unusual for two girlfriends competing for the affection of the same man to consult the same curandero/a. In this case, the curandero/a, has a professional obligation to maintain a client relationship just as if he/she were practicing in a licensed environment. Failure of exercising ethical discretion can produce tragic results for all involved. Authentic curanderos/as must maintain a high level of personal integrity, as well as uphold a personal oath between themselves and God.

143. PRAY FOR FATHER — *ORAR POR MI PADRE*

I came to you for prayers for my father's driving while intoxicated (DWI) case and for help to defeat his girlfriend who is mocking my family and my deceased mother. You told me to light a San Alejo candle to push away evil. The store where I purchase my candles ran out of San

Alejo and told me to use a candle called "to take away from," or *el retiro*. They said that it served the same purpose. The glass jar is turning black and the flame is very high. I was told this is because the candle is doing its job. Is that correct? Please keep us in your prayers now more than ever. My dad is now engaged to that woman and they are supposed to be leaving the area. We will see.

CURANDERO'S RESPONSE:

It is okay to use the *retiro* candle so long as you use a red one as opposed to a black candle. The difference is that the black wax will draw unclean or even evil spirits to execute the petition similar to the power of black magic. Red wax is a more powerful influence and the petition is carried out by divine and celestial spirits.

COMMENTARY:

In curanderismo, we frequently see aspects of sympathetic magic in use. That means the direct cause-and-effect association. In this case, the standard use of the San Alejo candle comes from the Spanish verb alejar, to get away from or push away. The saint's name, Alejo, is seen as the embodiment of the action desired.

The retiro candle is the same, but leaves the realm of saints out and delves into pure, unadulterated magic. The curandero wisely advises the petitioner to use the red candle, which is used for benign magic while the appropriately-named black candle is used for black magic and summons dark spirits for support. At all costs, one must always stay away from black magic and never seek to do someone physical harm.

144. GOING TO COURT — *CORRIENDO CORTE*

I am requesting your prayer for my entire family. I would also like to request your prayer for my son who is not with me because I have been separated from his mom for a year now. I have not seen my son ever since then and I really do miss him. I will go to court soon for child support and I really am looking forward to going because I really want my visitation rights as his father to be able to see and be with my son. He is five years old and he needs me. I love and miss him a lot, and he looks like me.

Another thing that I am having problems with is the law. I am on four-year probation for hanging out with the wrong friends. Now, I am the one paying the price and my friends are no longer friends. I feel as if I am on a chain that I cannot take off of me. It seems that every time I take a step forward in life, I end up taking two steps backward.

I need help to see how the world would be for me without feeling any worries, having my son by my side and the law off my shoulders. I pray to God for that to come true for me some day. Please pray for me that I may resolve my issues.

CURANDERO'S RESPONSE:

Please place fresh hen eggs, a head of garlic, lemons and a *piedra alumbre*, alum rock, or whatever you have or can find, and leave them on your home altar overnight. The following day, use all those objects to give yourself a *limpia,* or spiritual cleansing, rubbing the egg, or lemon, or garlic head over your body and saying one Our Father and making your petition. Do this in front of your altar. Pray Psalms 35 and 36. It can be done any day. Dispose of what you use for your cleansing by throwing it outside of your home and yard in the trash. Please keep me posted.

COMMENTARY:

Problems of life and family seemingly bury a person who cannot see the proverbial "light at the end of the tunnel." Cultural situations require cultural resolutions. In this case, the curandero recommends fresh hen's eggs, garlic, lemons or piedra alumbre, or alum rock, be placed on an altar overnight. These are items that are commonly used in cleansing in cases of susto, fright sickness, or mal de ojo, evil eye, and can be easily located. By placing them on the altar overnight, they are believed to pick up or absorb positive spiritual strength. Through these items, the limpia, spiritual-cleansing ritual, absorbs the bad spirits or negative thoughts from the person's body and transfers them to the objects. The tainted objects must be disposed of outside of the home; preferably at another location.

145. NO MORE JAIL — *NUNCA MÁS*

Thank you for all the work you have done on my mother's behalf. She is home and safe right now. I just pray and have faith that she will come out of this okay. I pray that she never goes back to jail or anywhere even worse.

I have been walking in my faith to the best of my ability. I pray and read my Holy Bible. I believe in the miracles God provides and I have been truly happy. My mother, father, my husband and I, and my two little sisters live in our house together.

One of my sisters is a senior in high school and I just know that she is going to be something wonderful some day. Please pray for her. We all worry about her. She is never home, is failing school, and feels her friends are the most important thing to her. Please pray for her protection. We really want her to realize how much we love her and how wonderful she is. She is beautiful and smart, she makes friends easily, and she is good to those friends. However, she does not show much respect to my parents, to her teachers or me.

She talks about dropping out of school. We want her to finish high school. She can graduate if she wants to and we know it. She says she hates us and never wants to come home. She says we fight with her all the time. How do we get her to understand and do the things that a young lady should do for her family and her school. We need your help and advice please.

I am attaching a picture of her in case you need it for your prayers. Thank you again for the help you are giving my mother. We love her so much and are so happy she is home.

I also wanted you to know that I have been drug free for a couple of months now. I think one of my biggest battles in life was drugs. I really let the drugs get a hold of me. I have turned my life around and, with the power of God; I will stay away from drugs for the rest of my life. Something that has been on my mind a lot, though, is that I took a drug screening about a month ago. I had not done any drugs for about a month before this screening. That should have been enough time for the drug to leave my system, but the night before the drug screening a friend of mine was able to bring me an instant drug screening test kit from her work. I tested positive for marijuana and cocaine.

Then, of course, the next day my probation officer gave me a surprise drug screening. It was not instant, though. It was sent off to the lab. That was nearly a month ago and I am scheduled to see her five days from now. Two weeks after that drug screening, I had another screening at my probation office and I passed it and was able to be dismissed from my probation.

I know I have messed up a thousand times in my life, but I have changed. I do not need to go to jail again to learn. This is not like all the other times. I enjoy my life with God. I do not want to do drugs ever again. I made a promise to never go through that again and I mean it. I know and believe fully that the Niño Fidencio has worked a miracle in my life. I know that God and my loved ones have forgiven me of my sins.

Now I just battle with the thought of my mistakes coming back to haunt me, and having to go to jail for that first drug screening if it was a bad screening. Please have mercy on me and pray for me to pass. Please light candles and work magic on my behalf so I can pass. I missed the holidays last year; due to my drug use, I was put in jail. I was there for all the major holidays and missed my baby sister's birthday for the third year in a row. I do not want to put my family through that again.

Thank you for your prayers and concern and please do whatever you can for me. I still have the prayers you sent me before and I will make sure to start praying immediately. I will make sure to take your advice for my sister's welfare and will make sure to believe in myself and the blessings that I am going to receive. Thank you and God bless.

CURANDERO'S RESPONSE:

I am proud of how well you are doing. I truly believe it was a demon that was keeping you on drugs and now that's over. Let me tell you something, you have to be aware of the promises you are making to me. Please, I always believed in you and I always knew you could do it. Now you have to believe in yourself. You are worthy of being blessed and loved by the spirit of the Santo Niño de Atocha who is one of many saints that protect prisoners and help people to stay out of prison. Pray Psalm 71 to keep people out of jail.

You are out of the dark and you will help me pull your sister out of the dark and into the light and happiness of the love of the Holy Spirit of the Lord and Creator. I shall continue to keep your mother in my prayers.

Regarding your sister, purchase a packet of dry rosemary and grind it into a powder. Sprinkle a teaspoonful of rosemary powder on the floor on all the corners of your sister's room and one spoonful under the mattress of her bed and leave it there. Call on the Holy Spirit to help you with your petitions for her.

COMMENTARY:

We conclude this section with another long-existing and ongoing case that is being "managed" by the curandero. Belief in God and spiritualism are not mutually exclusive with a person's falling into a life which places them at odds with the law. As in this case, the petitioner will most likely spend the rest of her life in and out of jail and abusing drugs. In between the intermittent episodes when she is out of the judicial system's revolving door, she tries her best to help her family, but always falls back. In this case, she is fearful her younger sister is following in her foolhardy footsteps. The curandero assures her she is genuinely loved by God and blessed by the Holy Spirit in an attempt to keep her on a straight path. The rosemary powder is a spiritual aid intended to protect her sister.

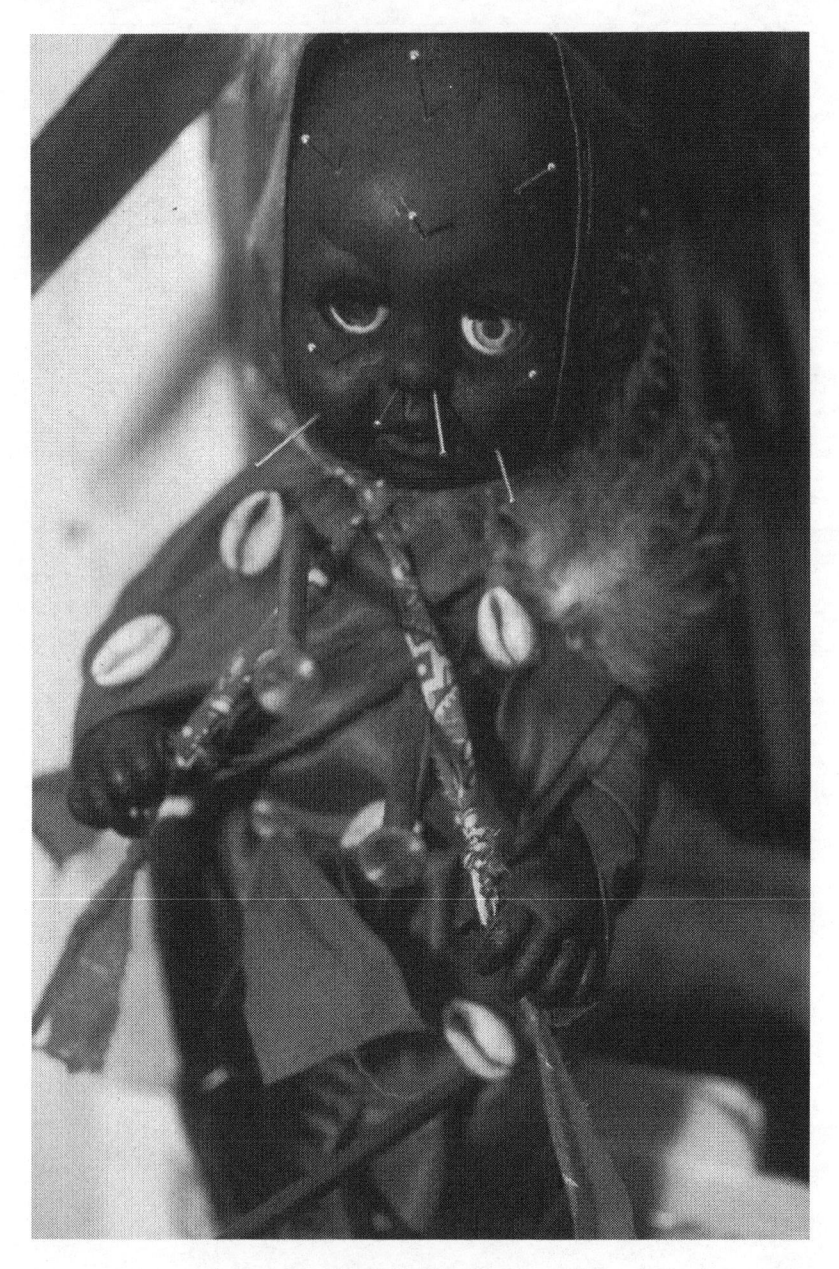

Mercado Sonora vendor displays a witchcraft doll intended to attract buyers to his shop. Witches require clients to purchase prepared dolls for the purpose of spell casting.
(Photo by José M. Duarte)

PART NINE

Healing the Evil Around Us: Witches, Spirits & Demon Possession

"Many Latinos consult curanderos because life is a constant search for the balance of extremes; religion versus folk religion; health versus illness; good versus evil, God versus devil; curandera versus bruja. The duality of the Latino cultural paradigm must be constantly nurtured and re-adjusted. If balance cannot be achieved, crisis, illness and even death loom in the near future."

– Antonio "Tony" Zavaleta, anthropologist

146. WITCHCRAFT SIGNS — *LAS SEÑALES*

How do I know if my problems are caused by a witchcraft spell?

CURANDERO'S RESPONSE:

To break the spell that has caused you such bad luck due to jealousies, envies and witchcraft that has been cast on you, recite the Prayer of the 12 Truths for nine consecutive days, cleansing your entire body with an alum rock. Burn the alum rock after the ninth day and study the rock as it burns, to see if you can see the face of the person who commissioned the witchcraft cast on you formed on the burning alum rock. Pray Psalm 40 to free you of evil spirits and witchcraft.

The Curandero's Prayer of the Twelve Truths

To all the stars in the heavens, I ask that you reveal the evil to me. I pray that the spell cast on me will be broken and that I might find the 12 truths that the Lord left for us in this world. I pray that I may be worthy of His love.

- One is the one Holy House in Jerusalem that the Lord left us.
- Two are the two tablets that the Lord gave Moses.
- Three is the Holy Trinity that the Lord gave us.
- Four are the four Gospels that the Lord gave us.
- Five are the five bleeding wounds the Lord suffered as He left the world.
- Six are the six candelabras that are burning on the altar of the Lord.
- Seven are the seven words that the Lord gave us.
- Eight are the eight pleasures that the Lord gave us.
- Nine are the nine months that the Lord was in Mary's womb.
- Ten are the Ten Commandments that the Lord gave us.
- Eleven are the eleven thousand virgins on the altar of the Lord.
- Twelve are the twelve apostles.

May the 13 rays of the sun illuminate my life, along with the 12 apostles; the eleven thousand virgins; the Ten Commandments; the nine months; the eight pleasures; the seven words; the six candelabras; the five wounds; the four Gospels; the Holy Trinity; Moses' two tablets; and the Holy House in Jerusalem. These are the 12 truths that the Lord left for us in the world. May I be worthy of the precious blood that His body shed for us.

COMMENTARY:

Curanderos believe that maladies originate from both natural and supernatural causes. Illnesses caused by nature may result from a perceived insult to God or a saint. Supernatural illnesses are caused by an agent like witches, or brujas, or warlocks, brujos. The curandero must first determine if an external agent is involved and this is accomplished by a combination of prayer and by the use of natural remedies.

If the remedy is unsuccessful, it is assumed that the illness or condition has a supernatural origin caused by a person on behalf of a petitioner. Here, the curandero has provided a prayer that can be used to identify and defeat a problem attributed to witchcraft. It is not always effective due to some very complicated and tenacious cases, but can be used in conjunction with other remedies with great success.

147. MOTHER IS CALLING ME — *ME ESTÁ LLAMANDO*

I have lived in the same house all of my life and I am now 65 years old. My grandmother, my mother and my father all died in the house where I live. It is a wonderful, loving house and I have never had any problems there, but recently I heard someone calling my name. They are calling me by the name my mother and grandmother used to call me, and at first I was scared. I knew it had to be one of them. What do you think I should do?

CURANDEROS RESPONSE:

This is a beautiful story you tell and you have nothing to fear. You do not have to fear the phantom, or *fantasma,* of your mother. You already know that there is nothing evil in your home. There are no wandering spirits, no devils in your home or in your life. What I sense is happening is either your mother or your grandmother has a message for you, or wants you to do something for them.

Light a candle on your home altar to Saint Vincent de Paul and ask him for spiritual tranquility and the next time you are called, call back: "what do you want? Give me a sign. Let me know what you want or leave me alone." This will work and you will both receive a message somehow and once you have completed the *manda,* or spiritual debt they assign you, they will leave you alone and return to the other side.

COMMENTARY:

It is a common belief in Latino culture that the diaphanous veil separating the physical world and the supernatural world is easily entered.

In fact, it is a major cultural belief that on November 2, el Día de los Muertos, the Day of the Dead, the portal to the ancestors is opened ever so briefly. Since ancestral worship is intrinsic in Latino culture, most are very cognizant of when their passed-on parents are trying to contact them. It is ill-advised to disregard these psychic signs. As the curandero suggests, simply speak out and ask for a sign from them. The ritual of calling out for a sign assists the living to appease the restless, deceased loved one.

148. THE SHE DEVIL — *LA DIABLA*

I want to ask you a question about this young man I know who works at our local flea market. He is very handsome and works for his aunt at her herb stall, or puesto de hierbas. He has jet-black hair and is always very *chiflado*, or spoiled, and very sure of his looks. All the girls around here just love him.

We all want him to be our boyfriend. But something very strange happened to him recently, and I wanted to know if it is really possible what they say happened. From one week to the next, his hair had streaks of gray in it and he became very nervous and shaky, even scared, or *asustado*. When I approached him, he turned away from me in fear.

He told the "flea market girls" that he was tricked by a heavy-set woman who came into his tía's *hierbería*, or his aunt's herb store, and charmed him. He said that she used his own tactics on him, turning herself into a beautiful young woman who charmed him into a mysterious night ride to a rural area out in the boonies, or *monte*, tricking him into making love to her. She revealed herself to him as a female devil, or *diablita*. She allowed all of the old women whom he had taunted before and ridiculed to torment him endlessly all night long and fulfilling their desires.

Is this possible? Could this really have happened to him to change him so completely? He is a nervous wreck and now he's afraid to even talk to us, the flea market, or *la pulga*, girls. I don't know if I should believe the story or not.

CURANDERO'S RESPONSE:

I try to tell people all the time that they must believe that evil is everywhere and that the devil is real. The head devil, Satan, has legions of little devils that do his bidding, and they are both male and female. He commands them to tempt us and to disrupt our lives. Those humans who are evil or mean to innocent people are especially vulnerable to demonic attacks. I can tell you that the story he tells is completely believable, and you should pity him.

His life has been changed forever because of his *chiflasón*, or spoiled behavior. He may never recover to become his old self, except for your prayers. Pray Psalm 131 for those who attract evil spirits. This is a good story that teaches us to always be aware of our actions, and that both angels and devils are watching us all the time.

COMMENTARY:

The personification of evil in the form of a devil or other demonic creatures is standard in all cultures. Most organized world religions teach people to be aware of their presence and stay away from them.

The most popular Christian iconography or representation of the devil as a red human form with horns and a pointed tail is rendered by the artist Carlos Gómez on this book's cover.

Many versions of pagan and Christian mythology also believe that Satan's minions, diablitos, or little devils, are able to command human beings to have sex with them. Human history is replete with examples of human and devil copulations.

149. EXORCISM — *EL EXORCISMO*

I almost called you this morning, but I think I will call you later or tomorrow morning about what I'm going to bring up.

I remember you telling me that when these strange things begin happening, you said that there were unclean spirits leading me down the wrong path. I got to thinking and pondering, and, most importantly, praying.

I have been having visions and dirty dreams about this girl I got involved with. I know that she suffers from many ailments and illnesses, such as anxiety, compulsiveness, and many other things.

Last night I went on the Internet and did some research on exorcism and possession and I found that there are experienced Roman Catholic priests that said that children who are unloved and neglected are extremely susceptible to possessions from evil or unclean spirits. I know for a fact that this was the case with this girl. She has complained to me that when she was a child her parents neglected her, and when she wanted to be loved and caressed. They always refused and pushed her away.

She and her mother told me that when she was only three years old, that her grandmother wanted her mother to buy the grandma's car and she always got really bad feelings about the car. Every time they were in the car, it felt as if death or an evil spirit was present in the car with her. They reluctantly bought the car from her grandma. Several months later her father was driving with the whole family in the car, and they were in a head-on collision with a drunk driver. The drunk driver was killed instantly as he flew through the windshield. Fortunately, her family survived.

I am convinced that the girl has many evil spirits in her body and her soul is desperately trying to fight them off. This fact manifests itself with all her illnesses trying to demoralize her. I also read that possession can manifest itself as depression, anxiety and sexual promiscuity.

All I ask from you is to please keep her in your prayers. She really needs to fight the dark forces that are bringing her down. Please let me know in your wise opinion what you think of this.

CURANDERO'S RESPONSE:

It is not uncommon or unnatural to dream about a person one becomes involved with. It is part of the transference of feelings by at least one of the two people and there is nothing wrong with that. There may be some truth to the statement that children who are unloved and neglected are extremely susceptible to possessions from evil or unclean spirits. The same could be said of children who are loved too much and who are paid too much attention. She could be just as susceptible to possessions from evil or unclean spirits.

If she has many evil spirits in her body as you believe she has, do you know if she has seen a priest or been examined for determination one way or another? Has she seen an exorcist to try to deliver her from such a state or condition? What has the medical or mental health profession done for her?

I have read and studied your e-mail, and I wondered how much professional help she has received, up to now? What other kind of help has she received, if any?

I need to know this before I can decide to develop a plan for treatment to try to help her recover. Begin to pray Psalms 29, 30, 31 and 59 for those who are possessed by demons.

COMMENTARY:

As the curandero points out, it is normal for the young man to have dreams about his female friend, as long as they are not bizarre. His dreams are not an indicator that the girl is possessed by unclean spirits. Latino culture espouses a spirit world of benign and evil spirits which play active roles in our lives. So, it is perfectly normal for this young man, who believes in unclean spirits, to wonder if demonic possession is a factor in the case of this girl. However, it would seem from the aforementioned facts he is reading way too much into the situation.

Very young children are known to have a much more acute sixth sense than most adults and it is unlikely that the young girl can remember very much about the purchase of a car when she was three. Because of the youth's strong belief in the spirit world, he is convinced that she retains many evil spirits. The curandero has been provided no evidence of this, and in fact, the problem may lie with the young man and not the girl.

He has no way of knowing what her actual condition is and is probably projecting his beliefs and apprehensions on her. His statement that the evil spirits are "manifested" through all of her illnesses, would lead us to believe that this is, in fact, an emotional situation which permeates his own life.

He may actually be trying to convey it to her in a kind of co-dependency situation.

Latino tenets routinely support and practice curanderismo; a belief system is thrust upon others within the circle of friends and/or family.

The surefire way to determine the facts about this situation is to take the young girl to a curandero who specializes in demonic possession for a detailed assessment. The curandero was very correct in asking the writer if the girl had been evaluated, either by a Roman Catholic priest or even by a psychologist. Before the curandero can develop a treatment plan, he will have to know her condition and history. Then, provide counseling while not reading too much into symptoms.

One of the negative effects of diagnosis of demonic possession and treatment by a curandero is that it produces a lifelong pattern of spiritual dependency resulting in a self-fulfilling prophecy. In fact, many times there is nothing actually wrong with the person. Most religions believe in evil or unclean spirits. Hence, belief in them means that they need to possess an unsuspecting and unprotected person. Finally, if a culture is so entrenched in the belief of spirit possession, then, that same culture must believe in and approve of, a person specializing in removal of evil spirits.

150. SMOKING OUT BAD SPIRITS—*EL SAHUMERIO*

I have noticed that both my home and business have been affected by the negative energies of certain persons who have visited them. Some of these persons, especially in my business, really wish me harm and I fear them and suspect them of doing witchcraft on me.

I remember as a young girl, my grandmother would perform a *sahumerio*, a smoking-house cleansing ritual, on our house after our hateful neighbor came into our home unannounced one time. I remember that my mother would burn some sort of incense and sprinkle prepared flower water around both our yard and home after our evil neighbor left.

Can you help me prepare and conduct this ritual because both my home and my business need it?

CURANDERO'S RESPONSE:

There are many products on the market for the purpose of cleansing and blessing a home or a business with a smoking incense concoction called a *sahumerio*. *Sahumerios* are used to rid the home of negative energies, evil influences, unclean spirits and bad emotions.

Sometimes a person might enter a home or business that is clearly unclean, or who leaves behind very negative forces. In cases like this, which are all too common, Holy Water from a church, or sometimes seven churches, is sprinkled around the outside and inside of the home or business. Successful house blessings require a *sahumerio,* or smoking-ritual cleansing, that could be a single ingredient or multiple ingredients. For example, a tree or plant resin incense, such as *copal,* mirra, or *estoraque,* or storax, leaf or bark incense as well as other parts of plants such as floral petals are mixed into a compuesto with other selected plants for a blending of all the different ingredients. Many persons pray to Saint Denis to assist in casting out demons.

Specially-selected liquid essences, including *siete machos* and ammonia are also mixed for powerful, aromatic magical blessings that cast out evil influences and attract the assistance of spirits of the light such as angels, saints and folk saints.

My own special blend of *sahumerio,* contains either *copal, estoraque,* or storax, *mirra,* incense along with bay leaves, rosemary, rose petals, ground cinnamon sticks, ground coffee and brown sugar moistened with essence of *narciso negro* or tobacco.

Another popular method of ridding a home or business of bad spirits or to give protection is to place a glass of water with *tomates marinos* in the home or business. These seeds are both male and female, and you must have one of each in the water.

I have found this to be a very powerful and effective cleansing, and blessing method with spiritual medicine. Always pray while applying the ritual to the house or business.

Businessmen and women should always protect themselves by asking their patron saints to intercede for them. Saint Homobonus is the patron saint for businessmen and Saint Margaret Clitherow is the patroness for businesswomen. His day is November 13 and her day is March 25.

COMMENTARY:

Spiritual cleansings of businesses or homes and their continuous protection are the most frequent rituals performed by curanderos/as. One of the most impressive experiences I have ever had was a request to bring a curandero to the home of a very infamous witch, or bruja, who had recently died. Her family was afraid to venture into her home until it had been cleansed of all its evil spirits. Not knowing what to expect, I don't think I have ever been so scared. In fact, the curandero had a very difficult time with the cleansing because it lasted four or five hours. He cleaned each nook and cranny of the tainted house, and when we finally left we could feel the difference. The house had been cleansed of all evil spirits.

151. OWLS AND OMENS — *LECHUZA Y BUEN AGÜEROS*

Last night I had a vision and I could see all the candles I had lit for Fidencio's spirit over the years. It was a magical experience. Then suddenly I noticed a bird flying in my darkened kitchen and it landed at the foot of my bed. I noticed that it was a white dove. I tried and tried to shoo it out of my house, but as I opened the back door a hummingbird flew into my kitchen.

I awoke to the sound of my son coughing. What does it mean? Does this have a spiritual meaning or special message for me?

CURANDERO'S RESPONSE:

First, I need total clarity from you. Did you have a vision that is a supernatural sight while awake, or did you have a dream while asleep? Angels often take the form of birds both good and evil. When they manifest to humankind, while awake or in their sleep, they are often seen as birds. Both doves and hummingbirds are considered good. The good ones are the Creator's messengers.

I believe that you are receiving a message, so you need to try to understand it. If it is a spiritual message, it will continue and the message will proceed through its own symbolism. Be sure to have a notepad next to your bed and write everything down that you dream. Only you can understand the Creator's messages, so be ready for them. I believe you should carry out ritual cleansings, or *limpias*, seven Fridays in a row and pray Psalm 23 to keep you safe from evil.

COMMENTARY:

It is normal for people to dream a cornucopia of spiritual images. Dreams are not always spiritual messages, but often they are. The curandero informs the petitioner that doves and hummingbirds are considered good omens, or buen agüeros, but there are also agüeros malos, or bad omens. Omen acceptance is part of every culture and, often, the person who believes that they have witnessed an omen will ask the curandero/a for an interpretation.

Most dreams, however, must be interpreted in sequence over time. A record of dreams is always a good idea and it assists the curandero, the dreamer and/or counselor with an accurate interpretation.

Owls, or lechuzas, are common symbolic entities in curanderismo. They do not always convey negativity, but they can. Curanderismo believes that evil witches can "shape shift," changing their form into that of an owl or other birds and animals. It's always advisable to cleanse oneself and each family member to rid the body and the home of negative influences. In this case, just to be sure, the curandero recommends repeating limpias, or ritual cleansings, for seven Fridays in a row.

152. SCARED OF THE UNSEEN — *EL MIEDOSO*

I am writing to you about a child. He seems to get scared very easily even though no one tries to frighten him. He sees things in the house that we cannot see that scare him. He gets so scared that he holds or loses his breath every time this happens to him, and it happens often.

In the beginning, he would get scared with any little noise, and now it can happen without any noise at all. When there is no one present, he jumps up or throws a kick, and then punches the air like if he is trying to fight off something or someone unseen. He is definitely seeing something we can't see.

Can you tell me what he sees? What is scaring him? What is he trying to fight off? Like I said before, after this occurs, he seems to lose his breath and looks like he cannot breathe. Can you please let me know what is scaring my nephew or more importantly, how can we help or protect him? Should we have our home and his room cleansed?

CURANDERO'S RESPONSE:

Is he an only child? How long has he been so easily scared? Do you think he has panic attacks or seizures? Have you tried treating him for fright sickness, or *susto*, or for some other trauma? Is he on any kind of medication? What is his age? Has he been checked by a physician? What does the doctor say about your nephew's condition?

It is important that I know these things. Is he allergic to anything? Please let me know as much as possible, so that I may be able to try to determine what's bothering him. Then I will see if there is something we might be able to do for his treatment and well-being from his symptoms. Pray Psalm 10 to overcome all evil spirits.

COMMENTARY:

Children are often believed to be able to see and hear things that as adults we cannot. This may be true, especially if the child is visibly fearful of things unseen. Once again, the curandero asks about any physical ailments. If no malady exists, then the curandero would prescribe that the child receive a ritual cleansing, or limpia, and that the home be cleansed spiritually as well, with a despojo or spiritual cleansing.

153. TOAD SPELL — *EL SAPO TONTO*

I am wondering if you can help me. A young girl has put a spell on my husband. She has a spell on him that makes him treat me very badly, and he refuses anyone but her. I know you may wonder how I know this, and I am not sure what to tell you. I just do.

The spell has gotten to the point where I just got fed up and walked out of the room to get away from him. I believe that is exactly what she wants me to do so that he will have a reason to leave me or have me leave him. Either way, the situation is desperate. We had a very good marriage before this woman showed up.

CURANDERO'S RESPONSE:

Please light a seven-day votive candle to San Alejo and another to San Ignacio de Loyola with your husband's photo under a clear glass of water between both candles to cleanse him of the spell that she has placed over him. Remember that at most *hierberías* there are pre-prepared candles and other products, like sprays, that can be used in the home against witchcraft.

COMMENTARY:

It is prevalent in Latino culture for spells to be used in fixing and breaking relationships. In many cases, if not most, they are harmless, but some are very evil.

In this case, the curandero recommends a primary-level reversing spell to determine if any evil is intended. Some spells, or trabajos, performed by competent witches, brujas may attempt serious harm or death to the party on which the spell has been cast.

In fact, there are documented cases of spiritual, supernatural warfare taking place between witches and curanderos that proceed for years without end or until one of them dies. In this case, the curandero recommended a first-level reversing spell to discover any evil intentions.

Once witchcraft spells have been created as "works," or trabajos, they are placed somewhere for safekeeping depending upon the requirement of the spell. Often, they are hidden or secretly buried in an intended victim's yard or business. Sometimes they are disposed of in water, like a river, or are thrown into the sea. Extremely evil works of witchcraft which are intended to take someone's life are often placed in cemeteries.

It is not uncommon for the witch, or bruja, to seal away the witchcraft job and sometimes items care placed in the mouth of a live toad and the toad's mouth is sewn shut. This action represents sure death for the innocent toad and the completion of the evil intent of the witchcraft spell.

154. THE MIND READER — *EL CLARIVIDENTE*

I would like for you to help me in my situation with my boyfriend, if you could. I told you in my last e-mail that he left me. Well, I have been talking to this person who can read people's minds. So far, everything she has told me has come true. She claims that she is not a witch and that she only uses her powers to help people. But it scares me a little because if she can cast good spells, she can certainly cast bad ones as well.

This mind reader told me that my boyfriend left me because he has a lot of stress in his life and that I give him more stress. He claims that I am a control freak. The mind reader told me that if we could take away all of his other stresses and leave only the one that I cause him, that it would not be enough to drive him away from me. But it sounds very strangely like witchcraft.

I don't want him in my life if I have to resort to witchcraft to get him. It is just so easy for him to blame all of his stress on me, rather than, for him to accept that all of these other problems are causing his stress, which I have nothing to do with. I just wanted to know if there is a way to help him clear his mind because I am afraid that he could have a nervous breakdown.

CURANDERO'S RESPONSE:

I shall try to do what I can for you. Why do you really think your boyfriend left you? What does this psychic spiritual advisor tell you is going to happen? Will she be able to help you with your dilemma and if yes, why are you contacting me? Did she ask you to change your behavior in order to get him to come back to you? Would he be willing to seek help?

Please send me a recent picture of him and of yourself, if you are willing for me to have them, so that I may keep both of you in my prayers. You may light a San Alejo and a San Ignacio de Loyola candle for their spirits to come to him and for you to cleanse yourself of confusion, evil and negative energies. Also, have either of you considered seeing a counselor?

COMMENTARY:

In the Latino community there are many people who claim to be able to cast spells to reunite lovers. It is never advisable to undertake this even though it may be very tempting. Many people you encounter will tell you that they have done it and that it has worked. This activity falls into the context of witchcraft; believed to be revisited upon the petitioner.

However, there is always a price to pay for delving into magic. You don't know nor understand the forces that are being utilized to bring about the desired effect and the heavy price you may pay. The returning sweetheart may exhibit negative personality changes as a result of the interference with his or her free will by the manipulating spirits.

155. DARK SHADOW — *UNA SOMBRA NEGRA*

My mom has been by recently to see you. She informed me that she had given you pictures of me and my boyfriend and that I could contact you if I needed to.

I am e-mailing you to see if you can help me out with a situation that has been taking place in my apartment. Ever since I moved in there, strange things have been taking place. I have trouble sleeping and I wake up every night around the same time, only to feel as though someone is staring at me from the doorway of my bedroom. On one occasion, I woke up as usual and saw a shadowy, childlike figure in the doorway. Then, a few nights later, my boyfriend was sitting on the bed and he felt a hand pressing down on his head but there was no one around. We were the only ones in the apartment.

We have also had very strange dreams. I dreamt that I was possessed by something evil. He has also had similar but more disturbing dreams. He had a dream that there was a little boy standing in the center of our bedroom and that he was trying to harm me. My boyfriend wanted to stop the little boy but could not grab anything. It was a ghost.

My boyfriend dreamt that his brother was in our apartment but it really was not him, it was something pretending to be his brother. About two weeks ago, my boyfriend woke up in the middle of the night and saw a dark shadow-figure standing over me with its arms raised. When he tried to reach for it, it disappeared. Last night he dreamt that his evil twin, or doppelganger, was pacing back and forth in front of our bedroom door staring back at him.

I would like to know if there is anything I could do to make all of this go away. I have tried Holy Water, but it only helps for about three weeks; then things start to happen again. If there is any advice as to what is causing this or how I can make this go away, please let me know. Any advice you can give us will be very much appreciated.

CURANDERO'S RESPONSE:

To cleanse the apartment and yourselves of ghosts or evil spirits or entities, burn incense, myrrh, and *copal* incense in the apartment to cleanse it and your physical persons as well. Getting rid of evil is often difficult, so enlist the help of San Mauricio, San Cipriano and San Cristóbal, all three are used to rid evil spirits. You must also perform repeated spiritual cleansings and pray Psalm 17 to stay safe from evil.

COMMENTARY:

Many persons believe that spirits, many times evil ones, can be invited into the home inadvertently. The spirits might enter attached to an object that one might acquire, say, at a second-hand store. Additionally, spirits will attach themselves to a person and be brought into the home.

Sometimes the spirit, which may be harmless, simply resides in the home and existed there years before you arrived. In any case, the home and the people who live there must be cleansed and only a competent curandero may adequately perform this ritual.

156. SPIRIT DOOR — *LA OUIJA*

I am in middle school, and in order to be popular you have to be in one of the groups in school. Most of the Latinos at my school are in the Chicano Club and they are really into the supernatural. I am learning a lot about the Aztec culture and how to perform their rituals.

Now, we are using the Ouija board to communicate with Aztec spirits and sometimes it gets really scary. I've talked to my mother about this and she thinks it's dangerous and wants me to contact you about it. What do you think?

CURANDERO'S RESPONSE:

The Ouija board is not a traditional item in Latino culture, but the Aztecs did have something similar. In the practice of *curanderismo* for the past 30 years, I have been approached by hundreds of Latinos with questions and issues in regard to their experiences with Ouija boards.

Each time I was consulted, people's inquiries were about how to get rid of evil spirits and all the problems brought about since the acquisition and utilization of the Ouija board in their home. Young and old, as well as everyone in the household, have declared to have had intolerable haunting and terrifying experiences. Others attest that they regret ever seeking spirits with the Ouija board.

What they discovered was seemingly endless torment and torture. One man informed me that he and his brother tried out the board, only to get into a gun fight the following day. Another family tried it only to discover the dark side of the spirit world coming through, bringing tragedy into their lives. I highly recommend that your club find another more traditional way to learn about Aztec culture and leave the Ouija alone.

COMMENTARY:

The Ouija board has been consulted since before the 17th century; perhaps even before then. Today, it is considered a modern parlor game based on an ancient form of divination. Even though it is common, many religions forbid their followers to use it since the Ouija can lead to potentially-dangerous life situations.

When curanderos/as work they are protected by a sacred precinct that they set up around themselves, and their clients. This sacred working space is usually approximate to their healing altar. Parlor games like the Ouija board and séances are dangerous because no protective area or zone has been set up. It is not uncommon for innocent participants to acquire unwanted spirits this way.

157. WORKING ME — *TRABAJÁNDOME*

Today, a woman came to my place of employment. She stopped at the guard shack and told them that I had told her to come and sell burritos, so they let her through and told her what building I was in.

When she walked in she asked someone to point me out to her. She did not know me and I do not know her. I certainly did not tell her to come and sell burritos. She did not know who I was and I felt sorry for her so I bought some of her burritos and ate them.

I now know that I was very stupid to do that. I am sure now that I ate some kind of witchcraft. The more I think about it, the more terrorized I become. I'm very scared because I realized that someone is trying to kill me by witchcraft. It is a very strange feeling. I am now imagining that something is growing inside me. She made it seem to the people at the guard shack that she knew me when she did not. It is obvious that someone sent her. Was she the messenger of death? Am I just being paranoid or is something very bad happening? Please help me or am I just freaking out over nothing?

CURANDERO'S RESPONSE:

This sounds very mysterious and horrible! Who do you think would do this to you? Maybe it was just her tactic to be allowed permission to enter certain gated work sites. Otherwise, she might never be allowed in. It is very probable that she knew exactly who you were, even though she pretended not to know you. In situations like this most often the messenger has been given your photo. You didn't meet the actual witch. You probably met a demon messenger. Are you positive you do not know who she is? It is very strange.

I do understand why you would feel sorry for her, which is part of the spell they placed on you so you would eat what they gave you. Do you understand why someone might be trying to do witchcraft on you? Someone gave her your name with instructions to sell you some burritos with poison or witchcraft powder in them.

Then on the other hand, it could be nothing. It sounds like you need to be very careful not to ever eat food from someone you don't even know. Someone may be trying to hurt you and it simply is not sanitary. It is very important that you let me know immediately if anything else happens. Say a special prayer to San Cipriano to assist you and pray Psalm 145 to keep ghosts and spirits away from you.

COMMENTARY:

This case is troublesome. It's quite evident someone visited the petitioner's workplace, lied to gain entry, and convinced the person to eat something of unknown origin. Latino culture in general, always tells its people never accept food from someone you do not know for fear that something has been placed in it with evil intent. The curandero offers good advice. When in doubt about food: always politely decline. If a person is hungry, it may be difficult to refuse but not if it's food you purchase. Caution and vigilance are always the best preventative measures.

158. WITCHCRAFT DOLLS — *MUÑECOS*

When I go to my local *hierbería*, herb market, I see a whole section with very ugly dolls. Some are made of cloth and others are made of wax. Some are genderless rag dolls and others are very anatomically correct female and male wax candle dolls. Whenever I ask the woman there about these dolls and what they are for, she instantly changes the subject. The most I have been able to get out of her is "if you don't know what they are for, then you don't need them."

I have gone to several mail-order websites which sell them in all types, sizes, materials and colors. I simply want a true explanation of what they are for and how they are used. Thank you.

CURANDERO'S RESPONSE:

The *hierbería* or *botánica* is first and foremost a business. Therefore, they live and die by sales. Sales are determined by the market and the things that people ask for. So *hierberías* and *botánicas* stock items for many different spiritual purposes, beliefs and traditions. The items stocked in these stores are for both *curanderismo* and for witchcraft, and the dolls and fetishes are for hexing. Both the cloth dolls, wax dolls or candles in human form are used in witchcraft and hexing rituals. They are not evil by themselves but when they are "worked," they can be very dangerous. Never touch one that you see or encounter with your bare hands. Pray Psalms 67 and 68 to keep evil from imprisoning you in a doll.

COMMENTARY:

Seeing a witchcraft doll in a store for the first time can be shocking, but what is more disconcerting is the discovery of these items after they have been prepared and used in a witchcraft spell intended to do someone harm. When they are completed, they may contain human hair and substances as well as personal clothing. As shown in the National Geographic documentary series "Taboo: Mexican Witchcraft," Latino witchcraft can and does seek to destroy marriages, and even kill. Not knowing what forces are used to bring forth the spell, these items of Mexican witchcraft should always be considered very dangerous.

159. I'M CURSED — *MALDICIÓN*

I believe I was cursed as an infant because my grandmother had many enemies. When I was about three years old, I woke in the middle of the night and saw a fireball over my baby bed. I remember it well. The next day, our house burned to the ground. I have had a lot of bad luck in every aspect of my life, personal, business and health. Doctors have told me repeatedly that there is nothing wrong with me, but I still have this feeling that I have inherited a curse. Please help me. I do not want to cry anymore or live in fear. I want to live a healthy, normal life and I would like to have some good luck for a change.

CURANDERO'S RESPONSE:

Thank you for your call and for your e-mail, and especially for your petition. It is likely that you are an extended recipient of your grandmother's curse. I have seen this many times where curses are passed on to children and grandchildren.

If your grandmother was cursed by her enemies, as you say, the curse falls on the rest of the family for generations to come.

The fireball you witnessed was a spirit messenger, either sent to warn you or to protect you from what was about to happen. You were, and probably still are, being watched over and protected by some entity; maybe the spirit of your grandmother. I believe you were born with a special mission in life, to serve others in some divine capacity. That is why you were not in the house when it burned down.

I would say that your survival is an example of Divine Providence and evidence that you are indeed protected. But Divine Providence is not good luck. They are very different things. I believe the doctors are correct, this is not a physical ailment, and it is a spiritual issue. I don't think that there is anything physically or psychologically wrong with you. You will have to protect yourself for the rest of your life from this curse, unless you can find someone powerful enough to break it.

COMMENTARY:

A family curse is a common thread within the Latino cultural and familial fabric. This is especially true in families with an ancestor or family member who practices or used to practice curanderismo or brujería. Curanderismo, as other cultural dogmas, definitely acknowledges that curses can be passed down from generation to generation.

160. THE WITCH — *LA BRUJA*

I read your e-mail and the reason I asked for your help is because I hoped you would help remove this woman from my ex-husband's home and, with God's help, he will come back home to me.

As I explained in my letter, there is this woman who has paid someone a lot of money so she can remain in my ex-husband's house. She is still paying someone to help her. As long as she is in the picture and doing these bad things, the situation between me and my husband will not improve. One day he is fine, and the next day he is different and will not even talk to me. That is why I need your help.

I need to remove this woman and all the witchcraft from my life. With God's help and Niño Fidencio, I have faith that things will improve. I just know it.

I am sorry if I did not fully explain myself about what I wanted earlier. I just want this woman to go away. I know in my heart that if she is gone, he will come home to me. This is the first time in all the years we have been together that this has ever happened. All I want to know is if you see any hope that things will get better, and if you can remove this woman from his house.

CURANDERO'S RESPONSE:

First, you must cleanse yourself with spiritual-blessing baths. Boil rice and use the water in your bath water for at least three Fridays in a row. Use the same boiled rice to sprinkle outside around your house, calling on the celestial spirits of light to favor you and approve your petition.

After that, you must burn a red wax candle with a glass of water over his picture at your bedside. You will call out his name three times near the glass of water in a longing fashion. Do this at 3 a.m. for as many early mornings as the candle is lit.

Soon after you do this, he will come to you. When he does, you will give him the same glass of water to drink out of. This will deliver him from all of her spells. Finally, you will light a Saint Michael the Archangel candle and implore the archangel to assist you to vanquish the other woman from this spiritual war you are in. If you are able to acquire any object of hers, burn it and then bury it in a jar in your yard. Once she is enclosed, she will never bother you again.

COMMENTARY:

Beware! Realize that the most common type of witchcraft is to experience a curse placed on a former spouse or lover. Many practicing witches are consumed by this business; casting no other spells, only those affecting relationships. Due to this ongoing witchcraft, it's always wise to be protected with a special amulet or talisman prepared by a magic ritual. Also, always be sure to cleanse yourself and your home; protecting the family unit and marriage in order to avoid problematic situations.

161. HOME SPIRITS — *ESPÍRITUS CASEROS*

Last night something very strange happened to me. I was reciting my evening prayer, when all of the lights, except in my son's room began to dim and flicker, on and off. Then, all the lights in the house totally went out. It was very scary, so we called the police and an electrician.

Then, there was a loud noise in our house and smoke began coming out of the floor. We saw sparks and lots of smoke, but there was no fire. It was weird.

Now, we are using the neighbor's power to connect to our house because we live in a rural area. Someone is going to try to connect our lights, but it has not happened yet. We felt like we were in a movie. Is there something we should be aware of? What do you think happened to us? Our house was the only one in the area that lost power. The whole thing had a kind of eerie feeling to it.

My son has been too afraid to return home and is staying with his grandmother and he has been missing school. I am sure at least I will have to cure him from *susto*. Please help me.

CURANDERO'S RESPONSE:

Please try to remember and tell me if anything like this has ever happened to you before. That is, in any other place that you have lived. Do you think it was a supernatural event or that you might have a ghost or spirit in your house? Why did you call the police? Don't you think it was just a problem with the electrical system under the house? I really do not think you have anything to worry about as far as ghosts are concerned. Am I picking something up spiritually?

I do not know why your son would be afraid to return home or why he would be missing school, unless you have taught him to fear the imagined supernatural. I don't think you are telling me the whole story. Did you ever stop to think he might not be coming home or be missing school for some other reason? A reason you know but are not telling.

Please light a candle to the spirit of Niño Fidencio, say your prayer and make your petition, and his spirit will help you. But most importantly, examine your conscience and tell the truth and face the facts as they really are.

COMMENTARY:

This is a classic curandero's cautionary tale. Try not to interject spiritual causes into ordinary everyday events. And do not teach your children to do that. If you do, it could become a behavioral pattern; forcing you into a life of constantly fearing the unknown when it's simply unnecessary. Be cautious and aware; but never fearful. Notice that the curandero must be rational when the petitioner obviously is not.

162. DARKNESS — *LAS TINIEBLAS*

It's me again, regarding my sister. Things are a little better with my nephew, but the situation is very stressful on my sister. Now, the doctors say she has arthritis in her neck from the whiplash she got when she was in a car accident last year. She's not doing well, and I also think someone did something very evil to her because she told me that she has seen a black shadow at the back door, and continues to see a *lechuza,* or owl, when dropping her son off at work.

My sister has been afraid to talk about her experiences, but now tells us that this black shadow person comes to have sex with her and she says that it's an ongoing experience. Please help me because I think someone is trying to drive her crazy. She is not herself and we need your help. Please e-mail me soon because this is very important.

CURANDERO'S RESPONSE:

I don't understand why you think someone would be trying to drive her crazy. All three of you should take a head of garlic and rub it all over your body, cleansing it of negative and evil forces and energies that bring about suffering and bad happenings to your sister. Say an Our Father when performing these cleansing rituals and say a special prayer to San Cristóbal, the patron saint against evil spirits. But most importantly, you need to settle down and find rational explanations for the things that you say are happening to her. Your sister must place a Holy relic above the head of her bed to ward off the errant incubus, or male devil she says is having sex with her.

Throw the head of garlic in the trash when you are done with the *limpias*. Repeat the *limpias* for seven consecutive Fridays. Start with one today, even though it is not Friday, for urgency reasons. Sprinkle rice and wheat seed with Holy Water around the house for protection and for prosperity. Do this the first day of each month. On the last day of each month, burn special *copal* incense in your home to further cleanse it. You should also consider a complete *sahumerio* or smoking *limpia*, of your home. This will cleanse the house of evil curses and negative energies that may have entered the home and especially the shadow man if he truly exists.

COMMENTARY:

Latinos frequently have latent recollections of events and experiences, especially if they are of a spiritual or supernatural nature. In this case, it was verified that the petitioner has suppressed memories of sexual abuse as a child.

From the testimony it seems that this woman has fully comprehended curanderismo and witchcraft most of her life. The appearance of a spirit (incubus or succubus) who has sex with someone is not uncommon in the life of a person encompassed by the supernatural. One aspect of the spirit world attracts others. The attraction, the sexual abuse, the repressed memories are not always benign. Especially in this case, it seems that the sister needs ongoing treatment and support.

163. EXORCISING DEMONS — *SACANDO DEMONIOS*

I am a Catholic, and recently our parish priest talked about persons possessed by demons and he says that the church has special rituals to cast them out.

I was talking to my friend about this, who is a Protestant, and she says that her church also performs exorcisms from time to time when her pastor believes that someone is demon possessed.

Can this be true? Have you ever seen such a thing? Can a *curandero* cast out demons also? I have heard that they can. Finally, how do you know when a person is demon possessed, are there any tests or signs?

CURANDERO'S RESPONSE:

Early in my experience as a *curandero*, a woman brought her niece for me to examine. Her niece had been ill and was under a doctor's care. The doctor had examined her and had run every kind of test, finding nothing wrong her. The young adolescent girl continued to be ill for seven months before she was brought to me.

On the surface, she seemed to be okay to me, but other than that, she was a little reluctant to see me or allow me to place my hands on her. She appeared to be uncomfortable or uneasy around me. I immediately sensed that there was something insanely evil deep inside her. I could see it looking back at me when I looked deep into her eyes. I blessed a Holy Rosary and a Cruz de Caravaca for her to wear around her neck. These blessed items would protect her against evil spirits.

I also asked that her aunt see to it that her niece drink a cup of tea daily made from three herbs: *peonía, tumba vaquero* and *perejil*. The concoction is intended to provoke the expulsion of the fluids that form in the stomach lining from the manifestation of any unclean spirit living in her body and making her ill. After my examination, her aunt drove the niece home, but before they arrived, the niece flew into an uncontrollable rage. In a terrible fit in the car, she tore the Rosary and Cruz de Caravaca from around her neck and threw them out the window.

Once home, her mother and aunts prepared the tea I recommended, and gave her a cup to drink. I was then called and asked if I was able to go to their home to perform a cleansing and healing ritual. Since I lived nearby, I was able to go and I arrived just a few minutes later. Entering the home, I gasped at what I saw. Several of her relatives were holding the girl down on the floor. It was then that I fully encountered what I had suspected from her initial visit. The young woman was demonically possessed and by a formidable demon.

I asked the family if they had contacted their family priest or minister. They indicated that a local priest had come by their home earlier in the week, but not prepared for what he found or trained as an exorcist, he quickly fled their house scared to death. They said that he would never come back. Knowing the priest personally, I called him and informed him of the situation with his parishioner. I told him I was going to pray for the girl and asked him for his blessing, for his prayers, and for my protection, and for that of the family. I performed the exorcism rituals on the girl as I have learned to do, and during this process I learned that she had started acting strangely after a visit to the cemetery with her aunts to pray at her grandfather's grave on Father's Day. That was seven months earlier.

I was told that at the moment when she passed through the cemetery's gate she accidentally stepped on a witchcraft object that had been placed on the ground.

After that, I was told that she appeared to be in a daze, in some altered state and became incoherent. During the exorcism sessions, I also learned that seven months before this event occurred, her parents were awakened in the middle of the night by their daughter's screams. She told them that two demons had come into her bedroom through a window and had sex with her.

I worked with this young girl, day in and day out, for more than four months. Finally, I was able to cast out a number of demonic spirits, asking each of them to identify themselves by name. Some of those, especially a very powerful and evil spirit, would keep returning to the girl's body refusing to leave permanently. This happened several times until it could no longer overcome the exorcism. The exorcism was eventually successful and the young girl was relieved from her torment, confusion, unrest and illness. A year later, she seemed to be fine and had no further incidences with evil spirits.

COMMENTARY:

Exorcising demons is an officially sanctioned rite of the Catholic Church. In Catholicism it is only performed by a person who is trained and approved by the bishop of a diocese. Exorcism is also a routine function of evangelical religions and their ministers, and a known practice of curanderos/as.

If you are interested in reading more about exorcism, there are several books written by Catholic priests, and others that have been recently published claiming that demonic possessions are gradually increasing worldwide. Therefore, the need for exorcisms and trained exorcists has also dramatically increased.

Another method which followers of curanderismo use to shun and cast out devils is to call upon the assistance of San Cipriano, San Alejo or San Ignacio. Then, they light a candle to San Miguel Arcángel and place it inside a vessel containing an inch of dirt along with an inch of Holy Water.

After a person takes their loved one to see a curandero for an exorcism that act should always be followed up by a trip to seek professional help as well. Very likely, the person will require ongoing assistance from both curandero/a and medical professional.

164. FREED OF DEMONS — *LIBERADO*

I do not know if the pastor is trying to heal me from witchcraft or from demonic possession, or both. The people gathered in a circle, holding hands, and he walked around the people, laying hands on people, commanding Satan to flee from us. The first time he prayed over me, it was as if my body was out of my control. I cried and I yelled and something made me want to vomit, but nothing came out but saliva.

At that time, he told me that I was a victim of witchcraft and that they probably gave me some tainted food made from witchcraft. The healing left me so drained that I could not do anything the rest of that day or night. The same thing happened the second time, except that when I tried to vomit, I vomited two drops of blood.

The last few times that he has prayed over me, my hands and my arms shook uncontrollably and tears flowed from my body, but I have not yelled like I did the first couple of times. Yesterday, my arm and hand shook, tears flowed, and mucous came out of my nose.

Earlier in my life, my body suffered a lot of broken bones from falls. I am a walking miracle. Many times, walking is painful, but I force myself to keep going. I feel as if my hands and my feet are tied. I feel kind of guilty about going to that church because I am a Catholic, but I feel that the laying-on-of-hands has helped me.

I still have not been physically able to do my apartment cleaning chores. Every effort of movement continues to exhaust me and I continue to forget things as well. I do feel better emotionally, even though I find myself crying uncontrollably more than usual.

I just wish I could find a job so that I can pay my rent and my bills because I don't have anyone that I can depend on to take care of me and it's best for me to be able to take care of myself, anyway. I think my ex-boss might be saying something negative about me. At times his behavior is very manic and talks off the top of his head without thinking. It makes me sad if he is doing that because he had sex with me. He used to be a priest and he should have some compassion left in him.

I will go to church to get some Holy Water and follow your advice for the next seven days. I hope that God will continue to bless you for your selfless decision to help me when you do not even know me. Please continue to keep me in your prayers.

CURANDERO'S RESPONSE:

It appears that the pastor suspects you are a victim of an evil influence. The question is will he be successful in breaking up or removing the evil influence that is tormenting you?

There are definitely signs of something wrong with you! Seek spiritual help from San Mauricio who is the patron saint of casting out devils. I feel you are a very proud person and you have difficulty in accepting help from others because those who have helped you have also abused you. You like to help others, but you usually do not like to receive help from others. Don't you think it is time for you to change at least until you can get back on your feet? Please tell me if you believe I am wrong.

I am keeping you in my prayers. I do not have to know you personally to care. I care very much when it comes to my fellow humans suffering pain or illness. Many of my fellowmen have cared for me without knowing me when I have been in need, and even if they had not known me, it is still the right thing to do.

I will pray for you to find a job or some help to sustain yourself honorably. You need to seek medical help if you are vomiting blood. Is the pastor willing to try to heal you from witchcraft? Can you apply for any assistance from organizations in your area? You may ask the pastor to provide you with Holy Water so that you may bathe with it and also drink it for at least seven consecutive days. Finally and most importantly, ask the pastor to baptize you in water and in the spirit.

COMMENTARY:

Many Latinos belong to evangelical churches in addition to practicing their beliefs in curanderismo. In this case, the evangelical community has attempted to cast out demons from the woman's body. She also claims to be a Catholic. Many evangelicals were raised as Catholics, as well as believing in curanderismo. Depending upon their spiritual circumstances, they often go back and forth from the Catholic Church to evangelical churches.

It is often poverty and lack of access to health care that causes a person to seek assistance anywhere support networks are available.

165. TORMENTED —*ATORMENTADO*

Is there a way that you can help me to understand the healing baths? I have been suffering for a long time and have been tormented by the devil all of my life. I can sense that my life is going to end soon. God has called me to do great things with my life, and healing me from this awful disease that has been cast upon me is one of the first things I'm going to accomplish with your help. If you think that you cannot help me, please let me know. I will stop contacting you. I will respect anything that you feel will help me.

CURANDERO'S RESPONSE:

You may try boiling rue, rosemary and basil, and bathe with the water on Mondays and Fridays at high noon. Do this for seven straight weeks praying and making your petition to the Lord God. Thank you for your kindness.

It will be a stronger healing if you are able to find and burn the San Alejo and the San Ignacio de Loyola candles for 40 straight days. You must place your photograph between both candles and a clear glass of water over your photo.

I pray you can be patient with me so that I may try to help you. If you are unable to be patient with me, I will understand and I will respect you for that and will step aside if you want me to. In addition, I must tell you, I make no promises. All I can do for anyone is try my best. If that is not good enough, then let that be the will of God. I, for one, will have to accept that.

COMMENTARY:

This is an intriguing case. First of all, the curandero did not answer the petitioner's question of "what are the baths for?" The curandero senses something else is at work here or the petitioner has a hidden agenda. While this may have been answered in another correspondence between the two, the petitioner is a suffering hypochondriac, and therefore, experiences imaginary maladies and suspects every remedy. Therefore, the petitioner will not rest until the question on the baths is answered. Simply stated, spiritual baths wash away negative energies.

Be wary of persons who have spent their lives living with hypochondria and who jump from one religion or from healer to healer. They can never be satisfied and never find relief because of their mental illness.

Because their lives are surrounded by their so-called physical ailments, they never want to hear the truth that it is all in their minds. Any healer, therapist, reader and/ or counselor can become exhausted or ill when a demanding hypochondriac visits too frequently. The hypochondriacs will wear the curandero out; then disappear when they feel that they have milked the healer for everything he/she has. Then they just move on to another curandero/a and are never heard from again. At some point, it becomes necessary to end the sessions to preserve the healer's own emotional and physical health.

166. GRANDMA IS A WITCH — *LA HECHICERA*

I am thankful for your response. Thank you for your suggested remedy for my previous request. I really like the remedy that uses the different waters and the goat's milk. I have a friend who can get me the sea and river water, but I will have to wait a few months for it to arrive.

I wanted to tell you about my grandma. A woman put a *brujería* hex on my grandma that will not allow her to ever go back to her home. If she steps a foot inside her hometown, she will surely die.

My grandma told me that a woman buried her hair and clothes in cemetery dirt and other evil stuff in a jar and buried it in my grandmother's hometown. That ritual act captures her spirit in that place until it is released.

My grandma is a famous *bruja*, witch, and she has been at war with other witches all her life. They are in a standoff right now, but have successfully prevented her from going home to die.

To make matters worse, I believe my grandma has used my photo and hair as well as my clothes to do witchcraft on me. She is upset that I don't want to be trained as a witch before she dies. It is even more evil than that. She wants me to carry on the war with the other *brujas*, witches, and I don't want that kind of life. So now, my grandmother has turned against me. I need help in defeating her because she is a very powerful and famous *bruja*. Thank you again.

CURANDERO'S RESPONSE:

First and foremost, stay away from your grandmother until you are able to resolve this issue with her. Yes, there are many possible ways of breaking witchcraft. I will prepare a very special and most powerful prayer to have witchcraft removed from you. Trust in your spirit.

To undo the witchcraft that has been done to you, you must take seven baths on seven consecutive Fridays. On the first Friday, bathe with water from a river. The second Friday, bathe with water from underground, like water from a spring or a well. The third Friday, bathe in rainwater. The fourth Friday, bathe in lake water. The fifth Friday, bathe with Holy Water, that must be from a Catholic Church. The sixth Friday, bathe with seven liters of goat's milk. The seventh Friday, bathe with three gallons of water from the sea. With each spiritual bath, you will receive a healing and by the seventh bath, the spell will be broken.

After seven weeks, your grandmother's witchcraft will no longer make you suffer and you will have defeated her. As a witch, she will know this and have more respect for you, but she is going to want to know my name and you should divulge that.

COMMENTARY:

In the United States and in Mexico, I have met persons who claim to have had grandmothers and grandfathers who were either healers and curanderos/as or witches/brujos/as. While this may be true, the descendant and their tales can become self-fulfilling prophecies in the lives of their descendants. The younger generation lives in the shadow of its ancestor and believes that it must carry on this war of the witches. This is simply not true. This leads to the absorbing of all sorts of spiritual and supernatural burdens, imagined health issues, and convoluted magical problems.

167. GUARDIAN ANGEL — *ÁNGEL GUARDIÁN*

I want to tell you about a dream I had a while back. I saw myself talking to Saint Michael the Archangel. I could not hear what we were talking about, but I remember seeing myself dressed in clothes similar to his with a sword and shield in hand and a helmet on my head just like a soldier. Then I looked into what seemed like a mirror and I had these huge white wings on my back.

I do not know what that dream meant, but I took it like I was being prepared for war. Then about a month and a half ago, I had another dream and I saw myself once again with Saint Michael the Archangel. I was holding a shield and a long sword in my hand with the wings on my back. I still could not hear what was being said to me.

What does all this mean? Is it just something crazy that I dreamed? I told my mom about it and I know this might sound funny, but I told her maybe it's time I have been chosen to fight a great battle. I know it sounds crazy, but that is the first thing that I could think of. You know what? She agreed with that.

What do you think it means? Please write back soon.

CURANDERO'S RESPONSE:

I remember you have e-mailed me before regarding your dreams about Saint Michael the Archangel talking to you. You have also talked to me briefly about this over the telephone on past occasions. It is obviously very important to you, as you have talked not only to me, but you have also consulted with the spirit of El Niño Fidencio.

It seems to me you have been influenced by the spirit of Saint Michael the Archangel. That is not bad, but it has a purpose and a responsibility you must learn. Sooner or later, the true purpose will be revealed to you. When you are ready you will probably hear or understand what is being said to you.

You might be having revelations of your spiritual origin and past spiritual existences. Or it's possible you may be having revelations that you are being chosen to fight a great spiritual battle against evil and wicked ways. It may mean you are being called by God to serve some undefined, as of yet, spiritual purpose. You may wish to consult about this matter again with the spirit of El Niño Fidencio.

COMMENTARY:

Individuals who grow up in and live within the spiritual sphere of curanderismo often have dreams where one or more of the spirits they recognize and see channeled, appear to them. This channeled spirit could be Saint Michael the Archangel, Pancho Villa, or even El Niño Fidencio and a slew of others. While it is possible that the spirit is talking to them, more than likely the subconscious mind is working on them during a deep sleep. A dream journal is always in order for proper analysis while also applying the scientific law, Occam's Razor, "the simplest answer is usually correct when given all the facts." Saint Michael could simply be this person's spiritual protector.

168. EVIL SPIRITS — *VEO LO MALO*

I am a woman that has suffered a great deal of hardship for the last 30 years. I have experienced seeing bad spirits all around me, all the time. I do not have the power to get rid of them myself. I have tried praying the Holy Rosary and many other prayers. These spirits have caused me to lose everything. At present, I am homeless and living in my car.

Please pray for me. Everything has gone wrong in my life and I am not sure why. I don't understand how I got this way. Please help me. I can see and I can hear at least three bad spirits talking to me right now while I am writing to you. They will not leave me alone and are threatening me. It is so bad that I cannot even get or keep a job anymore.

I always get turned down for employment wherever I go. I have no friends or family. Every time someone looks at me, it turns to hate. People say that I have a "demon possessed" look in my eyes. Why is that? Has a spell been cast on me?

CURANDERO'S RESPONSE:

You definitely need help. You need professional help, and you need to look for the nearest minister who can cast the demons out of you or they will surely kill you. You should place a pinch of cinnamon powder in your shoes before starting your day; calling on the spirit guide and protector and making your petitions. Do this ritual for 40 days in a row.

COMMENTARY:

Always be aware of individuals who claim to hear spirits or voices talking to them. Proper mental health evaluation is always important; especially if this behavior is affecting one's ability to live a normal family and work life. In this case, this woman must be referred immediately for a complete mental health evaluation. There are notable cases where a curandero/a has successfully managed mental cases of paranoid schizophrenia for years, but most often it is not possible without ongoing mental health care.

169. BEWITCHED — *EMBRUJADA*

Thank you for your kindness. I truly appreciate you and I will be patient. I'm just so used to people forgetting about or not caring at all about me. I'm so relieved I have your help and I'm thankful for your understanding. I'm at a difficult time in my life right now. I am trying my hardest to receive what the Lord has in store for me so I can begin my new life in the spirit.

I feel that this agonizing back and neck problem I have is the only way the devil has power over me. I'm growing spiritually and just surrendered my life to the Lord this year. I'm not giving up on my healing so the devil can have his way. My faith has grown so much and I have come a long way before I got in contact with you. I'm just tired of all the evil in the world and in my family.

CURANDERO'S RESPONSE:

I have you on my daily prayer list. I care very much about your spirituality and have great respect for you. If you have placed your life in the Lord's hands, the devil may tempt you, but he cannot touch you if you don't let him.

Evil will not go away. It must be defeated. It is one's own responsibility to have the faith, strength and valor to combat evil. You need to allow God to help you through those around you, and pray that God may bless those who hurt you. Pray that He allow those who can help you to be near you and set apart from you those who want to hurt you.

Find a special prayer to reverse the spell against you or a *rompe trabajo*, break a spell. You will know when you have found the prayer for you. Give yourself cleansing baths with healing herbs such as rosemary, mint, anise seed and star anise, basil and myrrh. Be sure to have a High John the Conqueror oil, spray or candle in your home and use it frequently by spraying it in the rooms that you are in the most such as your bedroom.

COMMENTARY:

People sometimes blame God for their bad luck or life's conditions. While bad luck will continue to be the most common blame, the truth is that people must think seriously about becoming spiritual while developing faith. Try not to allow evil to enter your thoughts and always remember that "an idle mind is the devil's workshop."

Some people believe that they inherently have bad luck or are salados, or salted. They are so convinced that they have bad luck, which they obsess over it, and that causes them to make bad decisions and worsens their situation. If one feels this way, one should wear an amulet or talisman to prevent it. Then, purchase candles and other objects in the hierberías to reverse bad luck. Sometimes they are easily taken advantage of by commercial curanderos. Always be aware of so-called curanderos who are only interested in your money.

170. AFRAID OF WITCHCRAFT — *ESPANTADO*

These last two days I have been very confused about God and I am very nervous. I have been seeking help from a man who practices Santería.

I feel that I am constantly being attacked by evil spirits and my schizophrenia has returned. This Brazilian man told me that I am a spirit medium and that is why I am suffering spirit attacks. He says that if I turn my back on my calling, I will go crazy, become *trastornado*. Please send some much-needed advice. I feel that I am also under attack by witches.

On the one hand, I am told that I am being called to become a *curandero*, while on the other; witches are trying to keep me from my spiritual development, or *desarrollo espiritual*. I do not even know what that is. Can you help me?

CURANDERO'S RESPONSE:

Seeking spiritual help from a variety of religious belief systems can lead to confusion and I think that is where you are. Keep the faith in a higher power, a supreme being you can always count on to be there for you in your hour of need. Place your life in God's hands and go on about living your life as best as you can. The sacred faith you place in Him will see you through your journey. You will be fine. I am your friend in prayer.

COMMENTARY:

There are many different religions and sects which surround us. Most offer support for humanity's multitudinous problems. In this case, the petitioner has encountered a practitioner of Afro-Brazilian or Afro-Caribbean practices.

Since these practices are based on spirit possession and trance-induced states, any cult that relies on spirit possession may be misdiagnosed as schizophrenic.

This petitioner claims to have schizophrenia and, therefore, is easy prey for cults. The santero probably thinks that the person is a trance medium in training but in fact has a mental condition. Since many of these practices are based upon trance-induced states, spirit possession, as well as drugged stupors, they resemble cults and not religions. Obviously, exceptions exist. Any group that insists that all members commit an act that causes fear, confusion and shame is highly destructive. Losing one's sense of self and connection to right and wrong is the first warning sign.

171. THE CONJURE — *EL CONJURO*

Some of my family members have put evil spells on me for about 30 years now and nothing I can do will take them off. Right now I am suffering from extreme jealousy, envy and hatred from anyone that sets eyes on me. It is a very complex spell. I have a very long list of people who hate me and want to do me harm. Please pray a special prayer for me. Please help me break these evil spells that have ruined my life.

CURANDERO'S RESPONSE:

You may start healing and reversing the evil spells by putting one tablespoon of salt and one ounce of rubbing alcohol in a pail of rain water, and bathe with that for nine straight Fridays. While you do this, complete your prayer to San Cipriano. You must pray to the healing spirits of light for blessings. Never give up. This might also be a spiritual test to see if you are worthy. Fight back against evil.

COMMENTARY:

Envy and jealousy amongst family members is very common. It is not unusual for family members to place or to arrange spells to be placed upon other family members and to carry on lengthy vendettas or to seek revenge, venganza. The fact that this person feels that everyone hates him is a sign of deep-seated problems and he believes he has been falsely judged, or perjuicio. Often, the failure to receive therapy results in the continued reaction or feeling that everyone is against them. Research has shown that counseling over time with a curandero can be a very effective treatment for an ongoing mental or emotional issue.

172. I'M SURROUNDED — *PERSEGUIDO*

I feel that there are those that wish for me to fail. I am about to begin working as a pre-kindergarten teacher, but I have already started off on the wrong foot. I believe that it is because people envy my success and the education that I have attained against all odds. No one else in my family is educated.

I have been cursed with bad luck with money and especially with love. I am a great believer that there are those who have the spiritual *don*, or gift. I know that the spirits can do both good and bad. Is there something that I can do to protect myself from envy and evil?

CURANDERO'S RESPONSE:

Cleanse yourself by doing a *limpia*, ritual cleansing, with a handful of *gobernadora*, creosote bush, or a bunch of fresh parsley, rubbing it over your entire body saying a prayer and making your petition to your spirit guide and protector, or guardian angel. Do this on the last day of each month.

COMMENTARY:

Many Latinos feel that they must consult a curandero if they suffer from loneliness and believe that the whole world is against them. All aspects of so-called bad luck are interpreted as evil spirits or spells cast against them when it is not necessarily the case. Sometimes life and challenges are our own soul's desire to grow strong. Cultural foundations are much stronger than educational achievements and one's personal level of educational achievement does not eliminate the need to enlist spiritual aid through a curandero.

173. CURSED — *ME MALDIJO*

Something has happened to me and I don't understand what it is or why it happened. I have had several sleepless nights. There are times when my ears are burning. If it's not one thing, it's another. All the clocks in my home have stopped working. All the wrist watches, as well as the clocks in the house have all stopped.

It's been a while that I've been looking for a job everywhere. I have applied for every type of job and nobody has called me. My money does not last. A woman I know told me that my ex-husband had done something so that my money would not last, and so that I would not advance in my job.

I want to know if this is true. She says that a bad spirit always follows me and it won't let me advance in anything I want to do. She says it dresses in black, is fat, and has a dark black hood. Can you tell if this is true? I continue to pray and have faith, but I'm so scared.

CURANDERO'S RESPONSE:

Start by burning incense in your house and also sprinkle Holy Water throughout the entire house. Cleanse yourself with a white candle. You can light it inside a good-sized can with about two inches of yard dirt at the bottom of the can. Place the candle in the dirt at the bottom of the can. When the candle burns all the way, take the dirt and throw it in a river where the water is running. Ask God to rid you of all the bad in you and to fill you with blessings.

COMMENTARY:

It is very common in Latin American cultures for persons to believe that they are being followed and/or pursued by evil spirits. Sometimes clocks and watches cease to function for persons who have had near-death experiences or when a relative has recently passed. The deceased relative wants to enlighten the living so they can realize that they are still loved and are being "watched over."

174. THE HEX — *EL HECHIZO*

I'm writing because I think someone has put a hex on me and I need help. I can be reached by e-mail. I contacted you several months ago concerning my problem with a spirit that was always around me. I am sad to report that I continue to face a series of misfortunes.

First of all, I broke three glasses within days of each other and that is a bad omen. I have not broken a glass in 30 years.

Then, I lost my job last month and I am still without a job. I am single and I do not have anyone to depend on except myself. I have depleted my savings and rent is due soon.

I was in a car accident and it was my fault. I sneezed and did not step on the brake soon enough, so I was in the middle of traffic that was not going in the same direction I was. I did not go through the red light but I stopped my car; hoping that the SUV coming would stop, but he did not. His wife was in the car with him and she will surely testify that it was my fault. I have no witnesses to support me, but it was my fault anyway.

I have gone before the judge three times but the police have not turned in the report. I will be going back today to see if I will be able to see the judge.

A few days after my accident, a woman ran into me and hurt me with an electric cart at a store. The store claimed that they were not responsible for my injury.

The woman tried to escape before the police could get there and she wasn't even shopping for groceries. She was only waiting for her daughter to do her shopping. She spoke only Spanish. A police report was made, but I doubt that the woman gave correct information. She didn't even say she was sorry. I was just standing at the checkout line minding my own business when she failed to control her cart. She hit me pretty hard on the back.

Early one morning this week, a policeman knocked at my door, because someone tried to pry the door of my car open and broke the window, trying to commit a burglary. I didn't have anything to steal, not even parking meter change. They got into the car and left the glove box open. A police report was made, but from what the policewoman said, it was someone that had been doing this for a long time and that they have no way to catch them.

What do you think is going on with me? No one can have this much bad luck without being hexed. Someone told me that I may need a *limpia*. I will look it up on the Internet but I do not know what that is or how it is done. All I know is that I have been in a state of shock for some time. I was hoping that the bad luck would end, but it has not. I still have the prayer for a person in need that you sent me. I have been praying a lot, but things keep happening. Do you have any suggestions?

CURANDERO'S RESPONSE:

May God bless you with a special healing. I will do all I can to help deliver you from this evil spell that someone has cast on you. It is very possible that there is a witch, or *hechicera*, who has special powers and/or is in league with the devil who is hexing you. *Hechiceras* are hired to cast spells, or *maldiciones*, or *salaciones* on people.

Please cut four red apples in quarters. Remove and collect all the seeds from the apple and place them under the mattress of your bed and leave them there. Boil the pieces of the four apples and bathe with the apple water saying a prayer and making your petition. Please let me know what happens. Boil seven heads of garlic and bathe with the water to remove negative energies, evil spirits and bad luck. Do this for three straight Fridays. Keep me posted.

COMMENTARY:

Not all Latinos are knowledgeable about curanderismo or its practitioners. They usually hear about curanderos by word of mouth or see their advertisements in the newspaper, television or on radio. However, the most popular referral is word of mouth. The best referrals are by people who respect and trust the curandero they have personally worked with. Hearsay or third-party references are not as direct as first-hand accounts.

In this case, the petitioner has consulted a curandero and does not feel that they have been helped. Disappointment in not having one's prayers or petition answered is very common. The curandero/a will always say that the petition is in the hands of God and that prayers which are not answered have in fact been answered, but not to the petitioner's liking.

In this question we learn about the concept of the sign. Does a breaking glass or another odd event constitute a sign from the spirit world? While it is not always so, in the realm of curanderismo the identification and interpretation of signs is very important. The so-called sign that a follower of curanderismo identifies will seem like nothing out of the ordinary to the lay person.

175. PINS AND NEEDLES — *ALFILERES*

Hello, brother. I'm writing again to let you know how things are going. We have been performing the egg cleansing ritual that you prescribed. Today is the third day in a row that we have performed the hex-breaking ritual with the egg on our poor innocent child. Each time we break the fresh egg after the *limpia*, or spiritual cleansing, the contents of the egg is rotten and full of little things that look like straight pins. It's ugly and horrible and stinks.

The truth is that we are very scared because we don't have any enemies that we know of. We don't have many friends either. We are homebodies and live in a small town. There are some people here that have animals such as cows and chickens, so I didn't have any trouble getting the fresh eggs.

I don't know who would hate us so much that they would want to cause extreme harm to a child. I understand that it could be coming from someone in our former town and the evil has followed us. However, one day I walked out of my house and noticed an egg had been thrown at my car. On another occasion, on the front door of my house, there was some kind of powder that looked like ashes. So it seems that someone here is trying to scare us or really has done something very awful to our child. I don't understand why, unless they have been sent from someplace else.

CURANDERO'S RESPONSE:

Get a hold of nine fresh farm eggs from someone you can trust. The ones they sell at the stores are not fresh. These have to come right from under the hen and in the morning if at all possible. Recite the Lord's Prayer as you pass the egg along the child's body in a sweeping motion early in the morning. The child could even be asleep. Be sure that you hold the egg in your right hand. Once you have done the sweeping, break the egg into a crystal glass or clear glass of water.

If the egg shows something that looks like straight pins in the water, that indicates that someone cursed him with something dreadful. If the egg looks all scrambled, it means that he is spooked, or something has scared him in the past or that he has been traumatized. If the egg is clear, that is real clean it means that he does not have any negative supernatural influences at this moment. If it has an appearance of an eye in the yolk, it means he has the evil eye. Regardless of whatever appears in the egg, continue the same ritual for a total of nine consecutive days. After studying the egg, you can dispose of it by flushing it down the toilet. But let me know on a daily basis what you see in the egg.

Let me know immediately if he hears voices, or if he is attacked by a spirit, or has visions or if he has any bad reaction of any kind. I also recommend that you bathe him in Holy Water from a Catholic Church for the same nine days that you cleanse him with the egg. Let me know if other family members in the same household begin to notice strange or unexplainable things.

COMMENTARY:

Nothing can be more frightening than encountering serious evidence of witchcraft in the form of a doll with needles, alfileres, or to "recognize" straight pins within the yolk of an egg that has been used in a cure, or limpia. While actual straight pins have been known to appear in egg yolks, apparently the questioner is talking about parts of the egg that look like pins.

Sympathetic magic is based upon making an association of two unrelated items and the belief that one causes the other.

Witchcraft objects should never be touched with a bare hand and always removed with gloves on. You should always consult a reputable curandero for expert advice. Making a small fire away from the house and burning the witchcraft dolls is a common remedy, but you must be very careful because the hex will try to "jump," or brincar, from the burning doll to a nearby human or animal; thus transferring and continuing the witchcraft. Then, the gloves which are worn during this process are subsequently burned as well.

176. CRAZY TODDLER — *EL LOQUITO*

My boyfriend and I have a three-year-old boy who is late in his development. He has had difficulty walking and talking and sometimes he is very quiet for hours. When this occurs, it is like he is locked inside his head. At other times, he is very hyper and uncontrollable. My boyfriend and I think he will be okay and will develop at his own speed. I know we overprotect him from his cousins.

Now that he is getting to the age where he could go to school, we are thinking of having him evaluated. When we mentioned this to my family, they just laughed and said that he is crazy and will never amount to anything.

We got really mad and offended about this, and our boy was watching and understands everything, began to yell and cry on the floor. He has feelings, you know? Then it got worse and they said he might be possessed by an evil spirit. We don't want our child growing up around people who are going to say these bad things about him. Do you have any advice for us?

CURANDERO'S RESPONSE:

There are many reasons why your child might act the way he does. These behaviors do not mean that there is anything wrong with him, but it is always good to check everything out. For example, *susto*, or fright sickness, evil eye, or *mal ojo*, and unclean spirit possession are all conditions that can afflict a child, but they do not mean that he is "crazy." You should always check with a medical doctor as well. Many children are being diagnosed with attention deficit hyperactivity disorder (ADHD), autism or any other childhood problem, but only a doctor can be sure of what he has if anything at all.

Often, a child who is unable to hear and unable to speak, or who seems to be developing slowly is suffering from some kind of trauma that caused fright, soul loss, or evil eye.

Think back in his life to when these behaviors began, was there anything that happened to him that you can remember? All these things can be corrected. At the other extreme, there is a possibility that someone is envious of you or your child. It could even be a family member who has cast a witchcraft spell on him. And yes, it could also be spirit possession, but, once again, all these things can be reversed.

It is a good idea to do two things. Have him cleansed by a reputable healer and evaluated by a child diagnostician. That is, whenever there are signs that something seems wrong with a child, the child should be immediately taken to a medical health care professional for examination, diagnosis, and evaluation. This will help the child and, at the same time, place you at ease.

Also have him spiritually cleansed, but most importantly, never allow your child to be in an environment where people, and especially strangers, are critical of him. If you allow this to continue, then as he grows, what they say about him will form his life's behavioral patterns, whether the comments are true or not. If everyone tells him he is crazy, then he will be crazy. Don't let this happen to your child.

COMMENTARY:

Witchcraft is a major and active force everyday in Mexico. Belief in and the practice of witchcraft in the major Latino communities of the United States is slightly less prevalent. However, with major migrations of people and news from Mexico available on television and other media, the practice of witchcraft has dramatically escalated in the last few years.

It is important to assist young couples with children to break away from these beliefs so that the new generation of Latinos/as is not influenced adversely. *If the environment is nurturing and not rife with negative news or name calling, bliss allows a child to develop normally and experience a pleasant upbringing.*

177. PROTECTING OURS —*PROTEGIENDO LO NUESTRO*

At both our home and at our business we are constantly finding the evidence of witchcraft, *brujería*, objects. Because we are successful, I don't think it will ever end, but is there something we can do to protect our home, our business, and our persons?

CURANDERO'S RESPONSE:

As a *curandero*, I like to practice what I preach. Some of the more popular items that are used for protection for the home, yard, property and business are the *sávila* plant, or aloe vera, which is placed at the entrance of the house or business. It is used to capture negative energies such as envies, jealousies and ill will from enemies as they pass by or enter the home or yard.

As the virtuous plants protect, they absorb negative and evil energies, which usually kills them. So, if your protective plant dies, you know that something evil attempted to get into your home or yard.

A woven strand of garlic heads three to four feet in length is usually placed over the door or near the entrance to the business as well. Never reuse that garlic in cooking; throw it away at the end of every year and get a new one.

Traditionally, and quite popular for the protection of the home, is the use of the San Ignacio de Loyola picture, or *estampa*, and the cross made from *palma bendita*, the blessed palm from Palm Sunday which is saved in the home, business and car throughout the year.

Horseshoes, glass containers with water and *tomate marino*, seeds found in the *hierbería,* are also commonly used protective amulets. The Jericho flower with sea shells and red flowers placed in the container will protect the business from bad luck.

For the home, a mixture of white rice, wheat germ and black mustard seed placed in Holy Water and sprinkled outside the home and in the yard will cleanse and protect the property. Always be certain to sprinkle it over the roof as well. This also "opens the door," *abre camino o puerta*, for the successful sale of the property if that is your wish. Make a written petition and say the appropriate prayers and it will come true. Florid water, *agua florida*, mixed with ammonia and a little bleach in Holy Water can be used as a floor wash or *despojo* in the home and sprinkled outside the entrance to the home for protection.

COMMENTARY:

One of the most common requests people make of a curandero/a, or a hierbera is for protective objects. There are literally thousands of objects and rituals used for this purpose, and each situation is different. Each solution has to consider the unique characteristics of the case.

178. FIXING THE GAME — *CONJURANDO EL FUTBOL*

I hope you can help me. I work in the front office of a professional soccer team and there are many Latinos around all the time, both men and women. Here in the office we find powders and oils, or *polvos y aceites*, and other uglier objects that have been placed at the entrance to our office, or in the locker rooms and sometimes, even buried on the field. Some of my co-workers and many of our athletes are scared by this.

For those from Latin American countries, this is business as usual. They believe it to be completely normal and some even participate by performing rituals to reverse hexes placed on our team. They say: "fight fire with fire."

I am not generally worried about what they do or what others are doing to us, but should I be? The general manager who is also Latin American says we should not worry because he has hired a powerful warlock, or *brujo*, in Los Angeles to reverse the spells that have been placed on us. What does that mean? I really don't know as much as I probably should about these things or what's happening.

A friend of mine who follows our team told me that he often finds the same kinds of objects at the entrances to his business that are even placed by persons inside his business. The objects are works of witchcraft, or *brujería,* and are intended to ruin his business.

Can this be true, do people actually do this to other people? More importantly, does it really work? How should I protect myself from whatever it does?

CURANDERO'S RESPONSE:

There are times when people show up here with all sorts of objects that they have found in their yards and businesses. All are strange, some are products of pranksters, but some are truly witchcraft items with ill will and produced with a real intent to harm. Some have attached to them the supernatural powers of the dark side.

This hexing is very common among Latinos and just as there are people out there who cast hexing spells. There are *curanderos* who reverse spells. It has become very popular for people to look for *brujos* to fix the outcome of a game, to make a business fail, to reverse the fortune of a political candidate, or to guarantee a drug deal. People try to use *curanderos* and *brujos* for just about anything.

Most often, people are just taken advantage of by unscrupulous persons who don't really know what they are doing, but suck them into the hexing game. We call them dabblers. But those who really know how to manipulate supernatural forces are more than willing for a price to assist in reversing the outcome of a game or a political campaign.

It is good to always be aware that these things exist. People who feel that they are the targets of ill intent may cleanse themselves with an egg, a lemon, an alum rock or with a handful of fresh herbs from the garden like *albahaca,* sweet basil. Often, all types of objects that have been "prepared" or used in a hexing ritual including liquids, oils, powders, dead animals, cemetery dirt, human feces, and many others things and objects which are then found in one's yard, home or business. Often they are never found because they are placed in cemeteries, thrown in rivers or the ocean or buried where you can't or don't find them. If encountered, they should never be touched with the bare hand in that they may have the power to harm and can transfer evil to an innocent person by contact.

Finally, you could go to your nearest *hierbería* and purchase a little book that discusses witchcraft spells so you can better understand.

COMMENTARY:

The practice of witchcraft, or brujería, is as popular now as it was hundreds of years ago. Because there are so many people who seek to use witchcraft against their neighbors, sadly, the practice of witchcraft is thriving.

Also, it is often reported in the media that evidence of witchcraft is associated with sports teams, businesses, homes, and political figures. This fact supports the contention that the practice is alive and well. Most often, it is intended to intimidate or scare, but sometimes, it is serious. The individual will contract a real witch or warlock in Mexico or some other place to cast deadly hexes and spells; usually evil ones.

The most gruesome case on record was the so-called satanic-gang killings on the United States-Mexico border 20 years ago when a Cuban American santero was using human sacrifice to "blind" (law stay away) law enforcement to his narcotic shipments through Mexico as well as across the border into the United States. It seemed to work for a while, but eventually resulted in the deaths of many and the imprisonment of others involved.

In the end, a "white" or good Mexican warlock assisted the federal authorities in reversing the evil power thus, bringing down the gang. In this case, fire and salt were used to win out over the evil.

179. HOLY DEATH — *LA SANTÍSIMA MUERTE*

I am praying more to the Lord than ever before. I feel His grace but I have a problem and I am scared that it will not be resolved. This is a matter of life or death. Please ask the Niño to help me pass my classes this semester so that I can pass the whole year and be promoted to my senior year in high school.

I made a promise to the Santísima Muerte that if I passed, I would not skip school, but I have missed a lot and I'm not feeling so good about my absences. I am afraid that our lady of the holy death will want to collect on my broken promise by claiming my life and taking my soul. I can't take the chance that the principal will excuse my absences so I want to ask the Niño to help me pass and to see if he can overcome La Santísima Muerte.

My mom doesn't understand this stuff or believe me, but I know you do. I have opened up to you more than to my parents because they don't believe in these things. I know that you understand these things and that I am truly scared. I talked to our priest, but he just told me it was all in my head. He doesn't understand or believe me either. I also know that making promises and breaking them is very serious business and I'm scared because that is what I have done.

I can feel that holy death has had enough of my absences because she has told me in my dreams to beware of my broken promise. I am afraid that I am going to die in exchange for being bad. I want to live, so can you please ask the Niño and see what he recommends and how to get out of this mess I got myself into. I know he can help me break my promise to the Santísima Muerte. He can talk to her in the spirit world and beg her to spare my life.

I just feel that my life is going down the tube. First, I was involved in a satanic cult, and now I've broken my promise to Holy Death. I'm all screwed up and very confused. To make matters worse, I cannot locate the woman who got me involved with the Santísima Muerte. Maybe she was a spirit and not a real person.

People are telling me that holy death is not like the Catholic Virgen and will kill me if I break my promise to her. I want to keep my promise but I'm only 17 and I'm not sure I know how to keep a promise. I'm scared and don't want to die.

The *bruja* I was seeing had me write my promises to La Santísima Muerte down on parchment paper, but none of them were about school or passing. They were about other terrible things that had to do with the devil and I am ashamed of doing that. She said that if I didn't keep the promises I wrote down, I will die. I really need to see Fidencio but I don't know if my dad will take me to see you and that is why I am e-mailing you.

I am afraid that Satan and holy death are coming for me soon to repay my promise with my life. Please ask the Niño to help me out of this situation. With all my faith I ask you to please help me pass my tests and the whole year, and to get out of my promises to holy death and to escape the grasp of the satanic cult I once belonged to. It's worse than a gang because they don't kill you with a gun. If I can get out of this one, I promise to be good all next year.

CURANDERO'S RESPONSE:

I am so sorry to hear your tragic story. Niño does not get involved with anyone who is committed to the Santísima Muerte. Niño recommends you forget about your involvement with the Santísima Muerte and with the satanic cult. Your faith in God and the Niño Fidencio should be sufficient to protect you from any evil. You do not have to be afraid of the Santísima Muerte, just have faith in God.

You must have faith that she cannot punish you if you break your promise to her. You are going to find out real soon that if you place your faith in God, He will fill you with the Holy Spirit, with courage and valor that can overcome anything like the holy death a million times over.

You need to forget all about the Santísima Muerte. Sweep her from your mind and do not think or talk about her. Do not ever mention her name out loud. That only gives her energy. Wake up and get a life and I will walk with you in the spirit to help you.

Try saying a reversing prayer. Instead of asking holy death to do something for you, why not ask in reverse, that something not be done. It might work.

COMMENTARY:

The cult of the Santísima Muerte has gained great popularity in recent years; originating in Mexico City and moving to the border and into Latino barrios in the United States (in South America called San la Muerte and differs from the Mexican version). The young man admits that he has been involved in a satanic cult with La Santísima Muerte and now seeks help from El Niño Fidencio.

Dabbling in the supernatural and with cults is extremely dangerous and the curandero appropriately indicates to him that he cannot and will not get involved. Recognizing that the young man is desperate, floundering, and without faith, the curandero attempts to allay his fears by asking him to invest faith in God.

So many young people these days place hope and faith in cults or evil spirits and then suffer the ensuing consequences when their lives collapse. There is always a price to pay when venturing to the dark side. Witchcraft seems like an easy solution to life's problems, but it opens up portals leading to demonic possession as well as other evil spirits.

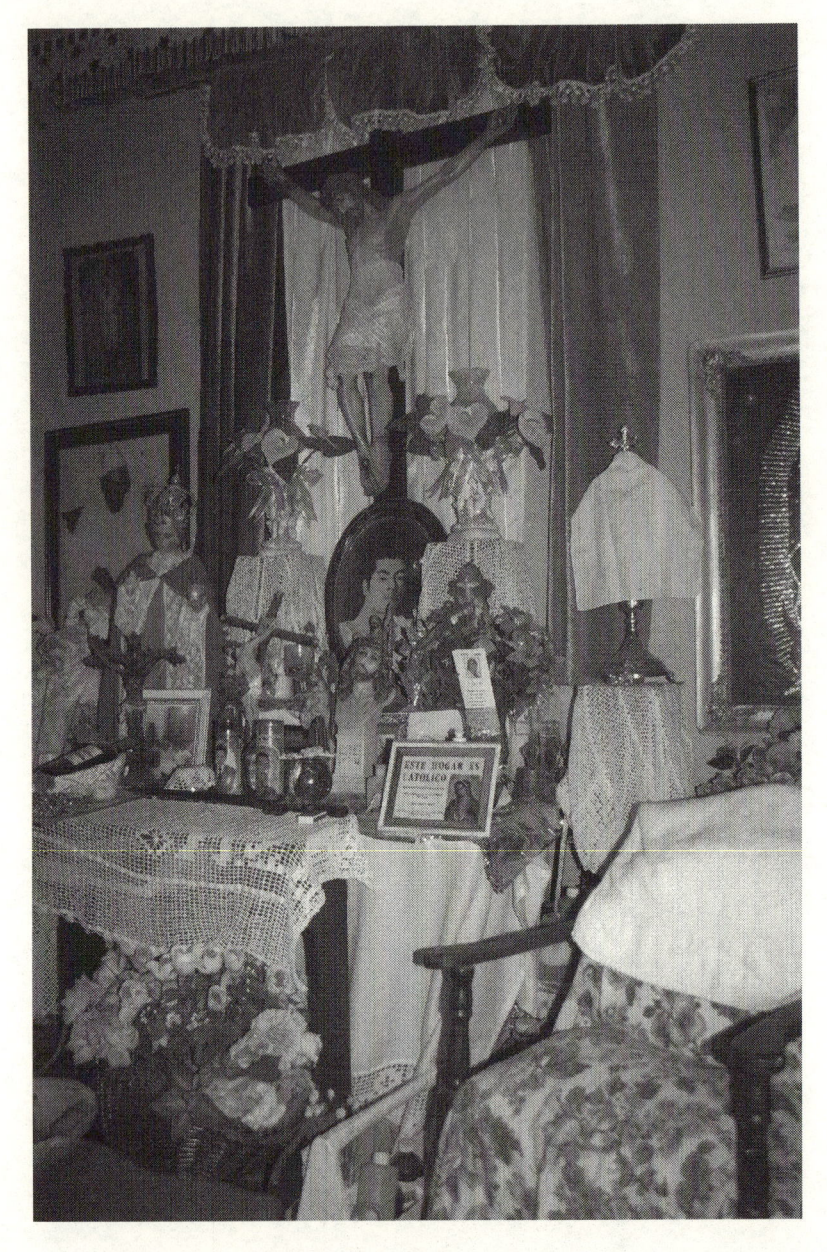

The miraculous altar of Ciprianita "Panita" Zapata de Robles in Espinazo, Nuevo León, México. (Photo by Zavaleta)

PART TEN

Giving Thanks: Prayers Answered and Miracles Received

"Let not your heart be disturbed. Do not fear sickness or anguish. Am I not here, who is your Mother? Are you not under my protection? Am I not your health? Do not grieve nor be disturbed by anything."

–Virgen de Guadalupe, 1531

180. PERSONAL PILGRIMAGE — *PEREGRINACIÓN PERSONAL*

I was born with a birth defect, and while it was not life threatening, it did have the potential to cause a lifelong disability if not corrected. My father and mother who were both Marines had few places to turn for help in the post-war years. My father's mother, my grandmother, asked my father to pray to the Virgen de Guadalupe, and to ask her to intercede with her Son, our Lord, asking for no less than a miracle for their baby boy. The miracle was granted, my experimental surgery was performed at the University of California at Los Angeles Medical Center in 1947 for no charge for the young Marine Corps family.

A couple of years later, my grandmother reminded her son not to forget the promise that he had made to the Virgen and that he was obligated to complete his promise and pilgrimage.

The miracle that was granted required my father to take his family on a pilgrimage into Mexico in order to fulfill his *manda*, or spiritual burden, and promise to the Virgen.

Half a century later and now that I'm 50 years old, my father and mother had never told me of my story of my surgery, miracle and our pilgrimage. Then, as a middle-aged man, I began having dreams and flashbacks of the trip we took when I was only three years old.

Wanting to know more about this aspect of my life and an explanation for the lifelong devotion I have to the Virgen de Guadalupe, I asked my aging and sickly father to tell me about it. It was only then that the fantastic story was told to me for the very first time. My father could remember only generalities, but not exactly where the place was that he took his young family and son.

I wanted to return there and to take my father back there before his death in an effort to repay my father for the faith he had so many years ago, and for asking the Virgin for my miracle. I asked the Niño Fidencio through his *materia*, or trance medium, how to get there.

The Niño Fidencio told me that he was familiar with my case and instantly revealed the pilgrimage location as El Chorrito in the northern Mexican state of Tamaulipas. So I made plans to take my father and my *materia* to El Chorrito.

The Niño told me that he had been waiting all these years for me to discover my story and that I should take my father there as soon as possible. So, within a couple of weeks, my father, my *materia*, her *guardia* and I made the trek southward from the Texas border to El Chorrito.

We had so much joy that day, as we visited there half a century later, and gave thanks for my miracle. Not long after that, my father died, but before his death, we were able to close the circle on the most important spiritual connection a father and son can have: love.

CURANDERO'S RESPONSE:

You have a beautiful story that points out the connection between Our Lady of Guadalupe and her helpers in heaven such as the Niño Fidencio. Your story is particularly touching for several reasons. The Niño Fidencio helps you to remember this important event in your life. He uses one of his *materias* to help you and you are able to take your father there thanking both he and the Virgen de Guadalupe for the miracle you received in your life and your lifelong devotion to her. Always remember to revere Saint James, or Santiago, the patron saint of pilgrims and celebrate his day July 25.

I am aware of countless stories of people who have a devotion to a certain saint or Virgen and are not sure why. Like you, others sometimes find out why, but in most cases they never do. You were lucky. Nevertheless, they do know that their devotion is real and profound.

COMMENTARY:

Latino culture is one of faith and deep devotion. Latinos revere the many aspects of the Virgen and the saints who serve as spiritual protectors; helping them cope with life's many dilemmas. Devotion to the Virgen of Guadalupe for example, is passed on generationally, as exemplified by this beautiful and heart-rending story. No doubt, this man will take his own children back along the same path to pilgrimage that began with his grandmother and his ancestors. Most Latinos do not make a distinction between saints of the Catholic Church and folk saints. However, both are equally valid and important to them.

181. GRANT US A MIRACLE — *DÁNOS UN MILAGRO*

This week my grandson is going to have a procedure to close a hole in his heart. Please pray for him. Please ask the Niño Fidencio for his procedure to come out alright and for him to be a healthy little boy. He is just an innocent little boy and we love him so much and we want him to live a happy and healthy life.

CURANDERO'S RESPONSE:

My prayers are with you, your family and your grandson. Modern medicine and heart procedures are so advanced; it is scientifically miraculous in itself. We must also appreciate the reality of divine intervention because it is also an essential human need for spiritual completeness, not only for the family, but especially for the patient in need.

COMMENTARY:

Never discount the power of divine intervention. Concurrently, we must understand and accept the reality of Divine Providence, which means that sometimes the lives of the most innocent are cut short. Prayer and faith provide personal assistance in cases like this. The curandero can provide guidance and constant prayer to support the family. Latino culture has developed, over the course of the past 400 years, a deep devotion for the saints and belief that God is active in our lives. This activity means that God answers prayers and delivers miracles to His faithful. The practice of medicine and the mestizaje of popular medical beliefs, both indigenous and European with their respective remnants, are still very visible in Mexican folk medicine today.

182. GOOD MEDICINE — *LA BUENA MEDICINA*

I have been the beneficiary of many of my grandma's home remedies and I won't ever forget how she insisted we shake out our shoes every morning before we put them on, to get rid of any scorpions that might have crawled inside. Sometimes one of us grand kids would scream and the scorpion would run across the floor until an older grandchild, with shoes on, would step on it and put it out of its misery. Since scorpions are common in desert areas, many children and adults with serious stings had to drive hours to a hospital if bitten by certain types of scorpions.

If we all went walking in the *campo*, or countryside, with my grandma, we felt safe. She always had a *rebozo*, or shawl tied over her shoulder with some fruit for us and her magical remedies if we needed them. When one of my cousins scraped against a *maguey* cactus, grandma was ready. The *maguey* cactus looks like a century plant or *yucca* plant with thick leaves, but has dry pointed leaves that can deeply scratch the fragile flesh of a youngster. It is pretty bad for an adult as well. My cousin fell into one when I was young and I remember what my grandma did for her. Grandma pulled out her pocket knife and sliced a lime in half and squeezed its juice onto the scratch then she massaged the whole area with the half of lime to keep the maguey poison from making her arm swell up.

In the *campo* the small rainbow cactus was covered with fine spines and easy to miss while walking but grandma was always ready. One of my cousins tripped, fell into a tiny bunch of rainbow cacti, the result was an armful of the tiny blonde needles that reflect the light spectrum and gives the little barrel-like plants the name of rainbow cactus. My grandma whipped out one of the braids of hair that comprised her bun and rubbed her loose hair in a circular motion on my cousin's arm until all the tiny spines disappeared. We thought it was magic! The truth is that the rainbow spines are too fragile to be removed by tweezers and human hair will pull them out of skin and then brushed out of the hair. Since they are not as thick as a human hair, there is something about human hair that grabs them when they come in contact with the hair shaft being rubbed against the spine-filled skin.

I have forgotten a lot of remedies, but if we were stung by a bee or wasp in the *campo*, or countryside, grandma would put a cup in our hands and tell us to go pee in it while she used the pocket knife like an old-fashioned straight razor and lay the blade almost flat against the skin, scraping the stinger out. Then she would pour the urine on the sting and it would neutralize the poison. Most people don't know that urine is sterile for the first minutes after it is expelled and grandma always rubbed it off and patted the area with a cloth that was doused with *pulque,* a homemade tequila-like brew that she had in a tiny bottle; carried in her *rebozo,* along with her many bandaging rags.

My question to you is do you know why she kept an aloe vera plant in the kitchen and why she made us drink raw onion juice if we had a cold?

Antonio Zavaleta and Alberto Salinas Jr.

CURANDERO'S RESPONSE

Your grandma was very wise indeed. Most of our grandmothers always kept aloe vera plants in the four corners of their yard as well as in their kitchen where meals were prepared. Drinking raw onion juice is an ancient and effective remedy for a head cold.

Your e-mail brings back fond memories for me as well, and I thank you for that. I remember that my aunt put raw onion and parsley into a blender and then strained the juice with cheesecloth and she would have us drink it when we started getting head colds or lung congestions. She also used the pulp for other remedies.

As you may know, the mesquite tree has many thorns that can easily puncture the skin even if the person is wearing leather gloves or chaps if they are on horseback. This thorn must be removed or it can cause blood poisoning and sometimes gangrene. The poultice my family used for the sores where the mesquite thorns were removed was the pulp from the onion and parsley mixed together with garlic and mustard seed mashed in a mortar and pestle then spread on the sore and bandaged. The folk would change the poultice regularly depending on how long the mesquite thorn had been in the skin and whether fever, delirium, and/or blood poisoning was present.

As for the aloe vera plant in the kitchen, the gel inside the leaves are commonly used for kitchen burns and the juice can heal scratches or kitchen cuts as well as calming stomachs that have frequent heartburn.

COMMENTARY:

Almost everyone has cherished childhood memories which are especially sweet when they involve remembering and learning under the direction of a grandmother or grandfather along with our cousins. Here the petitioner shares with us wonderful memories of her grandmother's remedies in a much simpler time. Memories from a time of innocence provide us with the framework for our sense of being, for our cultural realities and for our values.

The reality is that most of our grandmother's remedies can be verified as effective when compared to the "official" recipe book of the American

Pharmaceutical Association of the early 20th century. For example, medicated-nasal drops, whether mixed at home or at the corner pharmacy, consisted of oil of eucalyptus, oil of dwarf pine needles and menthol mixed in a light petrolatum liquid (*The Pharmaceutical Book*, page 18). This mixture is still used by curanderos today.

As we walk through life, sometimes we encounter a familiar scenario, a particular aroma or hear a sound or voice that stirs a dormant memory. Savor that moment! Your ancestors are conveying a special message just for you.

183. OUR LUCK CHANGED — *LA BUENA SUERTE*

We recently found out that the insurance check we were waiting for was mailed and that we will probably get it this week. It seems that with your help and Niñito Fidencio's help, our bad luck is starting to change to our favor. Even our car seems to be doing better and we haven't had to buy the part that we thought it needed.

My wife also wants to let you know about her grandmother. She still has that pain in her leg. She went to see the doctor and he gave her some medicine, but it didn't work for her. She has been applying different types of over-the-counter creams for pain, and sometimes they work and sometimes they do not. The doctor even had an x-ray done on her and everything seems to be okay. Every night at around 2:30 a.m., she wakes up with the pain. Do you have a remedy that she could use to get rid of this terrible pain?

CURANDERO'S RESPONSE:

I am glad that what El Niño Fidencio and I are trying to do for you seems to be changing your bad luck back in your favor. We can all thank God for His blessings on you. Without God's blessings, we would not be able to do anything for anyone.

Have your grandmother massage the pain area in her legs with lemon juice and then massage them with egg white. That should help her.

Keep using drops of the basil, or *albahaca* oil in your bath water and call on the spirit of Niño Fidencio to help with your financial needs and to change your luck. Also, please keep a Niño Fidencio candle on your altar on a regular basis. If you have trouble finding a Niño Fidencio candle, ask your *hierbería*, or herb store for the Santa Cruz de Caravaca candle.

To help your car, sprinkle some rice mixed with wheat seed and mustard seed in it to cleanse the vehicle of bad luck. I believe it breaks down due to envy and evil spirits causing all sorts of problems for you.

COMMENTARY:

Over the course of their lives, people develop deep faith in El Niño Fidencio, elevating him to folk-saint status. The petitioner refers to him using the diminutive term, Niñito or little boy child, a sign of profound respect and dedication practically on the same level as the Christ Child. Child status is also associated with innocence and the absence of sin.

In curanderismo, Catholic saints and folk saints alike are believed to influence the outcome of events, especially luck. Believers in curanderismo are certain that envy causes evil spirits to alter the outcome of events in our lives and the only effective method to overcome evil is to receive a spiritual cleansing.

184. PRAYING — *ORANDO*

I have been saying the following prayers you sent me for a while now. "Oh powerful spirit of Fidencio." "Niño Fidencio Síntora Constantino and, the "Oh Divine Spirit" prayers. However, I am not sure that I am saying them correctly or at the right time or using the correct candles for these prayers. I am also not sure what the proper situations are for each candle and each prayer.

I want to pray that I regain my confidence and that my strength returns to me. I pray that I will be sure to make the right decisions. I want to pray for my husband so that he can stop getting so angry and upset at work. I want to pray that the people who he works with will stop bothering him and will leave him alone. I want to pray for my sister's behavior to improve. I want to pray that she will respect her elders and do as she is told and that she will find a renewed interest in school, work and family. I get so upset with her because she is so disrespectful. Please continue to pray for me to have patience with her.

CURANDERO'S RESPONSE:

There is a special time for prayer, and the best time is when there is a special need. Prayer must come from within you, from the heart. There is prayer for the self to be recited alone. This is a private, personal prayer. There is also open, public prayer, and there are prayers for others. There are thankful prayers of gratitude. Prayer is most sacred and most powerful when one is fasting. Be sure to always consult a doctor before fasting.

The teaching of the Lord is that when two or more come together in His Holy name, He is there amongst you. *Curanderos* who work in the spiritual realm believe that the most special time for prayer is at 3 a.m. Below is a common prayer to Fidencio:

PRAYER: NIÑO FIDENCIO CONSTANTINO

Niño Fidencio Síntora Constantino, I come to you with faith and hope. I ask for your blessing, good health, enlightenment and strength. Please help me to resolve my financial and everyday problems. Cleanse me and keep me from all evil. Fill me with light, faith, hope and anoint me with the blessings of the Holy Spirit, Amen.

Afterwards, say one Our Father.

COMMENTARY:

Some form of prayer has always been an integral part of healing. In colonial Mexico professional prayers for hire or ensalmadores were believed to heal with prayers or Psalms. Today, curanderos/as frequently ask their clients to pray certain biblical Psalms as you have seen throughout this book.

Prayers are accepted anytime they are offered. Curanderos/as recommend specific prayers and candles for certain situations, but most people feel greatly relieved and improved by any prayer whenever recited. The curandero mentions that it is common to pray at 3 a.m., but this is principally a practice of the spiritist who believes that the veil between the physical world and the spirit world is thinnest at that hour.

185. GRANT ME STRENGTH — *FORTALÉCEME*

I am happy to meet you and I wish with all my heart that God and the Niño Fidencio will give you spiritual strength, so that you may continue to guide us and help us. I am praying for you. I bathed with the water of *ruda,* rue, *albahaca,* basil, *romero* and rosemary, but I forgot to buy the herbs for this Friday and I ask you if I can do this on Saturday? Does it matter? I feel desperate, and the fear of losing my job fills me with many doubts and emotional instability. I want to ask the Niño for strength, light and support to continue with the cycle of life, as God mandates. I have a profession and it has gone badly for me lately. I am convinced that I am bewitched, but I have faith and believe in miracles.

CURANDERO'S RESPONSE:

Thank you very much for your prayer. You should burn *copal* incense in your home for seven straight Fridays while praying the Our Father. Also, if you can, bathe with herbs. It must be Friday. Boil *ruda,* rue, *romero,* rosemary and *albahaca,* basil, and bathe with the water. The night before, strain the tea and then reheat it and bathe for seven consecutive Fridays praying the Hail Mary seven times. Read the prayers that I have sent you and say the prayer to the Holy Trinity to obtain and maintain a good job.

I am pleased that you have started your herbal-healing baths. I recognize that you have supernatural obstacles that stand in your way, but be strong because they will not win out over you. You must have faith and be more stubborn than those who would see you fail. Also, it is critical that you religiously complete your bathing rituals on Fridays as instructed. No other day will complete the requirements for the ritual and will negate its effects. You must understand that this is a matter of ritual and requires consistency. If you can maintain discipline, the Niño will provide you with all you need to live happy and content.

When you take these baths on the seven straight Fridays, be sure to also invoke the sacred name of Saint Michael the Archangel and ask for his protection. Invoke Saint Rafael the Archangel and ask him for health of body, soul and spirit. Invoke Saint Gabriel the Archangel and ask him for happiness. After your baths with herb water, say the prayers to El Niño Fidencio and ask for justice. Your situation is like a salacious assault, or wrongdoing, or like a curse that has befallen you and your life. But finally, if you do as I instruct, you will win out over evil.

COMMENTARY:

Within the pantheon of helpful spirits and entities, the archangels are considered the most powerful and are called upon for all sorts of difficult cases. There are many other entities also believed to intercede for us in our times of need. For example, the Archangel Rafael is the archangel of healing.

Spiritual baths and other prescribed regimens may be followed closely but don't necessarily have to be adhered to exactly unless they are parts of rituals or magical spells. In those cases, they must be followed exactly or they will not work. In this book the curandero has offered examples of many different saints to pray to and rituals that can be performed for their intercession.

186. SPIRITUAL ASSISTANCE — *AYUDA ESPIRITUAL*

I'm the person who spoke to you on the telephone this afternoon. It shocked me when you knew my last name without even knowing me. Like I told you, I'm new at this, but I am confident now more than ever that you can help me. I have been looking for spiritual help for a long time since things aren't going good for me.

I live in a circle that I can't seem to get out of. First, my life seems to get better for a little bit, but then, just as fast, it turns around to the negative again. I have looked for help but haven't found it. I know what is happening to me, but I can't find the solution. I hope you can help me. If you need more information about me or my condition, I will gladly send it to you. Thank you and I will expect a response soon.

CURANDERO'S RESPONSE:

I know you need a lot of help. You have always been and continue to be high and mighty, and at the same time not very trustful. Perhaps you have a reason. You have always looked for help and have come out being betrayed. Now everything looks too real and true to you. You don't know whether to believe in God or not. You find yourself very confused. I don't blame you. The cure you seek is in your own hands. In order for you to get rid of all your doubts it is totally up to you.

Yes, I'm going to reveal your solution. Your real problem is that you have no faith in God. Start to meditate with the Lord. Do this at three in the morning every day in prayer.

Also, do it every night for an hour until the spirit of God reveals Himself to you. Fast in the mornings for 40 straight days. Also, read Psalm 23 at noon for 40 consecutive days. After doing this, everything will be clear to you. Your true path will be revealed to you.

COMMENTARY:

People are often referred to curanderos/as by their family and friends, without ever having consulted one before. The physical appearance of the curandero/a, consulting room, or consultorio, as well as their rituals may seem extremely bizarre to a first timer. First impressions and the building of confidence are difficult. It takes time but definitely produces positive results. Frequently, people seek simple solutions to complex personal problems, relying on others instead of making meaningful changes in their lives. "God helps he who helps himself." The curandero can offer spiritual support but not for the person looking for a quick fix. The individual must take the situation seriously. There is no cosmic pill to transform life into a dream. Persons who refuse to confront the enemy within themselves and are so self-centered that to them, help means sucking all the energy out of the healer who offers it, will ultimately fail.

187. NIÑO IS LOVE — *NIÑO ES AMOR*

It has been many years since I first learned of the holy saint Niño Fidencio. I have read about his testimonies and his speeches. As he said, "invoke me three times and I will be with you, the messenger of the Holy Spirit." Being a man, it has been many years since I have had sexual relations with a woman and I have lost that interest. I reflect and say to myself, what is the reason for this since I still consider myself young at my age?

I ask and plead that you ask the most holy Niño Fidencio what to do to activate my interest in a normal relationship with a woman and to find a woman that can love me.

I cannot find one and sometimes solitude is good, but a man and a woman need to form as a generation of consequence only one flesh for happiness. I will await your polite response. I found you on the Internet. I am a Catholic and believe in God. I was baptized and confirmed and I remain grateful to your graceful attentions and wait for the Niño Fidencio to help me.

CURANDERO'S RESPONSE:

The Niño Fidencio was born on November 13, 1898 and died October 19, 1938. His fame and popularity was at its peak in 1928. Days after his death, he descended from the heavens spiritually fulfilling the order of the Lord Most High to continue attending his town and mission with the hopeless patients of the doctors.

In order to find your mate and true happiness, make your petition with great faith to God and the Archangel Saint Gabriel. The faith above all is very important since the spirit of the Niño Fidencio is very miraculous. The Lord gave to the Holy Spirit the authority and is manifested in the body of the Niño Fidencio to cure and help humanity. When the Niño died, his body was entombed right where he lay. His body was never removed from his house, and today that location is a major pilgrimage site for his followers.

The Niño Fidencio in life announced his death, and also advised his followers that his mission on earth was not finished. He announced that he would still continue to cure, but that they should be careful because there would be many who would pretend to be Niño Fidencio, but that he was only one and that he would not be in all of them.

Today, you see many Niño Fidencios just as he predicted so many years ago. In order to know if he is present in the medium, you should know that the Niño never charged for his treatments. He was poor and liked to walk without shoes and when his spirit is present you can feel the strength and see the miracles.

Never lose your faith and you may see God and the Niño manifested as a spiritual doctor to help you. Take baths and cleansings with water of *verbena, ruda,* or *romero,* and *albahaca* that is vervain, rue, rosemary and basil, for seven straight Fridays while praying and including petitions to the Holy Spirit.

COMMENTARY:

Persons of all ages turn to the Niño Fidencio to assist them in finding a loving and meaningful relationship. There are two other important concepts to take into consideration. First, some people who have a God-given healing gift, or don in Spanish, are not supposed to marry. They are just ordinary people like you and I. Spiritual healers often fall into this category as well.

Secondly, the union of love they seek can be spiritual with all the world's children as their own because they are "married" solely to their spiritual bond or path. This was the case of the Niño Fidencio who never married nor fathered children.

188. PROMOTED — *PROMOVIDA*

I want to give thanks to La Virgen de Guadalupe and to the Niño Fidencio for answering my petition and my prayers. I have been qualified for a promotion for several years, but never received one. My male co-workers, who are not any more qualified than I am, have always been promoted over me. I asked you what to do and you advised me to write a petition, to ask for a miracle, then to pray for it to occur. Now it has.

I have been granted a once-in-a-lifetime miracle and I know that now my career is on the rise. If I understood correctly, you told me that once my miracle was granted, it was my responsibility to fulfill my promise by making a pilgrimage to Mexico City to the shrine of the

Virgen de Guadalupe. I want to thank you for your help in showing me how to do this and to let you know that in December I will make the trip to Mexico to give thanks at the feet of the Virgen de Guadalupe on her day, December 12.

CURANDERO'S RESPONSE:

Yours is a wonderful story of having received a true miracle in your life. Most people pray for miracles, but are never aware if they were received even though we know that God hears our prayers. To ask, receive and be aware that you received a miracle from God, is a very special event and you are obligated to recognize it by giving back.

Giving back can be as simple as making a special little trip to a shrine near where you live or planning over a lifetime to make the big trip. Either way, always give back to God for a miracle received.

COMMENTARY:

The pilgrimage site of the Virgen de Guadalupe, the representation of Mary the Mother of God in the Americas, has become one of the world's most important Catholic shrines and pilgrimage destinations. Millions of believers undertake the difficult and costly trip to Mexico City yearly to give thanks for miracles granted in their lives.

189. GOOD TO US – *NOS TRATA BIEN*

As you know, I received my first unemployment check and it arrived just in time for us to catch up with our bills. I know that none of this would have been possible if we had not asked El Niño Fidencito to intervene in our case. The fact that I won my case when it looked like a totally unwinnable and uphill battle was due to your assistance.

The unemployment judge decided in my favor because my story was more credible, plus I had documented proof to back up my statements. My former employer was caught lying and they were reduced to only making allegations without any substantial proof or documentation to back up any of their statements.

My last job interview went really well. All I have to do is wait for the results of my background check. I am not really concerned about it and I should be working again soon. I know that all this was done through the love and assistance of the Niño Fidencio.

You know that my wife is not a believer in the spiritual world. She is skeptical about all this and it is so frustrating to me that she is not a believer or gives any credit to you and the saints.

Today when my wife got to work, they asked her if she would be able to work a double shift, all day and all night. This has never happened before because the company she works for just does not do it. She will not be home until midnight or after but we will make an extra $200. We desperately need it right now, so I have to let her do it. This windfall is more proof to me that God is taking care of us and that Fidencio is truly a loyal spirit and that he will go to great lengths just to make sure that his faithful servants are taken care of.

CURANDERO'S RESPONSE:

The spirit of El Niño Fidencio is with you, brother. I am happy you attribute your court victory regarding your unemployment benefits to your faith in El Niño Fidencio. Your wife, not being a believer in matters of your faith, brings friction to your marriage, but don't allow it to be a problem in your marriage. I know that it bothers you a lot, but you need to know that it bothers her as well. Your faith tests her faith, be certain of that. Try to reach some kind of compromise or middle ground with each other.

COMMENTARY:

One of the most popular petitions curanderos receive is for assistance at work or with obtaining a job. The world of work can be a treacherous place that exists outside of the emotional safety net of family and home. At work one commonly encounters envidia, or jealousy. One encounters persons who lie and tempt one's spouse. The spiritual world has been called upon to protect and keep loved ones safe in the workplace.

190. GARDEN OF HEALING — *JARDÍN DE CURACIÓN*

I'm writing you back because I was remembering my great aunt and how she raised me after my mother passed away. You had given me several ways to protect my house, and the garlic braid hanging next to the doors going outside brought back many wonderful memories. Thank you for the pleasure that those memories have given me, as well as your wise advice.

My great aunt had a wonderful green thumb and the adobe wall that surrounded the house was filled with old juice and vegetable cans that were nailed onto the wall. My auntie made small holes in the can bottoms and filled them with earth. She rooted geraniums, started seedlings, and grew kitchen herbs. One whole side of her house was planted with corn and elephant garlic, at least that is what she called it. I think others might say it was *ajo macho*, or male garlic, because it was the biggest head of garlic cloves and it had very tall green straight leaves like green onions or scallions. Anyway, it looked really huge to me as a young girl and I loved watering the corn and garlic as much as the bounty of flowers because their bright colors made me happy.

Once a year we would pick the garlic and she would make big four-foot-long braids and she would have me pick red, hot pink and white geraniums, lavender and purple petunias, as well as yellow, orange and red zinnias. All the beautiful colored flowers would be woven into the garlic wreath and hung to dry under the *enramada*, or shade arbor, so as the flowers dried, they would retain their bright colors and the green garlic stems would turn as gold as dried wheat. When the garlic strands were ready, we would say a prayer as we tied red satin ribbons into bows on each end. The prayer was a blessing for our home, but I don't remember it being the same each time because I was allowed to add my own little prayer at the end of auntie's prayer.

At night, after supper, we would build a fire inside a 55-gallon drum at the back of the lot where a gate prevented our goats and chickens from entering the garden. It was our trash-burning barrel made of metal. Auntie would stand up on a kitchen chair and pull the garlic strands from the previous year down from above the front and back doors to the house. Then, she would put them in the fire, watching them burn until they were ash. Only then, would we hang the new blessed garlic and flower strands above the front and back doors on the four large nails that made them rest on an arch above the doorway.

Auntie explained to me that the old strands had protected our home for a year and were laid to rest. Since they had done their job well, it was time for a new generation of garlic and flowers to take their turn.

I wanted to ask you why she always insisted that the garlic in the kitchen never be braided and why she called it eating garlic that was kept in a covered ceramic pot with air holes on the side and was never to be placed near the kitchen window?

CURANDERO'S RESPONSE:

Thank you, sister, for the wonderful story of family history, I am glad that my answers about protecting your home have been helpful.

When garlic strands are used for protection, they are used to absorb negativity and jealousy inside or outside the home. That is their purpose. It was ingenious of your great aunt to make the strands ornamental because no one would take them apart to use a clove or two for cooking. The ugly thoughts or feelings of others are absorbed into the garlic strands and, if eaten, can make one very sick, especially if the family is a target of other people's envy or witchcraft. Your auntie was right. They must be replaced once a year and burned. I suspect that the garlic-and-floral braid was placed in an arch to resemble a church door or her connection to the archangels. As far as the eating garlic goes, it will dry out the juicy cloves if it gets too hot in the sun and rot if it gets too moist. Most garlic pots sold in cooking stores have vents on the sides so that the garlic will not mold in moist, humid or rainy climates.

COMMENTARY:

This book is now finished and we hope that it has given you as many fond memories as it has given us an enduring pleasure in writing it for you. Culture is rich and alive in our lives and we must never forget who we are, where we come from and who our ancestors were. After all, they are constantly keeping vigilance over us, fully expecting us to do the right thing.

All who have contributed to this book hope and pray that all the questions posed, answers given and explanatory commentaries triggered pleasant memories and/or actualized spiritual food for thought. Also hopefully, it stimulated remembrances of family remedies you may have marveled at, wondered about and maybe even forgotten through the years.

Treasure this little book. In the future, it may be the only place you will find this information consolidated into one source. Pass it along to your children. Consider it your personal spiritual-and-cultural reference book handed down to you from your grandmothers and other ancestors. (The previous story was submitted by Jamie Sams.)

Antonio Zavaleta and Alberto Salinas Jr.

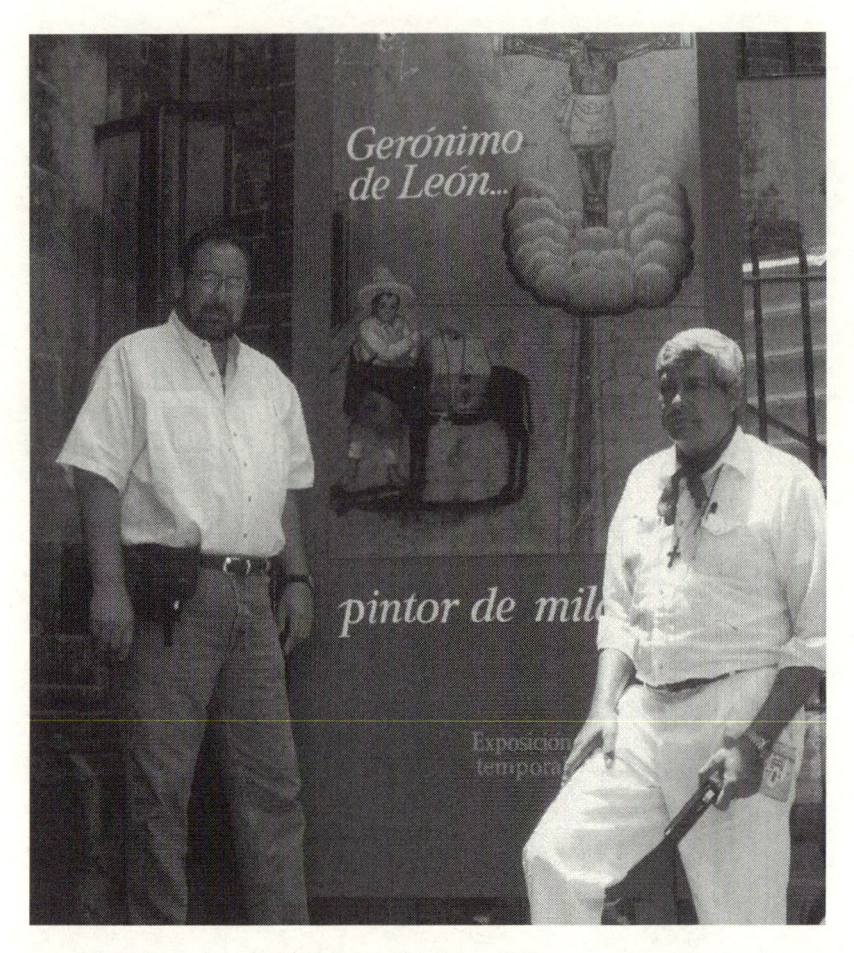

Authors, anthropologist Tony Zavaleta and *curandero* Alberto Salinas Jr. are seen at the entrance to the ex-voto museum at the Basílica de la Virgen de Guadalupe in Mexico City. (Photo by José M. Duarte)

Authors' Notes

Curandero Conversations: El Niño Fidencio, Shamanism and Healing Traditions of the Borderlands is a product of the El Niño Fidencio Curanderismo Research Project at The University of Texas at Brownsville and Texas Southmost College, and is co-authored by anthropologist Antonio N. Zavaleta, Ph.D., and *curandero* Alberto Salinas Jr.

This ongoing *curanderismo* research project was established in 1988 and operates the most comprehensive website on Latino folk healing and *curanderismo* on the Internet (http://vpea.utb.edu/elnino/fidencio.html).

The project utilizes time-honored methods in field anthropology, including ethnography and video-ethnography; participant observation-based field work in Espinazo, Nuevo León, México as well as many other locations in Mexico and throughout the United States-Mexico border.

As the lead anthropologist and project director Dr. Zavaleta has studied *curanderismo* along the United States-Mexico border for more than 40 years and the Fidencista movement for 25 years. Dr. Zavaleta provides the commentary which follows each of the 190 original questions and *curandero's* responses.

In 1995 the research project began interviewing Edinburg, Texas-based *curandero* and independent Fidencista, Alberto Salinas Jr. His ethnographic profile is important because as a bilingual, Mexican American male *curandero* he is unique. The majority of *curanderas* are female Spanish-speaking monolinguals. The *curandero's* responses in the book are provided by Salinas.

Salinas became a *curandero* in the tradition of the Niño Fidencio, after a brief career in public service; fulfilling a lifetime calling to spirituality.

Born with a gift of healing, or *don,* he is descended from several generations of native healers. As a *curandero* in the age of technology, he employs a mixture of indigenous healing rituals, spiritual cleansings, *limpias,* healing baths, *baños,* medicinal plants, or *plantas medicinales,* as well as the use of his healing hands combined with prayer. Salinas continually searches for new esoteric information that might somehow assist those seeking his help.

Because of his unique level of biliteracy and technological ability, Salinas was provided with an Internet-ready computer for the purpose of corresponding with the project. After more than 20 years of practicing one-on-one consultations at his healing center in the lower Rio Grande Valley of Texas, he began consulting via e-mail. This new and innovative aspect of his healing mission rapidly became a major component of his daily consultations.

By 2007 he had logged more than 7,000 e-mail consultations. Many e-mail consultations are ongoing and have established deep personal relationships between client and *curandero.* Salinas' Internet clients consult with him regularly and repeatedly.

It should be noted that as an authentic Mexican American *curandero,* Salinas plays a major and incalculable role in the health-care safety net of his extended community. As in the many examples you have read, Salinas provides a variety of services because of his knowledge of folk remedies, traditional herb use and esoteric Latino practices. Additionally, he developed informal skills in counseling as a result of the need for such support by his clientele requesting his help. Salinas does not charge for his services, but does accept discretionary donations. He leads a very modest life; returning most of the donations to his healing practice.

From the outset it was apparent to the El Niño Fidencio Curanderismo Research Project that Salinas' thousands of e-mail consultations represented a treasure trove of information on *curanderismo*. These recorded consultations also offer a rare view into the lives of Latinos and others. The analysis of this vast collection of e-mail exchanges serves as the foundation of this book.

Curandero Conversations serves to assist the average person to understand what *curanderos* do and why people seek their help with health and personal problems. It further serves as a descriptive guide for professional health care, religious and social-service providers, as well as many individuals who interact with Latinos in professional settings.

This book is a sorely-needed resource for understanding the cultural realities and health disparities of millions of Latinos in the United States today.

Curandero Conversations further seeks to clarify, for health and social-care providers, the importance of the role that cultural competencies play in provider interaction with Latinos and other cultural minorities. It attempts to fill the gap in cultural competencies related to the Latino population because there isn't anything which is easily available to them in regards to *curanderismo*. Health and social care providers must understand these aspects of Latino culture in order to better serve the Latino community.

The format of the e-mail exchanges and commentaries by Dr. Zavaleta serve as mini-case studies for professionals. They are learning opportunities. A chance to experience and study the many assorted types of cases they may encounter in their work with Latinos but never experience with valuable background information; including input from a healer and anthropologist. These additional perspectives provide a rare opportunity for contextualized mini-cases based on real-life experiences.

Additionally, *Curandero Conversations* provides the reader with a priceless view into the not widely seen or completely understood world of *curanderismo*. This is especially true in that it provides us with an attempt to understand the mysterious world of El Niño Fidencio, Mexico's most famous *curandero*. The followers of Fidencio, called Fidencistas, practice a unique blend of folk Catholicism and *curanderismo*.

Fidencismo is not fully recognized or accepted by the medical profession or the Catholic Church. In reality it operates simultaneously in the community with modern medicine and Catholicism.

While often misunderstood by religious officials, health-care providers and social service workers, the practice and utilization of *curanderos/as*, thrive in the United States and Mexico and throughout Latin America today. The Latino population, irrespective of socioeconomic level or education, maintains a widespread cultural belief in folk religion and folk medicine.

Wherever Latino populations are found the number of persons who consult *curanderos*, spiritualists, card readers, herbalists and many other alternative practitioners in the Latino community grows annually.

Curanderismo never serves as a substitute for the qualified advice and treatment by medical doctors, social care or religious professionals. However, understanding *curanderismo*, its beliefs and rituals, provides critical assistance to the interaction between professional caregivers and Latinos in real-time scenarios.

Studies in cultural competency have clearly shown that consultation with *curanderos/as*, when practiced alongside modern medicine, social, psychological and religious counseling, bridges the gulf of misunderstanding that exists between these two different, and at times opposing, belief systems.

While numerous religious symbols are introduced and discussed in this book, the book is not about religion nor does it promote religious beliefs or the recommendation of one belief system over another. Religious symbolism is an essential part of *curanderismo* and is an everyday cultural reality for most Latinos.

While the book abounds with folk remedies prescribed by a *curandero*, this book suggests that we learn from them not use them. This book does not suggest or promote that people in need visit a *curandero*. What this book does is provide you with the most comprehensive glimpse into present-day *curanderismo* currently available.

The popularity of *curanderismo*, in all its aspects, is especially due to the burgeoning Latino media industry. The events occurring in Puerto Rico or in Colombia today appear on Spanish-language newscasts in the lower Rio Grande Valley of Texas, Chicago, and Los Angeles the same day. Hence, the Spanish language is a special cultural bond that most Latinos share and the spiritual world is the glue that binds them.

Curanderos/as practicing their local site-based, healing arts are now complemented by the availability and anonymity of Internet consultations. The boundaries of distance, access and culture in consultations are obliterated by the Internet. People in need of spiritual help and healing, who would never actually visit a *curandero* in person, consult online with impunity. The privacy of Internet use has assisted in increasing the use of *curandero* consultations especially in times when health care is more difficult to access.

In the United States, medical education has generally failed to meaningfully and systematically incorporate an understanding of cultural competency in its curricula as it relates to Latino populations. There are, however, acknowledged exceptions and the federal government along with many university health-science centers, and health-related organizations have championed the notion of teaching and implementing cultural competencies in recent years.

In spite of all that we have learned about the importance culture plays in the delivery of health care, Latinos continue to be one of the least understood groups in the American health care delivery system.

Each year the American population grows more culturally diverse. We must ask and answer the question, "Should health-care professionals be concerned about mastering cultural competencies related to Latinos in their practice?"

In general, Latino populations are faced with limited resources and this has exacerbated their need to access alternative and complementary health-care delivery systems.

Health-care professionals must construct and accept new and effective health-care models that take culture into consideration in treating Latinos as well as all immigrant populations.

The success of future health-care delivery systems requires that modern medicine and culturally-appropriate alternatives be incorporated into a new functioning paradigm where understanding *curanderismo* is a key concept.

Modern medicine should take a position of open-mindedness relative to *curanderos*. Medicine's position should be one of scientific inquiry and not of intolerance. Medical practitioners should be continuously vigilant of patients' beliefs, values and behaviors; seeking knowledge on the cultural issues that shape individual health models.

Cultural beliefs are critical in diagnosing disease, epidemiology, ethno-pharmacology, and complementary health practices. Medical and social service providers should develop the communication skills necessary to elicit information from patients and their families as well as to comprehend their personal beliefs.

Information empowers medicine in participatory decision-making regarding health-care delivery. Only when cultural systems and the medical field cooperate will the health-care delivery system be competently able to provide essential health care needed by Latinos, along with other underserved and/or economically-marginalized populations.

Appendix I
Cultural Competency

"Practitioners in this country also face many unique obstacles to the level of care they would like to deliver. Some of these obstacles involve cultural misunderstandings and miscommunications with patient populations whose languages, experiences and backgrounds differ from those of their providers."

– Quality Health Services for Hispanics:

The Cultural Competency Component, 2001

Cultural Competency Resources

Please note: The following Cultural Competency Resources have been selected from among the hundreds that can be found on the Internet. The majority are public domain Federal Government sites. All site links have been provided. Many more resource links are available in addition to those referenced here. They are intended to assist you to understand and to develop Cultural Competency materials for your office, clinic, social service agency or classroom. Appropriate attribution is given including the link where the materials in their complete form may be located.

Cultural Competency Resource 1

Where to go first for Cultural Competency information

Health Resources & Services Administration and Cultural Competency

- U.S. Department of Health & Human Services, Health Resources and Services Administration, Study on Measuring Cultural Competence in Health Care Delivery Settings. http://www.hrsa.gov/culturalcompetence/measures/sectioni.htm

- The U.S. Department of Health & Human Services, Office of Minority Health, National Standards on Culturally and Linguistically Appropriate Services (CLAS)

- http://www.omhrc.gov/templates/browse.aspx?1vl=2&1vlID=15

- U.S. Department of Health & Human Services, Health Resources and Services Administration, Transforming the Face of Health Professions through Cultural and Linguistic Competence: The Role of the HRSA Centers of Excellence. ftp://ftp.hrsa.gov/competence.pdf

- U.S. Department of Health & Human Services, Health Resources and Services Administration, the Bureau of Primary Health Care, the Office of Minority Health, and the Substance Abuse and Mental Health Services Administration, Quality Health Services for Hispanics: The Cultural Competency Component. ftp://ftp.hrsa.gov/hrsa/qualityhealthservicesforhispanics.pdf

Important Bibliographies on Cultural Competency on the Internet

1- CulturedMed, Culturally Competent Health Care bibliography selected and compiled by Jacquelyn Coughlan,

2- http://www2.sunyit.edu/library/html/culturedmed/bib/cultcomp/index.html

3- CulturedMed, Culturally Competent Health Care bibliography for Hispanic Groups, selected and compiled by Jacquelyn Coughlan, http://www.sunyit.edu/library/culturedmed/bib/hispanic/index.html

4- CulturedMed, Culturally Competent Health Care bibliography for Women and Children, selected and compiled by Jacquelyn Coughlan, http://www2.sunyit.edu/library/html/culturedmed/bib/womenandchild/index.html

5- Health Resources and Services Administration Study on Measuring Cultural Competence in Health Care Delivery Settings, http://www.hrsa.gov/culturalcompetence/measures/sectioniii.htm

6- Transforming the Face of Health Professions Through Cultural and Linguistic Competence Education: The Role of the HRSA Centers of Excellence, ftp://ftp.hrsa.gov/competence.pdf

7- Quality Health Services for Hispanics: The Cultural Competency Component, ftp://ftp.hrsa.gov/hrsa/qualityhealthservicesforhispanics.pdf

A very complete list of websites with many useful resources

8- http://www.nyc.gov/html/doh/downloads/pdf/qi/qi-ccpriority-resources.pdf

Cultural Competency Resource 2

Understanding Culture

Culture is defined many ways. This definition is from the HRSA report on Cultural Competency, "The thoughts, communications, actions, customs, beliefs, values, and institutions of racial, ethnic, religious, or social groups. Culture defines how health care information is received, how rights and protections are exercised, what is considered to be a health problem, how symptoms and concerns about the problem are expressed, who should provide treatment for the problem, and what type of treatment should be given. In sum, because health care is a cultural construct, arising from beliefs about the nature of disease and the human body, cultural issues are actually central in the delivery of health services treatment and preventive interventions."

HRSA Cultural Competency Final Report p. 4

What does Competency Mean?

The HRSA Editor's note states that the term competency "refers to the ability to perform effectively based on requisite attitudes, skills, and knowledge." The writers of the HRSA report on Cultural Competency are clear to note that one of the most important competencies is linguistic competence. HRSA 2005, p. 10

Cultural Competency in Health Care and the Social Services

Cultural and linguistic competence is a set of congruent behaviors, attitudes, and policies that come together in a system, agency, or among professionals that enables effective work in cross-cultural situations. 'Culture' refers to integrated patterns of human behavior that include the language, thoughts, communications, actions, customs, beliefs, values, and institutions of racial, ethnic, religious, or social groups. 'Competence' implies having the capacity to function effectively as an individual and an organization within the context of the cultural beliefs, behaviors, and needs presented by consumers and their communities.

http://www.omhrc.gov/assets/pdf/checked/finalreport.pdf

Why Cultural Competencies are Important

1- Perception of illness and cause varies by culture

2- There are culturally diverse belief systems relative to health and illness

3- Culture influences health seeking behaviors and attitudes

4- Culture influences individual preferences to health care

5- People have had varying personal experiences in the health care system

6- Environmental conditions influence cultural practices, beliefs and perceptions

7- Health care providers from the culturally and linguistically groups are limited

The Cultural Competency Standards are intended to be used by:

1- Policymakers

2- Accreditation and credentialing agencies

3- Purchasers

4- Patients

5- Advocates

6- Educators

7- The health care community in general

Quality Health Services for Hispanics: The Cultural Competency Component, p.9

National Standards for Culturally and Linguistically Appropriate Services in Health Care Final Report, 2001, p.4

National Standards for Culturally and Linguistically Appropriate Services in Health Care: Preamble

The following national standards issued by the U.S. Department of Health and Human Services' (HHS) Office of Minority Health (OMH) respond to the need to ensure that all people entering the health care system receive equitable and effective treatment in a culturally and linguistically appropriate manner. These standards for culturally and linguistically appropriate services (CLAS) are proposed as a means to correct inequities that currently exist in the provision of health services and to make these services more responsive to the individual needs of all patients/consumers. The standards are intended to be inclusive of all cultures and not limited to any particular population group or sets of groups; however, they are especially designed to address the needs of racial, ethnic, and linguistic population groups that experience unequal access to health services. Ultimately, the aim of the standards is to contribute to the elimination of racial and ethnic health disparities and to improve the health of all Americans.

The CLAS standards are primarily directed at health care organizations; however, individual providers are also encouraged to use the standards to make their practices more culturally and linguistically accessible. The principles and activities of culturally and linguistically appropriate services should be integrated throughout an organization and undertaken in partnership with the communities being served.

The 14 standards are organized by themes: Culturally Competent Care (Standards 1-3), Language Access Services (Standards 4-7), and Organizational Supports for Cultural Competence (Standards 8-14). Within this framework, there are three types of standards of varying stringency: mandates, guidelines, and recommendations as follows:

CLAS mandates are current Federal requirements for all recipients of federal funds (Standards 4, 5, 6, and 7).

CLAS guidelines are activities recommended by OMH for adoption as mandates by federal, State, and national accrediting agencies (Standards 1, 2, 3, 8, 9, 10, 11, 12, and 13).

CLAS recommendations are suggested by OMH for voluntary adoption by health care organizations (Standard 14).

http://www.omhrc.gov/assets/pdf/checked/finalreport.pdf pp.3-4

Cultural Competency Resource 3

Cultural Competence Standards 1 through 3 are recommended for adoption by the federal government.

http://www.omhrc.gov/clas/

Culturally and Linguistically Appropriate Standards (CLAS 1-3)

Standard 1 Recommended

Health care organizations should ensure that patients/consumers receive from all staff members, effective, understandable, and respectful care that is provided in a manner compatible with their cultural health beliefs and practices and preferred language.

Standard 2 Recommended

Health care organizations should implement strategies to recruit, retain, and promote all levels of the organization a diverse staff and leadership that are representative of the demographic characteristics of the service area.

Standard 3 Recommended

Health care organizations should ensure that staff at all levels and across all disciplines receives ongoing education and training in culturally and linguistically appropriate service delivery.

http://www.omhrc.gov/assets/pdf/checked/finalreport.pdf

Cultural Competency Resource 4

The following material outlines the importance of language in the delivery of health services for cultural competency Standards 4 through 7. All are mandated for adoption by the Federal government.

http://www.omhrc.gov/clas/

The Importance of Language in the Delivery of Service

Culturally and Linguistically Appropriate Standards (CLAS 4-7)

Standard 4 Mandated

Health care organizations must offer and provide language assistance services, including bilingual staff and interpreter services, at no cost to each patient/consumer with limited English proficiency at all points of contact, in a timely manner during all hours of operation.

Standard 5 Mandated

Health care organizations must provide patients/consumers in their preferred language both verbal offers and written notices informing them of their right to receive language assistance services.

Standard 6 Mandated

Health care organizations must assure the competence of language assistance provided to limited English proficient patients/consumers by interpreters and bilingual staff. Family and friends should not be used to provide interpretation services (except on request by the patient/consumer).

Standard 7 Mandated

Health care organizations must make available easily understood patient-related materials and post signage in the language of the commonly encountered groups and/or groups represented in the service area.

Cultural Competency Resource 5

The following material outlines the importance of both organizational support and cultural competence for Standards 8 through 14. Standards 8 through 13 are recommended for adoption by the federal government while standard 14 is to be adopted voluntarily.

Organizational Support for Cultural Competence

Culturally and Linguistically Appropriate Standards (CLAS 8-14)

Standard 8 Recommended

Health care organizations should develop, implement, and promote a written strategic plan that outlines clear goals, policies, operational plans, and management accountability/oversight mechanisms to provide culturally and linguistically appropriate services.

Standard 9 Recommended

Health care organizations should conduct initial and ongoing organizational self-assessments of CLAS-related activities and are encouraged to integrate cultural and linguistic competence-related measures into their internal audits, performance improvement programs, patient satisfaction assessments, and outcomes-based evaluations.

Standard 10 Recommended

Health care organizations should ensure that data on the individual patient's/consumer's race, ethnicity, and spoken and written language are collected in health records, integrated into the organization's management information systems, and periodically updated.

Standard 11 Recommended

Health care organizations should maintain a current demographic, cultural, and epidemiological profile of the community as well as a needs assessment to accurately plan for and implement services that respond to the cultural and linguistic characteristics of the service area.

Standard 12 Recommended

Health care organizations should develop participatory, collaborative partnerships with communities and utilize a variety of formal and informal mechanisms to facilitate community and patient/consumer involvement in designing and implementing CLAS-related activities.

Standard 13 Recommended

Health care organizations should ensure that conflict and grievance resolution processes are culturally and linguistically sensitive and capable of identifying, preventing, and resolving cross-cultural conflicts or complaints by patients/consumers.

Standard 14 Voluntary Adoption

Health care organizations are encouraged to regularly make available to the public information about their progress and successful innovations in implementing the CLAS standards and to provide public notice in their communities about the availability of this information.

http://www.omhrc.gov/clas/

Cultural Competency Resource 6

National Center for Complementary and Alternative Medicine (NCCAM)

National Institutes of Health – U.S. Department of Health and Human Service
http://nccam.nih.gov/about/plans/2005 and http://nccam.nih.gov/timetotalk/

Introduction

Patients and their health care providers need to talk openly about all of their health care practices. This includes the use of complementary and alternative medicine (CAM).

The National Center for Complementary and Alternative Medicine (NCCAM) at the National Institutes of Health has launched an educational campaign—Time to Talk—to encourage the discussion of CAM use. As the Federal Government's lead agency for scientific research on CAM, NCCAM is committed to providing evidence-based CAM information to help health professionals and the public make health care decisions.

Why Talk?

To ensure safe, coordinated care among all conventional and CAM therapies, it's time to talk. Talking not only allows fully integrated care, but it also minimizes risks of interactions with a patient's conventional treatments. When patients tell their providers about their CAM use, they can better stay in control and more effectively manage their health. When providers ask their patients about CAM use, they can ensure that they are fully informed and can help patients make wise decisions.

In a nationwide Government survey, nearly 50 percent of all adults age 18 or older reported using some form of CAM (excluding prayer) during their lifetime, and 36 percent of adults reported CAM use in the past year; people age 50 to 59 were among the most likely to report using CAM. However, in a survey of people age 50 or older, less than one-third of those who reported using CAM have discussed it with their physicians.

CAM is defined as a group of diverse medical and health care systems, practices, and products that are not presently considered to be part of conventional medicine. CAM includes products and practices such as herbal supplements, meditation, chiropractic care, and acupuncture.

Communication between Clients and Providers about CAM Use

Of those age 50 or older who use CAM, more than two-thirds (69%) did not talk to their physicians about it.

The most common reasons cited by respondents who had seen physicians but had not discussed CAM with them were that the physician never asked (42%), they did not know they should (30%), and there was not enough time during the office visit (19%).

More than one-half of respondents (56%) who had talked about CAM with their physician said they—not their physician— had initiated the CAM discussion.

Topics Discussed with Providers

For respondents who talked with their providers about CAM, the topics most frequently discussed were the effectiveness of a CAM therapy (67%), what to use (64%), how a CAM therapy might interact with other medications or treatments they receive (60%), advice on whether or not to pursue a CAM therapy (60%), and the safety of a CAM therapy (57%).

Tips to Start Talking

Patient Tips for Discussing CAM with Providers

When completing patient history forms, be sure to include all therapies and treatments you use. Make a list in advance.

Tell your health care providers about all therapies or treatments— including over-thecounter and prescription medicines, as well as herbal and dietary supplements.

Take control. Don't wait for your providers to ask about your CAM use.

If you are considering a new CAM therapy, ask your health care providers about its safety, effectiveness, and possible interactions with medications (both prescription and over-the-counter).

Provider Tips for Discussing CAM with Patients

Include a question about CAM use on medical history forms.

Ask your patients to bring a list of all therapies they use, including prescription, over-the-counter, and herbal therapies, and other CAM practices.

Have your medical staff initiate the conversation.

Cultural Competency Resource 7

1. The following material is adapted from the Kleinman physician-anthropologist model for understanding the relationship between culture and health are as outlined in, Transforming the face of health professions through cultural and linguistic competence: the role of the HRSA Centers of Excellence, 2005; and from, Kleinman A. Patients and Healers in the Context of Culture. University of California Press. Berkeley, CA; 1980.

   This material is particularly important in understanding curanderismo.

   ftp://ftp.hrsa.gov/competence.pdf

The Kleinman physician-anthropologist model

1- What do you think has caused your problem?

2- Why do you think it started when it did?

3- What does your sickness do to you; how does it work?

4- How severe is your sickness?

5- Will it have a short or long duration?

6- What kind of treatment should you receive?

7- What are the most important results you hope to receive from treatment?

8- What are the chief problems you sickness has caused you?

9- What do you fear about your sickness?

ftp://ftp.hrsa.gov/competence.pdf   pp.70-71

Cultural Competency Resource 8

The following material is adapted from three Commonwealth Fund articles on Cultural Competence cited below. They are intended to further provide the reader with resources for the development of a cultural competence program.

Essential Principles of Cultural Competency

1- Community representation and feedback are essential at all levels of the organization

2- Cultural competency must be integrated into all existing systems of a health care organization, particularly quality improvement efforts

3- Changes made must be manageable, measureable and sustainable

4- Making the business case is a critical element for change

5- Commitment from leadership is a key factor to success

6- Staff training is necessary on an ongoing basis

Taking Cultural Competency from Theory to Action, 2006, Ellen Wu and Martin Martinez, The Commonwealth Fund

http://www.commonwealthfund.org/publications/publications_show.htm?doc_id=414097

Barriers to Culturally Competent Care

1- Lack of diversity at all levels in the health care workforce

2- Lack of on-going training at all levels in the health care workforce

3- Lack of appropriate cross-cultural communication between the patient and the provider

4- Lack of appropriate outreach to the culturally diverse community

5- Failure to institutionalize a culture of cultural competency in the clinical setting

6- Failure to employ at all levels a culturally diverse workforce

7- Failure to implement change

Cultural Competence in Health Care Emerging Frameworks and Practical Approaches, Joseph R. Betancourt, 2002, The Commonwealth Fund

http://www.commonwealthfund.org/usr_doc/betancourt_culturalcompetence_576.pdf?section=4039

Cultural Competency in the Future

1- Health care organizations should employ principles of patient-centeredness and cultural competence to ensure care is individualized and equitable

2- Researchers should use and refine measures of cultural competence and patient-centeredness, and explore the impact of their unique and overlapping components on patient outcomes

3- Educators should develop multidisciplinary programs to improve the patient-centeredness and cultural competence of health professionals

4- Health care organizations should measure and track patient-centeredness and cultural competence as part of their efforts to delivery high-quality care

5- Patients should provide feedback to health care systems by participating in surveys and focus groups, for example, to ensure that organizations attend to patients' diverse needs and preferences

The Role and Relationship of Cultural Competence and Patient-Centeredness in Health Care Quality, 2006, The Commonwealth Fund, Mary Catherine Beach, Somnath Saha, and Lisa A. Cooper

http://www.commonwealthfund.org/publications/publications_show.htm?doc_id=413721

Cultural Competency Resource 9

The following material is adapted from, Bridging the Cultural Divide in Health Care Settings: The Essential Role of Cultural Broker Programs, It was developed for the National Health Service Corps, Bureau of Health Professions, Health Resources and Services Administration of the U.S. Department of Health and Human Services by the National Center for Cultural Competence, Georgetown University Center for Child and Human Development, Georgetown University Medical Center in 2004

The goal of the Cultural Broker Project is in keeping with the NCCC's overall mission to "increase the capacity of health care and mental health programs to design, implement and evaluate culturally and linguistically competent service delivery systems." p.1

The following is intended to be an overview and to give the reader a sense of what the Cultural Broker Program is and how it functions. For a complete review of this important material please see:

http://www11.georgetown.edu/research/gucchd/nccc/documents/Cultural_Broker_Guide_English.pdf

http://www11.georgetown.edu/research/gucchd/nccc/documents/Cultural_Broker_Guide_Spanish.pdf

The Cultural Broker Program

1- The cultural broker is a liaison

2- The cultural broker is a cultural guide

3- The cultural broker is a mediator

4- The cultural broker is a catalyst for change

The Benefits of a Cultural Broker

1- Assess the values, beliefs, and practices related to health in the community

2- Enhance communication between patients/consumers and other providers

3- Advocate for the use of culturally and linguistically competent practices and in the delivery of services

4- Assist with efforts to increase access to care and eliminate racial and ethnic disparities in health

The Benefits to the Patient/Consumer

1- Patients/consumers who have positive experiences with cultural brokers will be more likely to continue to access services, which potentially improves health outcomes and reduces health disparities

2- Patients/consumers will recognize the health care setting's commitment to deliver services in a manner that respects and incorporates their cultural perspective

3- Patients/consumers may be motivated to seek care sooner when they know that providers understand and respect their cultural values and health beliefs and practices

4- Patients/consumers may be able to communicate their health care needs more effectively and better understand their diagnoses and treatment

5- Patients/consumers who benefit from this approach may also encourage others within their community to access and use services. This approach has the potential to positively impact the health of the entire community

Benefits to the Health Care Provider

1- Health care providers will be able to elicit more in-depth information what will assist with accurate assessment, diagnosis, and treatment

2- Health care providers will be able to communicate diagnosis and interpret risks associated with different treatment options more effectively

3- Health care providers may be more effective in serving patients/consumers who have chronic diseases and conditions that may require a higher degree of self-management

4- Health care providers who communicate effectively with patients and consumers may experience a greater degree of satisfaction in their work, particularly when they see improved health status and outcomes

5- Health care providers can become more knowledgeable of and connected to the communities they serve

Benefits to the Health Care Setting

1- Health care settings can create a reputation for being committed and inclusive community partners, which improves access and use

2- Health care settings can increase the use of preventive services to minimize the use of cost-prohibitive emergency care

3- Health care settings can increase cost effectiveness in service delivery by decreasing return visits from patients/consumers who did not clearly understand treatment protocols

4- Health care settings may be able to reduce potential liability through improved communication

5- Health care settings can engender mutual respect and trust within the communities they serve, which assures sustainability

Guiding Principles for Cultural Broker Programs in Health Settings

1- Cultural brokering honors and respects cultural differences within communities

2- Cultural brokering is community driven

3- Cultural brokering is provided in a safe, non-judgmental and confidential manner

4- Cultural brokering involves delivering services in settings that are accessible and tailored to the unique needs of the communities served

5- Cultural brokering acknowledges the reciprocity and transfer of assets between the community and health care settings

Cultural Competency Resource 10

IMPROVING THE CAREGIVER/PATIENT RELATIONSHIP

Original materials written and compiled by the American Medical Student Association (AMSA), re-printed with permission. http://www.amsa.org/programs/gpit/cultural.cfm

1. Do not treat the patient in the same manner you would want to be treated. Culture determines the roles for polite, caring behavior and will formulate the patient's concept of a satisfactory relationship.

2. Begin by being more formal with patients who were born in another culture. In most countries, a greater distance between caregiver and patient is maintained through the relationship. Except when treating children or very young adults, it is best to use the patient's last name when addressing him or her.

3. Do not be insulted if the patient fails to look you in the eye or ask questions about treatment. In many cultures, it is disrespectful to look directly at another person (especially one in authority) or to make someone "lose face" by asking him or her questions.

4. Do not make any assumptions about the patient's ideas about the ways to maintain health, the cause of illness or the means to prevent or cure it. Adopt a line of questioning that will help determine some of the patient's central beliefs about health/illness/illness prevention.

5. Allow the patient to be open and honest. Do not discount beliefs that are not held by Western biomedicine. Often, patients are afraid to tell Western caregivers that they are visiting a folk healer or are

taking an alternative medicine concurrently with Western treatment because in the past they have experienced ridicule.

6. Do not discount the possible effects of beliefs in the supernatural effects on the patient's health. If the patient believes that the illness has been caused by embrujamiento (bewitchment), the evil eye, or punishment, the patient is not likely to take any responsibility for his or her cure. Belief in the supernatural may result in his or her failure to either follow medical advice or comply with the treatment plan.

7. Inquire indirectly about the patient's belief in the supernatural or use of nontraditional cures. Say something like, "Many of my patients from ___ believe, do, or visit___. Do you?"

8. Try to ascertain the value of involving the entire family in the treatment. In many cultures, medical decisions are made by the immediate family or the extended family. If the family can be involved in the decision-making process and the treatment plan, there is a greater likelihood of gaining the patient's compliance with the course of treatment.

9. Be restrained in relating bad news or explaining in detail complications that may result from a particular course of treatment. "The need to know" is a unique American trait. In many cultures, placing oneself in the doctor's hands represents an act of trust and a desire to transfer the responsibility for treatment to the physician. Watch for and respect signs that the patient has learned as much as he or she is able to deal with.

10. Whenever possible, incorporate into the treatment plan the patient's folk medication and folk beliefs that are not specifically contradicted. This will encourage the patient to develop trust in the treatment and will help assure that the treatment plan is followed.

Cultural Competency Resource 11

The following material is adapted from, Quality Health Services for Hispanics: The Cultural Competency Component, a collaboration between the Health Resources and Services Administration (HRSA), Bureau of Primary Health Care (BPHC), the Substance Abuse and Mental Health Services Administration (SAMHSA), the Office of Minority Health (OMH), and the National Alliance for Hispanic Health (formerly known as the National Coalition for Hispanic Health and Human Services Organizations).

This material is intended to, "help health care professionals better understand, and more effectively respond to the growing needs of over 30 million Hispanics in the United States. It should facilitate greater access to, and utilization of, health and human services for this patient population, as well as provide useful suggestions on improving one-to-one provider-patient interactions."

The following are considered key cultural concepts in understanding and teaching about the delivery of services to Latino culture.

1- Family   Familia: Latino culture is family centered

2- Religion   Religión: Health care cannot be separated from religion

3- Respect   Respeto: Always respect the elders in Latino culture

4- Familiarity   Familiaridad: Treat Latinos as you would treat friends

5- Trust   Confianza: Latinos respect trust, give it and gain it

6- Kindness   Amabilidad: Always be kind, friendly and genuine

7- Fatalism   Fatalidad: Latinos believe that happenings have ordained reason

8- Beliefs   Creencia: Respect all Latino beliefs

9- Dignity   Dignidad: Treat Latinos with dignity no matter how humble

10- Spirituality Espiritualidad: The Latino world of understanding is based upon belief in God and the supernatural

Understanding the Latino Family

1- Understand the importance of the Latino extended family as a support network

2- Understanding that the family reaches beyond blood and marriage to the most important friends and ritual kin

3- Never underestimate the importance of the opinion of family members regarding ones health and treatment choices

4- Understand that the parental tie to children never ends and that parents always exert influence through life

5- Latino parents have more influence over their adult children than do their children's spouses

6- When there is a health crisis the Latino family is always consulted first

Latino Social Realities

1- Latinos are often referred to alternative forms of treatment at the same time that they see doctors. The two systems work side by side

2- Older generation Latinos are adverse to the health care system and will do anything not to participate. This is especially true of adult males

3- Latinos simply do not conceptualize seeking help for emotional, psychological or psychiatric problems

4- For Latinos the male group or *palomilla*, and the ritual kin such as godparents called compadres and comadres are always sought out for opinions on major life events first

5- Latino males are notoriously non-compliant in following treatment and in taking their medications

6- Latinos will always associate a supernatural cause with illness and will seek spiritual attention

7- Almost all Latinos have some sort of home altar where family patron saints are revered and where promises are made

8- Most Latinos will defer to authority and speak very little

9- In Latino culture males are regarded as the head of the family but in reality the mother is the functional head of the family

10- The male Latino authorization is always required for a medical procedure on the women and children in his family

11- The Latino couple tends to dominate its children's lives both in and outside of the home

12- Latino children are always expected to look out for one another and especially for the younger and the sisters

13- Latino feelings of guilt have a religious origin and while there is an increasing number of evangelicals among Latinos, most are Catholics

14- Latinos will practice their Catholic faith, evangelical faith and folk-faith simultaneously

15- All Latino socio-economic levels will rationalize and opt for folk healers if the need is great enough

16- Sessions with folk psychiatrists are just as valid and functional for Latinos as sessions with professional therapists

17- Often the Latino world view revolves around a constant struggle of good against evil, mitigated by the saints

18- Latinos will respond if you speak to them in Spanish. Be careful not to make the mistake of assuming that all Latinos speak Spanish as their primary language

19- Always respect personal space by maintaining a comfortable and respectful distance, make Latino patients and all patients feel comfortable during consultation

20- Be sure to always make eye contact with Latinos when talking to them, maintain a pleasant tone of voice and take care that your touch does not offend.

Appendix II
Important Internet Resource Links

Important Internet Resource Links
Listed by the Number of the Question in the Book

Note to the Reader: The authors made every effort to assure that these Internet links were functioning at the time of publication but Internet links come in and out of service. They are provided to you as a resource and as a point of departure for your extended search for information.

#6 <u>Explore: The Journal of Science and Healing</u> by Dr. Larry Dossey's official website see: <u>http://www.dosseydossey.com/larry/default.html</u>

#6 Official site for Noticias de Antropología y Arqueología (Anthropology and Archaeology News), see: <u>http://www.naya.org.ar/forms/suscripcion_almas.htm</u>

#6 & 67 From Spiritual Emergency to Spiritual Problem: The Transpersonal Roots of the New DSM-IV Category, <u>http://www/spiritualcompetency.com/jhpseart.html</u>

#12 For a description of the history and use of the Caravaca Cross see: <u>http://www.caravacadelacruz.org/la_cruz/origen.html</u>

#13 Official website for the El Niño Fidencio and Curanderismo Research Project at the University of Texas at Brownsville, see: http://vpea.utb.edu/elnino/fidencio.html

#13 Experience Spiritual Healing with El Niño Fidencio and Alberto & Lidia Salinas, see: http://www.elninofidencio.com/index.html

#13 An Essay on Cultural Diversity, Alternative Medicine, and Folk Medicine by David J. Hufford, Ph.D. see: http://www.temple.edu/isllc/newfolk/medicine.html

#13 Sobadora or Sobador, Mexican Health Beliefs, see: http://answers.google.com/answers/threadview/id/328593.html

http://www.pshm.org/curanderismo.shtml

http://www.proz.com/kudoz/spanish_to_english/medical_general/2018531-huesero.html

http://en.wikipedia.org/wiki/Curandera

#14 Mother Herbs and Agro Products

http://www.motherherbs.com/abortifacient.html.

#14 Papa Jim's Botanical a retail store and catalog company furnishing the world with the products they need located in San Antonio, Texas, see:
http://www.papajimsbotanica.com/

#14 Lucky Mojo is both an online magic shop and a real magic store located in Forestville, California, see: http://www.luckymojo.com/luckymojocatalogue.html

#14 Original Products Corp located in Bronx, New York stocks all your mystical supply needs, including talismans, books, herbs see: http://www.originalprodcorp.com/

#14 The Dispensatory of the United States of America Twentieth Edition (1918), see: http://www.swsbm.com/dispensatory/usd-1918-complete.pdf

#14 The United States Pharmacopeia (USP) is an official public standards–setting authority for all prescription and over–the–counter medicines and other health care products manufactured or sold in the United States, See: http://www.usp.org/

#14 Botánica de los Orishas Cubanos in Miami Florida, see: http://www.botanica-de-los-orishas.com/toc-sp.html

#14 Directory of Services, Botanicals and Other Shops, see: http://ilarioba.tripod.com/botanicas.htm

14 Ethics in Herbal Medicine, see: http://www.siu.edu/~ebl/leaflets/ethics.htm

#14 Herb Glossary and botanical terms. http://www/motherherbs.com/herb-glossary.html

#15 Sociedad de Río Negro online site, see: http://www.rionegro.com.ar/arch200302/s16g08.html

#15 Official site for de la difunta Correa-San Juan, Argentina, see: http://www.visitedifuntacorrea.com.ar/

#15 Wikipedia Site for Ceferino Namuncurá who was a saintly religious student and the object of a Roman Catholic cults of veneration in northern Patagonia and throughout Argentina, see: http://www.en.wikipedia.org/wiki/Ceferino_Namuncur%C3%A1

#15 Article for Ceferino Namuncurá, un santo manpuche, "The Soul of the Indian" in Santiago de Chile, see: http://www.mapuche.info/news02/merc010826.html

#15 Los Angeles Times, archive for Saturday July 30, 2005 article on "Unveiling the life of a folk saint" Teresa Urrea, Santa Teresa de Cobora, see: http://articles.latimes.com/2005/jul/30/entertainment/et-urrea30

#15 The Miami Herald, archive for December 16, 2001, for residents along U.S. Mexican border find strength in local folk saints, see: http://www.latinamericanstudies.org/religion/juan-soldado.htm

#15 An article on Juan Castillo Morales, the unofficial patron saint for the impoverished Mexicans who sneak illegally into the United States in search of a better life, see: http://www.zermeno.com/J.C.Morales.html

#15 Reditus: A chronicle of aesthetic Christianity, shows article on folk saints in the Catholic Church, see: http://arturovasquez.wordpress.com/tag/folk-saints/

#15 Article in Wikipedia the free encyclopedia on Allan Kardec he was a pseudonym of the French teacher and educator Hippolyte Léon Denizard Rivail (Lyon, October 3, 1804 – Paris, March 31, 1869), who is known today as the systematizer of Spiritism, see: http://www.en.wikipedia.org/wiki/Allan_Kardec

#15 For centuries men and women have been unexplainably inspired to speak and set down on paper words that were "not their own," see: http://www.spiritwritings.com/kardecspiritstoc.html

#15 Website for Spiritual Magnetic School of the Universal Commune, A.C. Mexican National Council, Escuela Magnético Espiritual de la Comuna Universal a.c. Consejo Nacional Mexicano en el nuevo milenio (e.v.), see: http://www.joaquintrincado.com.mx/

#15 Subscribe now to receive CDROM on miraculous souls and popular saints and other devotions, Almas Milagrosas, Santos Populares y Otras Devociones, see: http://www.naya.org.ar/forms/suscripcion_almas.htm

#15 Understand more about San Alejo, see: http://www.devocionario.com/santos/alejo_1.html

#16 Liturgy Training Publications, The Liturgical Year Calendar, see: http://www/ltp.org/

#16 When you need special help, St Jude of Thaddeus prayer, see: http://www.johntoddjr.com/151%20Sanjudas/sanjudastadeo.htm

#16 St. Jude of Thaddeus the patron saint of desperate cases, see: http://www.catholic.org/saints/saint.php?saint_id=127

#16 Ask Sister Mary Martha, see:

http://asksistermarymartha.blogspot.com/2007/03/patron-saint-of-everything-you-need.html

#17 For types of mental illness see: http://www.webmd.com/mental-health/mental-health-types-illness

#17 Baylor College of Medicine Multicultural Patient Care, see: http://www.bcm.edu/mpc/special-hl.html

#18 For Folk Medicine in Hispanics in the Southwestern United States see: http://www.rice.edu/projects/HispanicHealth/Courses/mod7/mod7.html

#18 For grandma's pharmacy, or la botica de la abuela, see: http://www.ciao.es/sr/q-la+botica+de+la+abuela+opinion+821564

#18 Herbs have been used as medicine for the treatment of diseases and conditions for many thousands of years, see: Folk Remedies Natural Health at: http://www.folkremediesforyou.com

#18 Antique medicines contained everything from arsenic to opium, see: http://www.webmd.com/a-to-z-guides/features/look-back-old-time-medicines

#18 Henrietta's herbal homepage for cataplasma, see: http://www.henriettesherbal.com/eclectic/kings/linum_cata.html

#19 Faith healers especially popular among Hispanics, see: http://www.txstate.edu/news/news_releases/external_news/2003/01/faithhealers012703.htm

#19 Articles on Latino conversion to Protestantism include, see: http://www.hispanic5.com/more_hispanics_leaving_catholicism_for_evangelical_protestantism.htm

#19 There is a religious revolution taking place in the Latino community in the U.S. and Puerto Rico today. Recent studies on Latino religion in the U.S. and Puerto Rico have shattered all previously held stereotypes that to be Latino is to be Roman Catholic, see: http://jaar.oxfordjournals.org/cgi/content/citation/67/3/597

#19 Changing Faiths: Latinos and the Transformation of American Religion Pew Hispanic Center and Pew Forum on Religion & Public Life, see: http://pewhispanic.org/reports/report.php?ReportID=75

#19 An article in The Los Angeles Times archive for Sunday March 08, 1998, Latin American Faith Healing draws many adherents in LA., see: http://articles.latimes.com/1998/mar/08/local/me-26813

#19 Fifty things that you should know about tongues and healing see: http://www.biblebelievers.com/jmelton/tongues.html

#23 The Rider-Waite tarot deck is the most popular tarot deck in use today in the English-speaking world (the Tarot de Marseille being the most popular deck in the Latin countries), see: http://en.wikipedia.org/wiki/Rider-Waite-Smith_deck

#23 The baraja (literally deck/pack of cards) is a Spanish set of playing cards with some resemblance to the 52-card Anglo-American-French deck, but is usually made up of only 40 cards, see: http://en.wikipedia.org/wiki/Spanish_deck

24/31/55/57/111/126// 135/143 Most of us have performed our first act of candle magic by the time we are two years old, see: http://www.ecauldron.com/candlemagick.php

http://www.religions-and-spiritualities-guide.com/candle-magics.html

Religious and spiritual guide, see: http://www.religions-and-spiritualities-guide.com/support-files/spiritualcandlecolourmeaning.pdf

#25 Amulets and Talismans see: http://www.paganshopping.com/Merchant2/merchant.mvc?Screen=CTGY&Category_Code=A1

#27 Posadas and Pastorela, see: http://www.mexconnect.com/mex_/travel/ldumois/ldcposadas.html

#28/181 Miracles or Milagros, see: http://www.collectorsguide.com/fa/fa052.shtml

#29 And finally a must read is: Telling Stories, Building Altars Mexican American Women's Altars in Oregon, see: http://www.historycooperative.org/journals/ohq/107.4/ricciardi.html

#29 Cultural riches, Mexican home altars, see: http://www.pbs.org/independentlens/newamericans/culturalriches/art_altars.html and http://www.washingtonpost.com/ac2/wp-dyn/A52812-2004Jan3?language=printer or http://www.altarshop.com/home-altars

#30 Our Lady of Guadalupe, Patroness of the Americas, see: http://www.sancta.org/

#30 Patron Saint Topics, see: http://www.catholic-forum.com/saints/patron00.htm

#30 Patron Saints see: http://www.scborromeo.org/patron_s.htm

#30 Santo Niño de Atocha, see: http://en.wikipedia.org/wiki/Santo_Ni%C3%b1o_de_Atocha

#31 The doctor's book of home remedies for children: Introduction to home remedies for children, see:
http://www/mothernature.com/Library/Bookshelf/Books/50/1.cfm

#31 Home remedies for children: treating common illnesses with natural home remedies see: http://www/homemademedicine.com/children.html

#32 Mollera caída (sunken fontanel) is another folk illness which affects infants, see: http://altmed.creighton.edu/MexicanFolk/mollera_caida.htm or http://www.rice.edu/projects/HispanicHealth/Courses/mod7/caida.html

#33 For a Latina, becoming a mother can be a moment of great pride and joy; yet, becoming a mother in a country other than her own can be scary and confusing. For more, see:
http://www.nchealthystart.org/aboutus/maternidad/vol2no4.htm or http://books.google.com/books?id=-mry9Fs6CRQC&pg=PA54&lpg=PA54&dq=partera+folk+healing&source=bl&ots=f9Hlvo6xi_&sig=GG0_GxDWc0MxVUnc30uy4y5dCPs&hl=en&sa=X&oi=book_result&resnum=1&ct=result

#34 Empacho is a gastrointestinal illness which can affect anyone but is commonly seen in children, to learn more, see: http://altmed.creighton.

edu/MexicanFolk/Empacho.htm or http://www.rice.edu/projects/HispanicHealth/Courses/mod7/empacho.html

#36 The natural care reviews, remedies for earaches, see: http://naturalcurereviews.com/remedy14-3-earache.html and http://www.youqa.cn/html/Alternative_Medicine/medicine/1630.html
http://loteriachicana.net/2008/04/29/backyard-remedies/

#37 Santo Ignacio de Loyola founder of the company of Jesus (Jesuits 1491-1556), see: http://www.corazones.org/santos/ignacio_loyola.htm

#38 At Little flower's American Folk Remedies they specialize on Native American book, music and art online, see: http://www.geocities.com/littleflowers_remedies/?200820

#38 Earth clinic folk remedies, ailments from A-Z, see: http://www.earthclinic.com/cures.html

#38 For health 911 folk remedies website, see: http://www.health911.com/remedies/rem_indx.htm

#38 Online archive on American Folk Medicine of UCLA, see: http://www.folkmed.ucla.edu/

#39 For cerebral palsy help information see: http://www.cerebralpalsyhelp.com/?crtag=Google2 or http://www.ninds.nih.gov/disorders/cerebral_palsy/cerebral_palsy.htm

#40 The national institute neurological disorders and stroke center, see: http://www.ninds.nih.gov/disorders/spina_bifida/spina_bifida.htm

#41 Article on anger management for children, see: http://ezinearticles.com/?Children-Anger-Management-Tips&id=132222

#41/176 The National Institute of Mental Health for Attention Deficit Hyperactivity Disorder (ADHD) is a condition that becomes apparent in some children in the early school years, see: http://www.nimh.nih.gov/health/publications/adhd/complete-publication.shtml

http://www.psychiatrictimes.com/display/article/10168/55206

#42 Dr. Larry Dossey official website, see: http://www.dosseydossey.com/larry/therapies.html

#42 /43 Medline plus trusted health information for you, article on kidney disease, see: http://www.nlm.nih.gov/medlineplus/kidneydiseases.html

#43 Archives of pediatrics and adolescent medicine, see: www.archpediatrics.com

http://aapgrandrounds.aappublications.org/cgi/content/extract/8/4/37

http://wjn.sagepub.com/cgi/content/abstract/30/5/588

http://jama.ama-assn.org/cgi/content/abstract/288/1/82

Parasites http://www.kidsgrowth.com/resources/articledetail.cfm?id=81

Children's parasitic diseases http://www.cdc.gov/ncidod/dpd/kids.htm

Giardiasis http://www.familysurvey.com/parent/infections/stomach/giardiasis.html

#46/47 Harborview Medical Center, University of Washington, herb drug interactions fall 2004, see: http://ethnomed.org/clin_topics/herbal_medicine/herb-drug_rev.pdf http://www.herbmed.org/herblist.asp?varAll=All&varName=Scientific

http://www.mayaherbs.com

http://www.dragonriverherbals.com/Pages/catalog.html

#46 http://www.swsbm.com/ManualsMM/MatMed5.pdf

#47 Understanding the theory behind Greco-Arabic medicine, see: http://www.traditionalmedicine.net.au/chapter2.htm

#48 Jamie Sams website, Emerging Worlds of Progressive Medicine, see: http://www.emergingworlds.com/ch_stories_detail.cfm?Content=46

#50 The National Cancer Institute has plenty of information see: http://www.cancer.gov

For the American Lung Association, see: http://www.lungusa.org

#52 The National Institute of Diabetes and Digestive and Kidney Diseases (NIDDK) conducts and supports basic and clinical research on many of the most serious diseases affecting public health, for more information, see: http://diabetes.niddk.nih.gov/dm/pubs/neuropathies/

http://www.diabetes.org/home.jsp

http://www.diabetes.org/communityprograms-and-localevents/latinos.jsp

http://www.sclda.org/

http://www.diabetes.org/for-health-professionals-and-scientists/latino-presentation.jsp

http://www.diabetes.org/for-health-professionals-and-scientists/latino-presentation.jsp

#54 Family doctors on-line for skin rashes and other changes, see: http://familydoctor.org/online/famdocen/home/tools/symptom/545.html

#56 Herbal Preparation, see:
http://www.soulhealer.com/herb%20properties.htm

#58 The Los Angeles times archive for Thursday November 20, 2003, see article where faith healer pleads guilty to unlawful medical practice, see:
http://articles.latimes.com/2003/nov/20/local/me-faith20

#60 Susto is a folk illness that is similar to fear or anxiety in Western medicine, see: http://altmed.creighton.edu/MexicanFolk/Susto.htm

http://www.rice.edu/projects/HispanicHealth/Courses/mod7/susto.html; http://en.wikipedia.org/wiki/Susto

#61/146 Envy or jealousies, see: http://en.wikipedia.org/wiki/Invidia

#62/ 151/ 167 Symbols are the language of dreams and acquiring the ability to interpret your dreams is a powerful tool, see: http://www.dreammoods.com/dreamdictionary/

#67 American Association of Psychiatry, see: http://ajp.psychiatryonline.org/cgi/content/full/159/9/1603 and http://ajp.psychiatryonline.org/cgi/content/abstract/151/6/871

#68 Culture competency Q and A on death and dying, see: http://www.minoritynurse.com/features/health/05-04-04b.html

Changing the way you feel about grief and loss in Latin American Countries, see: http://www.beyondindigo.com/articles/article.php/artID/200089

#69 Wearing a scapular see: http://www.newadvent.org/cathen/13508b.htm

#70 A 2005 article in WebMD®, reported on an article published in the Archives of Disease in Childhood, September 2005, Vol. 90. "Crying Behavior Recorded in 3rd Trimester Fetuses," documents that fetuses do cry as Latinos have always known, see: http://www.webmd.com/baby/news/20050913/babies-may-start-crying-while-in-womb

#73 Arturo Vásquez is a native of Hollister, California, who spent five years in religious life as a seminarian and a monk. He graduated from the University of California, Berkeley with a bachelor's degree in Latin American Studies, see:
http://arturovasquez.wordpress.com/2008/07/22/el-aire-basura

#73 See Sherry Field's: "Pestilence and Head colds: Encountering Illness in Colonial Mexico," Columbia University Press 2008, for more explanation, see:
www.gutenberg-e.org/fields

#74/ 176 In the Western world, people usually do not make a distinction between illness and disease, like evil eye, susto, aire, for more information see: http://anthro.palomar.edu/medical/med_1.htm http://www.sfbardo.com/maldeojo.htm or http:en.wikipedia.org/wiki/Evil_eye

#77 /139 Professional counseling after sexual abuse, see: http://www.americanhumane.org/protecting-children/ http://www.nlm.nih.gov/medlineplus/childabuse.html

http://www.crosscreekcounseling.com/sexual_abuse.html

http://early-childhood-development.suite101.com/article.cfm/child_molestation_prevention

#80 Learn more about St. Anthony of Padua, see: http://www.americancatholic.org/Features/Anthony/

#/81/ 150 /178 Sahumerio or aromatic smoke, see: http://www.terra.cl/astrologia/index.cfm?pagina=temas&id_cat=15&id_reg=604568

#83 Saint Joseph is popular among Sicilian-Americans, see: http://www.luckymojo.com/saintjoseph.html

#84/144 For a definition on a barrida, the ritual of cleansing or sweeping, in which a person is swept from head to toe, see: http://medical-dictionary.thefreedictionary.com/barrida

#85 Christian Apologetics and Research Ministry, The Psalms, see: www.carm.org or http://www/carm.org/kjv/Psalms/Psalm.htm

#91 Substance Abuse and Mental Health Services Administration, see: http://www.samhsa.gov/ or http://www.samhsa.gov/matrix2/topics.aspx

#91 SAMHSA works to improve the quality and availability of substance abuse prevention, alcohol and drug addiction treatment, and mental health services, see:
http://ncadistore.samhsa.gov/catalog/productDetails.aspx?ProductID=17503

#117 Look for lucky products and la suerte at the luckymojo site and others, see: http://www.luckymojo.com

#127 Catholic online, saints and angels, see: http://www.catholic.org/saints/saint.php?saint_id=308 or http://www.newadvent.org/cathen/10275b.htm

#135 Augustine's Spiritual Supplies shop, see: http://www.augustinespiritualgoods.com/courtcase_page.htm

#146 The national geographic online, see: http://channel.nationalgeographic.com/series/taboo

Curandero Conversations

#146 New age publisher in tarot, witchcraft, magic, shamanism, and astrology, see: http://llewellyn.com

#148 Succubus, see: http://en.wikipedia.org/wiki/Succubus

#149 Tracy Wilkinson's, The Vatican's Exorcists: Driving out the Devil in the 21st Century, see: http://www.catholic.org/international/international_story.php?id=21056

http://home.newadvent.org/cathen/05709a.htm   http://www.exorthodoxforchrist.com/exorcism_&_catholic_priests.htm

http://www.trosch.org/chu/exorcism.htm

#149 /163 A simple exorcism for priests or laity, see: http://www.holygrail-church.fsnet.co.uk/exorcism.htm

#149/165 Catholic exorcist demonic influences is strong in today's world, see:
http://www.catholic.org/international/international_story.php?id=21056

#149 Exorcism and Catholic priests, see: http://www.exorthodoxforchrist.com/exorcism_&_catholic_priests.htm

#149 American folklore top 10 spooky stories see: http://www.americanfolklore.net/folktales/tx3.html

#156 Thought and action, the Ouija board, see: http://catholic-perspective.blogspot.com/2008/07/ouija-board-brings-demonic-possession.html

The danger of the Ouija board by Dan Corner, see: http://www.evangelicaloutreach.org/ouija.htm

#158 Witchcraft dolls see:
http://www.calastrology.com/voodoo.html   http://images.google.com/images?hl=en&rlz=1T4ADBF_enUS237US239&resnum=1&q=voodoo+dolls&um=1&ie=UTF-8&sa=X&oi=image_result_group&resnum=1&ct=title

#168 Mental Illnesses, http://en.wikipedia.org/wiki/Schizophrenia

#169 Witchcraft spells, see: http://www.witchcraftspellsnow.com/

#170 Umbanda see: Afro-Brazilian religion or http://en.wikipedia.org/wiki/Umbanda

#179 For the most recent information on La Santisima Muerte see: http://fmso.leavenworth.army.mil/documents/Santa-Muerte/santa-muerte.htm

#184 For prayer book information see: http://www.catholicdoors.com/prayers/novena.html

#180 Mary's Gardens Home Page, Flowers in Spanish, http://www/mgardens.org/S-FOL.html

#180 New Advent, catholic encyclopedia article on miracles, see: http://www.newadvent.org/cathen/10338a.htm

New advent, catholic encyclopedia, article of divine providence, see: http://www.newadvent.org/cathen/12510a.htm

For Mexican cultural profile, language, history, politics, greetings and displays of respect, see: http://ethnomed.org/cultures/hispanic/mexican_cp.html

The Professional Forum offers the latest research papers, medical articles, and protocol documents relating to chronic illnesses and stealth viral infections see: www.emergingworlds.com

Medscape and Medicine is the largest online community of physicians and healthcare professionals today, see: http://medscape.com/viewarticle/525639

The day of the dead a Mexican celebration, see: http://www3.niu.edu/newsplace/nndia.html

Appendix III
A Border Herbal

"He causeth the grass to grow for the cattle, and herb for the service of man: that he may bring forth food out of the earth."

–Psalm 104:14

Note to the Reader:

The following Border Herbal contains 542 of the most common medicinal plants used and prescribed by *curanderos* along the U.S.-Mexico border. Dr. Zavaleta and his staff have studied and catalogued medicinal plants for more than 35 years.

Several things are important to note: The plant names, spellings, and their multiple uses differ from region to region. The primary source for the herbal is the Official Pharmacopeia and Dispensatory of the United States and Mexico.

The authors have done their best to verify names, spellings, Latin names and uses for the reader. There can be no guarantee that they are correct but we believe that they are. We also believe that this is the only source that contains the English names, the Spanish names, the Latin names and the uses for this number of plants used in *curanderismo*.

Antonio Zavaleta and Alberto Salinas Jr.

The information is compiled from hundreds of sources. Please use it with care and always see a doctor. The medicinal plants listed below are intended for educational purposes only and not for medical purposes.

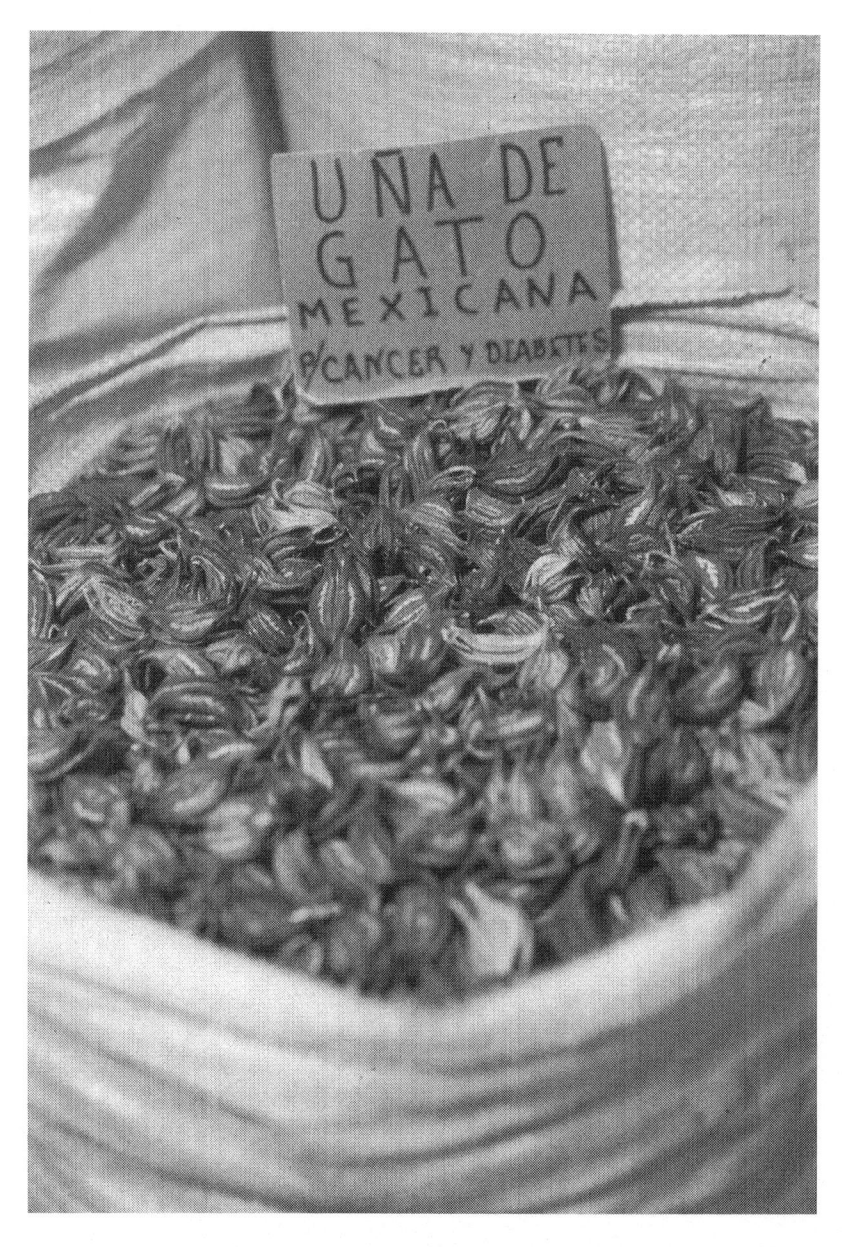

Vendors at the Mercado de Sonora sell medicinal plants wholesale and in bulk for distribution and resale in the hierberías throughout the nation and abroad.
(Photo by José M. Duarte)

	English Name	**Spanish Name**	*Botanical Name*	**Used to Treat**
1	Acacia	Acacia	*Acacia greggii*	Muscle pain, superficial wounds
2	Aconite	Acónito de Nepal	*Aconitum napellus*	Flu, cold symptoms
3	Agrimony	Agrimonia	*Agrimonia parviflora*	Purify the blood, colds, fevers, diarrhea
4	All Heal	Valeriana	*Prunella vulgaris*	Digestive disorders, wounds, sores, ulcers, fever, diarrhea
5	Alfalfa	Alfalfa	*Medicago sativa*	Kidney, urinary tract, indigestion, arthritis
6	Almond	Almendra	*Prunus amygdalus L*	Digestive system, urinary tract, asthma
7	Aloe Vera	Sábila	*Aloe barbadensis*	Burns, wounds, rheumatism, gastric ulcers
8	Alpine Lichen	Parmeliaceae	*Parmelia acharius*	Sore feet, burns, cuts
9	Amaranth	Amaranto	*Amaranthus spp.*	Heart problems
10	Ambrosia	Hierba Amarga	*Ambrosia artemisiifolia*	Insect bites, rheumatic joints, fevers, nausea, intestinal cramps, diarrhea
11	American Alum Root	Heuchera	*Heuchera americana*	Sore mouths, stomach pain, sore eyes
12	American Coffee Bean Tree	Árbol de Café	*Gymnocladus canadensis*	Sore throat, cough, tonsillitis
13	American Spikenard	Aralia	*Aralia racemosa*	Respiratory system, cough, rheumatism, asthma
14	American Wormseed	Epazote	*Chenopodium ambrosioides*	Intestinal disorders, calms nerves, worms wounds
15	Anacacho Bauhinia	Pata de Vaca	*Baubinia congesta*	Controls diarrhea
16	Angelica	Angélica	*Angelica archagelica*	Cramps, bronchial congestion

17	Angel's Trumpet	Florifundio	*Datura stramonium*	Arthritis, asthma
18	Anise	Anís	*Pinpinella anisum*	Stomach cramps, sore muscles, cough
19	Annatto	Achiote	*Bixa orellana*	Skin inflammations, insect bites
20	Antelope Horns	Inmortal	*Asclepias asperula*	Respiratory disorders
21	Apache Plume	Ponil	*Falugia paradoxa*	Hair, cough
22	Apple	Manzana	*Pyrus malus*	Gout, liver, constipation
23	Apple Mint	Mastranzo	*Menta rotundifolia*	Sore throats, stomachache, bee stings
24	Apricot	Albaricoque	*Prunus armeniaca*	Asthma, cancer, eye, cough
25	Areca Palm Nut	Areca	*Areca catechu*	Digestion, sore throat, cough
26	Arizona Poppy	Contra Yerba	*Kallstroemia californica*	Eye irritations, sore throat
27	Arnica	Arnica	*Arnica montana*	Sore muscles, bruises, wounds, hemorrhoids
28	Artichoke	Alcachofa	*Cynara scolymus*	Liver, diabetes
29	Aspen	Alamo Temblón	*Populus tremuliodes*	Appetite, headaches, fevers, diuretic, skin
30	Astragalus	Astrágalo	*Astragalus membranaceus*	Urinary and respiratory tract
31	Avocado	Aguacate	*Persea americana*	Menstrual, headache, muscle strain, aphrodisiac
32	Awnless Bush Sunflower	Cuájalo	*Simsia calva*	Stomachache
33	Aztec Marigold	Caléndula Azteca	*Tagetes erecta*	Fever, stomachache
34	Balsam of Peru	Bálsamo Peruviana	*Toluifera pereirae*	Flu, strep throat, rashes, wounds, lice
35	Balsam Root	Balsamorhiza	*Balsamorhiza sqittata*	Sore throat, colds, bronchitis
36	Banana	Platano	*Musa genus*	Potassium

#	Common	Spanish	Scientific	Uses
37	Barley	Cebada	Hordeum vulgare L	Diarrhea, gastritis, healing ointments
38	Basin Sagebrush	Chamizo Hediondo	Artemisa tridentata	Rheumatism, aches, pains
39	Bay Berry	Arbol de la Cera	Myrica californica	Cough, dysentery, congestion
40	Bay Laurel (Bay leaves)	Laurel	Lauris nobilis, litsea	Sore throat, colic, insomnia, earache
41	Bean	Frijol	Phaseolus vulgaris	Headaches
42	Bearberry	Cáscara Sagrada	Rhammus purshiana	Laxative, purgative, tonic, antibacterial
43	Bear Grass	Sacahuista	Nolina microcarpa	Veins, rheumatoid arthritis
44	Bee Brush	Quebradora	Aloysia gratissima	Bladder infections, bronchitis, colds
45	Beet Plant	Betabel	Beta vulgaris	Skin problems, digestive, headaches
46	Belladonna	Belladanna	Atropa belladonna	Neuralgia, headache, ulcer, inflammation
47	Benzoin	Benjuí	Styrax benzoin	Minor sores, skin protection
48	Beth Root	Rizoma	Trillium erectum	Hemorrhage, respiratory, insect bites
49	Bilberry	Arándano	Vaccinium myrtillus L	Digestive disorders, urinary tract
50	Birch	Abedul	Betula alba	Kidney and urinary tract
51	Birthwort	Aristoloquia	Aristolochia clematitis	Sweating, insect bites
52	Bistort	Bistorta	Polygonum bistorta	Hemorrhoids, nose bleeds, diarrhea, bruises
53	Bitter Orange	Naranja Agria	Citrus aurantium	Abdominal pains, coughs, nerves, insomnia
54	Bitter wood	Cuasia	Quassia amara	Dysentery, bile, indigestion, lack of appetite

#	Common	Spanish	Latin	Uses
55	Blackberry	Zarzamora	*Rubus strigosus*	Inflamed gums, mouth ulcers, diarrhea
56	Black Cohosh	Cohosh Negro	*Actaea racemosa L*	Menopausal symptoms, breast cancer
57	Black Cumin	Comino Negro	*Nigeooa sativa L*	Asthma, bronchitis, colic, flu, impotence
58	Black Mulberry	Mora Negra	*Morus nigra L*	Fever, eye sore, throat
59	Black Mustard	Mostaza Negra	*Brassica negra*	Epilepsy, toothache, bruises, colic, rheumatism
60	Black Nightshade	Yerba Mora	*Solamum nigrescenas*	Edema, fever, cough, heart disease, hemorrhoids
61	Black Pepper	Pimienta	*Piper nigrum*	Heartburn, gas, diarrhea, constipation
62	Blessed Thistle	Cardo Bendito	*Cnicus benedictus (L)*	Heartburn, digestive system
63	Blood Root	Sanguinaria	*Sanguinaria canadensis*	Skin cancer, warts
64	Blue Cohosh	Caulophyllum	*Caulophyllum thalictroides*	Rheumatism, menstruation, indigestion
65	Blue Flag	Iris Versícolor	*Iris virginica*	Uterus, chronic rheumatism
66	Bold	Boldo	*Peumus boldus*	Headache, cold, liver, sore muscles
67	Boneset	Eupatorio	*Eupatorium*	Fever, rheumatism, pneumonia
68	Borage	Borraja	*Borago officinalis*	Fever, cough, sore throat, kidney, urinary tract
69	Bougainvillea	Buganvilia	*Bougainvillea glabra*	Cough, bronchitis and asthma
70	Bottle Gourd	Chilicote	*Lagenaria siceraria Molina*	Headaches, baldness

71	Brazil Wood	Brasil	*Harmatoxylum brasiletum*	Diarrhea, rheumatism, kidney, dental, fever
72	Brazilian Cocoa	Guarana	*Paullinia cupana*	Drowsiness, weight loss
73	Bricklebush	Prodigiosa	*Brickellia cavanillesii*	High blood sugar, excess bile, diabetes
74	Brittle Bush	Incienso, Yerba del Vaso	*Encelia farinosa*	Gum problems, toothache, fever, arthritis
75	Brook Mint	Poleo	*Mentha arvensis*	Stomach irritations, nausea, diarrhea, insomnia
76	Broomweed	Escoba de Rosita	*Gutierrezia texana*	Menstruation
77	Bryony	Brionia	*Bryonia dioica*	Severe headaches, arthritis, swollen joints
78	Buchu	Buchü	*Barosma betulina*	Urinary tract infections, inflammations, gout, nausea, flatulence, diuretic
79	Buckeye	Ojo de Venado	*Macuna sloanei*	Amulet
80	Buckthorn Bark	Frangula	*Rhamnus frangula*	Relieves constipation, rectal problems
81	Buffalo Gourd	Calabacita	*Cucuribita foetidissima*	Intestinal parasites
82	Burr Marigold	Aceitilla	*Bidens pilosa*	Colic
83	Burro Brush	Yerba del Burro	*Hymenoclea sp*	Arthritis, rheumatism, intestinal worms
84	Burdock Root	Lappa	*Arctium minus*	Eczema, acne, boils, bites, burns, bruises
85	Butcher's Broom	Rusco	*Ruscus aculeatus L*	Jaundice, kidney infection, urination, fever

86	Butterfly Bush	Salvia Real	*Buddleia americana*	Stomach disorders, pimples, cough, colds
87	Butternut	Nuez de Cuba	*Juglans cinerea*	Rheumatic, arthritic joints, headaches, constipation
88	Button Bush	Jazmín Uvero	*Cephalanthus occidentalis*	Indigestion, constipation, liver, gallbladder
89	Button Snakeroot	Yerba del Sapo	*Eryrrgium*	Menstruation, kidney, rheumatism
90	Cabbage	Repollo	*Brassica oleracea*	Acid reflux, joint pain
91	Cabbage Rose	Rosa de Castilla	*Rosa centifolia*	Mild laxative
92	Cachane	Cachane	*Senecio cardiophyllus*	Puerperal fever
93	California Poppy	Copa de Oro	*Eschscholtzia californica*	Insomnia, anxiety, spasmodic cough, cuts
94	Campeachy Wood, Logwood	Palo de Campeche	*Haematoxylon campechianum*	Diarrhea, stimulant
95	Camphor Tree	Alcanfor	*Cinnamomum camphora*	Sore muscles, wounds
96	Camphor Weed	Arnica Mexicana	*Heterotheca subaxillaris*	Hemorrhoids, bruises, sore muscles, bronchitis
97	Canada snakeroot	Jengibre Salvage	*Asarum canadense*	Digestive problems, swollen breasts, colds
98	Canadian Fleabane	Pazotillo	*Conyza canadensis*	Insomnia, anxiety, spasmodic cough, cuts
99	Candlewood	Ocotillo	*Fouquiera splendens*	Varicose veins, hemorrhoids, fatigue
100	Cannabis	Marijuana	*Cannabis hemp*	Pain reliever, arthritis, asthma, epilepsy, glaucoma, muscle relaxant
101	Canyon Ragweed	Chícura	*Ambrosia ambrosioides syn.*	Menstrual cramps

102	Capers	Alcaparras	*Capparis spinosa L*	Arthritis, cancer, cataracts, dysentery
103	Caraway Shrub	Alcaravea	*Carum carvi*	Dyspepsia, hysteria
104	Cardamom Seed	Semilla de Cardamomo	*Elettaria cardomomum (L)*	Appetite, nausea, vomiting
105	Carnation	Clavel	*Dianthus caryophyllus*	Indigestion, gas, bloating, cough
106	Carob Tree	Algarroba	*Ceratonia siligua*	Infantile diarrhea, obesity, gastritis
107	Castor Bean Plant	Higuerilla	*Ricinus communis*	Constipation, colds, fever, bruises
108	Catechu	Gambir	*Uncaria gambir*	Diarrhea
109	Cayenne Pepper	Berberé	*Capsicum frutescens*	Circulation, heart disease, sore throats
110	Cat Claw	Uña de Gato	*Uncaria tomentosa*	Gastric ulcers, tumors, intestinal ailments, gastritis
111	Catnip	Cataría	*Nepeta cataria*	Insomnia, fever
112	Cedar	Sabino Macho	*Juniperus sp*	Urinary tract, fever
113	Celandine	Celedonia	*Chelidonium majus*	Warts, fungous growths
114	Celery	Apio	*Apium graveolens var.*	Kidney, cough, colds
115	Century Plant	Maguey	*Agave salmiania*	Digestive disorders arthritis, cuts, wounds, mouth sores
116	Centaury Herb	Tlanchalagua	*Centaurium*	Used to induce weight loss
117	Chaff-Flower (Prickly)	Tánguis	*Achyranthes aspera L.*	Fever, malaria, heat stroke, headache
118	Chamomile	Manzanilla	*Matricaria chamomile*	Nervousness, acid indigestion, gas, colic pain
119	Chaparral, Creosote Bush	Gobernadora, Hediondilla	*Larrea tridentata*	Insect bites, ringworms, urinary tract problems

120	Chaste Tree	Aceitunillo	*Vitex mollis*	Pulmonary ailments, menstrual problems, diarrhea
121	Cheeseweed Mallow	Malva de Castilla	*Malva parviflora*	Boils, coughs, ulcers in the bladder
122	Cherry	Cereza	*Prunus avium*	Cystitis, bronchial, edema
123	Chestnut Leaves	Hojas de Castaño	*Castanea dentata*	Cough, heart trouble
124	Chickweed	Pamplina	*Stellaria media*	Painful urination, intestinal inflammation
125	Chicory	Achicoria	*Intybus sativum*	Tonic, appetite stimulant, bruises, impotence, diabetes
126	Chinch Weed	Manzanilla de Coyote	*Pectis papposa*	Stomachache, gastrointestinal cramps, diarrhea
127	Cinnamon	Canela	*Cinnamomium zeylanicum*	Flu, rheumatism, indigestion, nausea, hangover
128	Cinquefoil	Cincoenrama	*Potentilla simplex*	Hoarseness, sore throat, sores, rashes, irritated skin
129	Citron	Cidro	*Citrus medica L*	Asthma, bronchitis, dyspepsia, lumbago, seasickness
130	Clematis	Barba de Chivo	*Clematis virginiana*	Headaches, sore throat, colds, skin sores
131	Clove	Clavo	*Syzgium aromatic syn.*	Toothache, nausea
132	Cocoa	Cacao	*Theobroma cacao*	Burns, eye, wounds
133	Cocklebur	Calcitrapa	*Xanthium strumarium*	Cystitis, diarrhea, rhinitis, sinusitis, cuts and scrapes
134	Cockspur	Espino Blanco	*Acacia cornigera*	Stimulant, fever reducer
135	Coconut	Coco	*Cocos nucifera*	Amoebae
136	Colchicum Root	Cólquico	*Colchicum autumnale*	Joint pain, gout

137	Colombo	Calumba	*Jateorrhiza palmata*	Digestion, gas, nausea, diarrhea
138	Common Basil	Albahaca	*Ocimum basilicum*	Digestive disorders, nervousness, menstrual cramps
139	Common Comfrey	Sueldo	*Symphytum officinale*	Skin infections, insect bites, wounds
140	Common Fig	Higuera	*Ficus carica*	Antiseptic, laxative
141	Common Ivy	Yedra	*Hedera helix*	Coughs, bronchitis, sore or watering eyes, skin problems
142	Common Juniper	Enebro	*Juniperus communis*	Painful urination, colds, fever
143	Common Lantana	Cinco Negritos	*Lantana camara*	Rheumatism, snakebite, insect bites
144	Common Plantain	Lantén	*Plantago mayor*	Dysentery, wounds, canker sores
145	Common Sage	Salvia	*Salvia officinalis*	Stomach gas, sore throat
146	Common Tansy	Hierba Lombriguera	*Tanacetum vulgare*	Intestinal worms, menstrual bleeding, skin diseases
147	Condurango Bark	Bejuco del Cóndor	*Marsdenia cundurango*	Calms stomach, reduces nausea
148	Copaiba	Copayero	*Copaifera reticulate*	Respiratory disorders, athlete's foot
149	Copalchi	Copal Chií	*Coutarea latiflora*	Kidney ailments, diabetes, fever
150	Copperleaf	Yerba del Cáncer	*Acalypha lindheimeri*	Indigestion, dysentery, wounds, bruises, muscle pain
151	Cordyceps	Tochukaso	*Cordyceps sinensis*	Cough, anemia, impotence, infertility
152	Coriander	Cilantro	*Coriandrum sativum*	Toothache, impotence, anxiety
153	Corn Silk	Barba de Maíz	*Zea mays*	Cystitis, incontinence, PMS

154	Cottonwood	Alamo	*Populus angustifolia*	Arthritis, diarrhea, dental problems
155	Cow Parsnip	Grande Berce	*Heracleum sphondylium*	Laryngitis, bronchitis, toothache, epilepsy, colic
156	Cranberry	Aírela	*Vaccinium macrocarpon*	Urinary tract infection
157	Crown Beard	Añil del Muerto	*Verbesina enceliokes*	Hemorrhoids, chapped lips, spider bites
158	Crucifixion Thorn	Chaparro Amargosa	*Castela emoryi*	Dysentery, liver
159	Cubeb Berries	Cubeba	*Piper cubeba*	Asthma, bronchitis, indigestion, coughs
160	Cucumber	Pepino	*Cucumis sativas*	Diuretic, emollient, purgative
161	Cudweed	Gordolobo	*Gnapalium spp.*	Colds, bronchitis, asthma, diarrhea
162	Cultivated White Oats	Avena	*Avena sativa*	Osteoporosis, hyperactive children, stress
163	Culvers Root	Leptandra	*Veronicastrum virginicum*	Liver disorders, stomach disorders, fevers
164	Cupid's Flower	Cabello de Angel	*Lpomoea qualoclit Linn.*	Hemorrhoids, constipation
165	Curly Parsley	Perejil	*Petroselinum crispum*	Water retention, premenstrual syndrome, insect bites
166	Custard Apple	Chirimoya	*Annona cherimola*	Sore muscles, diarrhea, ringworm
167	Cypress	Cedro	*Cupressus sempervirens*	Warts, wounds, infections, bronchitis
168	Damiana	Damiana	*Turnera diffusa var.*	Bedwetting, impotence
169	Dandelion	Diente de León	*Taraxacum officinale*	Liver, kidney congestion, skin eruptions, water retention

170	Date Palm	Palmera de Dátiles	*Phoenix dactylifera L*	Asthma, cough, fever, estrogen deficiency, toothache
171	Deadly Nightshade Leaf	Hojas de Belladona	*Atropa belladonna*	Headache, menstrual symptoms, peptic ulcer
172	Deer Weed	Yerba del Venado	*Porophyllum spp.*	Indigestion, colic
173	Desert Anemone	Yerba Mansa	*Anemone tuberosa*	Depression, urinary system
174	Desert Barberry	Alegrita	*Mahonia trifoliata*	Bacterial, food poisoning
175	Desert Broom	Yerba del Pasmo	*Baccharis L.*	Stuffy nose, insect bites,
176	Desert Cotton	Algodoncillo	*Gossypium thurberi*	Back and pelvic pain
177	Desert Hollyhock	Yerba del Negro	*Sphaeralcea angustifolia*	Eye irritations, sore throat, skin irritations
178	Desert Willow	Mimbre	*Chilopsis linearis*	Indigestion, yeast infections, cough, skin infection
179	Devil's Claw	Espuela del Diablo	*Harpagophytum procumbens*	Pain, skin problems, joint pain, sores, ulcers
180	Digitalis	Digital	*Digitalis purpurea*	Circulation
181	Dill	Eneldo	*Anethum graveolens*	Poor lactation
182	Dog Grass	Triticum	*Agropyron repens*	Arthritis, rheumatism, gout
183	Dog Weed	Parralena	*Dyssodia pentachaeta*	Gastritis, indigestion, colic
184	Dogwood	Cerezo Silvestre	*Cornus officinales*	Fever, headache, exhaustion
185	Dong Quai	Dong Quai	*Angelica Sinesis*	Menstrual and puerperal disorders
186	Donkeys Tail	Cola de Borrego	*Sedum morganianum*	Eye wash
187	Dragon Blood Powder	Siete Raíces	*Daemomorops draco*	Cuts and abrasions

188	Drake's Foot	Contryerba Blanco	*Psoralea pentaphylla*	Food poisoning, fever, chills, stomach flu
189	Dry Poblano Pepper	Chile Ancho	*Capsicum baccatum*	Cholesterol and triglyceride
190	Dwarf Pennyroyal	Poleo Chino	*Hedeoma oblongifolia*	Fevers, menstrual cramps, indigestion
191	Eggplant	Berengena	*Solanum melongena*	Blood cholesterol, high blood pressure, burns
192	Elder Flower	Flor de Saúco	*Sambucus mexicana, nigra*	Complexion, colic, intestinal gas, colds, laxative
193	Elecampane	Nula Campana	*Linula helenium*	Pneumonia, cough, asthma, bronchitis
194	Elephant Tree	Copal	*Busera jorullensis*	Fever, gums, spider bites
195	Ephedra (Ma Huang)	Efedra	*Ephedra sinica*	Bronchial asthma, cold, cough
196	English Marigold	Caléndula	*Calendula officinalis*	Eye infections, sore throat, fever, wounds, earache
197	Eucalyptus	Eucalipto	*Eucalyptus globulus*	Cough, bronchitis, asthma
198	Euphorbia (Spurge)	Yerba de Golondrina	*Euphorbia pilulifera*	Asthma, respiratory infections
199	European Mistletoe	Muérdago, Injerto	*Viscum album (L)*	Seizures, headaches
200	Evening Primrose	Yerba del Golpe	*Oenothera kunthiana*	Wounds, bruises, urinary tract
201	Evergreen Ash	Fresno	*Fraxinus udhei*	Constipation, diuretic, fever
202	Eyebrights	Eufrasia	*Euphrasia arguta*	Runny nose, congestion, eye
203	False Unicorn Root	Helonias	*Chamalirium*	Infertility, morning sickness
204	Fava Bean	Habas	*Vicia faba L.*	Alcoholism, cancer, estrogen
205	Fennel	Hinojo	*Foeniculum vulgare*	Digestive disorders, intestinal gas, menstrual cramps

206	Fenugreek	Fenogreco	*Trigonella foenum-graecum L*	Baldness, diabetes, dyspepsia, cholesterol
207	Fern	Cola de Zorra	*Cheilanthes elegans*	Stomach swelling
208	Feverfew	Altamisa Mexicana	*Tanacetum parthenium syn.*	Migraines, stomachache, menstrual cramps, colds, flu
209	Field Poppy	Amapola	*Papaver rhoeas*	Nerves, insomnia, cough
210	Filaree	Alferillo	*Erodium cicutarium*	Urinary disorders, sore throat, wounds, arthritis
211	Firecracker Bush	Trompetilla	*Bouvardia ternifolia syn.*	Snake, stings, dysentery
212	Flat-Top Buckwheat	Colita de Rata	*Eriogonum fasciculatum*	Bladder problems, wounds, diarrhea, sore throat
213	Flax	Linaza	*Limum usitatissimum*	Burns, abscesses, cough
214	Flower Hay	Flor del Heno	*Tillandsia usneoides*	Toothache, stomach pain, kidney, gallbladder
215	Four - O'clock	Maravilla	*Mirabilis mulitflora*	Arthritis, rheumatism, bruises
216	Four -Wing Salt Brush	Chamizo	*Triplex capeskins*	Fever, stomachache, diarrhea
217	Frankincense	Francoincienso	*Boswellia sacra flueck*	Dysentery, fever
218	French Rose	Rosa de Castilla	*Rosa gallic*	Infantile diarrhea, inflamed gums, throat, fever
219	Fringe Tree Bark	Chionanthus	*Chinonanthus virginicus*	Mild laxative action, wounds and sores
220	Garden Heliotrope	Valeriana	*Valeriana ceratophylla*	Insomnia, nervousness
221	Garden Nasturtium	Mastuerzo	*Tropaeolum majus*	Anemia, mouth sores
222	Garden Thyme	Tomillo	*Thymus vulgaris*	Cough, indigestion, toothache

223	Garlic	Ajo	*Allium sativan*	Toothache, indigestion, gas
224	Gay Feather	Cachana	*Liatris*	Sore throat, tonsillitis
225	Gentian Root	Genciana	*Gentiana gentianella spp*	Digestive function, appetite
226	Geranium	Geranio	*Pelargonium spp.*	Diarrhea, headache, sores
227	German Chamomile	Manzanilla	*Matricaria chamomila*	Menstrual cramps, colic, indigestion, insomnia
228	Giant Hyssop	Toronjil	*Agastache mexicamum syn.*	Nerves, insomnia, digestive disorder, menstrual cramps
229	Ginger	Jengibre	*Zingiber officinale*	Stomachache, indigestion, nausea, fever
230	Ginseng	Ginseng	*Panax ginseng*	Energy and sense of well-being
231	Goldenrod	Vara de San Jose	*Solidago virgaurea*	Water retention, congestion
232	Goldenseal	Sello de Oro	*Hydrastis candensis*	Sore eyes, hepatitis, dyspepsia fever
233	Golden Shower	Caña Fistula	*Cassia fistula*	Rheumatism, ulcers, fever, skin disease
234	Gourd Tree	Cirián	*Crescentia alata*	Diarrhea, cough, asthma
235	Grape	Parra	*Vitis vinifera*	Diarrhea, hemorrhage, hemorrhoids
236	Great Mullein	Verbasco	*Verbascum thapsus*	Burns, diarrhea, colic
237	Greek Hay	Fenogreco	*Alholva trigonella*	Constipation, diabetes, cholesterol
238	Green Gentian	Cebadilla	*Swertia radiata*	Constipation, indigestion
239	Green Tea	Té Verde	*Camellia sinensis L*	Mild stimulant, diuretic,
240	Greenbrier Root	Cocolmeca	*Phaseouls spp.*	Kidney pain, infertility

241	Ground Cherry	Costomate	*Physalis lobata*	Obstruction in the intestines
242	Guava	Guayaba	*Psidium spp.*	Diarrhea, dysentery, wounds, sore feet
243	Gum Arabic	Acacia	*Acacia senegal*	Headache, skin irritations, diarrhea, coughs
244	Gum Asafetida	Asafétida	*Ferula assa-foetida*	Bronchial, allergic asthma, cramps, constipation
245	Gum Myrrh	Myrrha	*Commiphora molmol*	Asthma, bronchial, coughs, constipation
246	Gum Weed	Yerba del Buey	*Grindelia phanactis*	Colds, cough, sore throat, kidney
247	Hand Flower Tree	Flor de Manita	*Chiranthodendron pentadactylon*	Nervous system disorders
248	Hawthorn	Espino	*Crataegus laevigata*	Abdominal pain
249	Hemlock Spruce	Abeto	*Abies canadensis*	Coughs, colds, gastric irritation
250	Henbane	Beleno Blanco	*Hyoscyamus niger*	Urinary tract infection, kidneys
251	Henna	Alcana	*Lausonia inermis L*	Toe nail fungus
252	Herb of God	Hierba del Sueño	*Calea zacatechichi*	Induces sleep
253	Hibiscus	Jamaica	*Hibiscus sabdariffa*	Fever, eye infections, sores, wounds
254	Holywood	Gayacán	*Guajacum sanctum*	Blood in stools
255	Hop Tree	Cola de Zorrillo	*Ptelea trifollata*	Lack of appetite, indigestion
256	Hops	Humulas	*Humulus lupulus*	Sedative, antiseptic properties, reduce inflammation
257	Horehound	Marrubio	*Marrubium vulgare*	Bronchitis, asthma, indigestion,

258	Horse Balm	Centinodia	*Collinsonia canadensis*	Laryngitis, chronic bronchitis, indigestion
259	Horse Chestnut	Castaño de Indias	*Aesuculus hippocastanum L*	Congestion, backache, arthritis
260	Horsemint	Mastranzo Nevado	*Mentha longifolia (l)huds.*	Cold, dermatitis, impotence, pain, rheumatism
261	Horse Nettle	Especie de Solano	*Solanum carolinense*	Convulsive disorders, epilepsy
262	Horseradish	Rabano Picante	*Cochlearia armoracia*	Urinary tract infections, bronchitis, sinus congestion, coughs
263	Horsetail	Cola de Caballo	*Equisetum arvense*	Kidney stones, wounds, skin diseases
264	Horseweed	Simonillo	*Conyza confussa*	Bile, diarrhea, colitis, hemorrhoids
265	Houseleek	Siempreviva	*Sedum sp*	Intestinal irritation, sores, burns, headaches hemorrhoids
266	Hummingbird Flower	Espinosilla	*Loeselia mexicana*	Fever reducer
267	Hyacinth Bean	Frijol de la Punzada	*Dolichos lablab*	Headaches
268	Indian Cockle	Cocculus	*Cocculus indicus*	Ringworms, scabies
269	Indian Mallow	Hierba de la Francesa	*Abutilon incanum*	Leukorrhea
270	Indian Paintbrush	Santa Rita	*Castilleja arvensis*	Kidney problems, wounds, measles, cough
271	Indian Plantain	Matarique	*Psacalium decompositum*	diabetes, arthritis, rheumatism, wounds
272	Indian Root	Yerba del Indio	*Aristolochia mexicana*	Snakebite, infections
273	Indian Tobacco	Lobelia	*Lobelia inflata*	Tumors, ulcers, leg sores
274	Ipecac	Ipecacuana	*Cephaelis ipecacuanha*	Vomiting

275	Irish Moss	Chondrus	*Chondrus crispus*	Coughs, bronchitis, indigestion, gastric
276	Jerusalem Thorn	Palo Verde	*Parkinsonia aculeata*	Fever, indigestion
277	Jimson Weed	Estramonio, Toloache	*Datura stramonium*	Asthma, intestinal cramps, diarrhea
278	Jojoba	Jojoba	*Simmondsia chinensis*	Cuts, burns, rashes, diarrhea
279	Juliana	Cuachalate	*Juliana adstringens*	Wounds, gum problems, infertility
280	Jumping Cholla	Velas de Coyote	*Oputia fulgida*	Urinary tract, peptic ulcers, gastritis
281	Kava	Kava	*Piper methysticum*	Anxiety, tension, alcohol
282	Kidney Wood	Palo Azul	*Eysenhardtia polystachya*	Kidney disorder, urinary tract disorders, toothache
283	Kidneywort	Hepatica	*Anemone hepatica*	Fevers, colds, liver disorders
284	Kino	Kino	*Pterocarpus marsupium*	Diabetes, obesity, joint pain
285	Kola Nuts	Kola	*Cola nitada*	Depression, morning sickness, migraine headaches
286	Lady Skipper	Flores de Belin	*Cypripedium sp*	Toenails
287	Larkspur Seed	Espuelas de Dama	*Delphinium ajacis*	Wounds, piles, colic, lice
288	Lavender	Alhucema	*Lavandula spica*	Colic, indigestion, and nerves
289	Leadwort	Yerba de Alacrán	*Plumbago scandens*	Wounds, ulcer, cuts, edema,
290	Lemon Balm	Abejera	*Melissa officinales*	Insomnia, anxiety, muscles
291	Lemon Tree	Limón	*Citrus aurantifolia*	Diarrhea, colds, respiratory cuts, sores
292	Lemon Grass	Zacate de Limón	*Cymbopogon citratus*	Digestive, sedative

293	Lemon Scented Verbena	Cedrón	*Aloysia triphylla*	Upset stomach, menstrual cramps
294	Lentils	Lenteja	*Lens culinaris medik*	Alcohol syndrome
295	Lettuce	Lechuga	*Lactuca sativa lomgifolia*	Digestive tract, circulatory system, respiratory tract
296	Licorice	Orozuz	*Glycrrhiza glabra*	Cough, wounds, gastrointestinal ulcers
297	Lilac Tree	Arból de Lilia	*Syringa vulgaris*	Burns and malaria
298	Lily of the Valley Root	Lirio de los Valles	*Convallaria majalis*	Fevers, diuretic, sedative
299	Limber Bush	Sangre de Drago	*Jatrpha dioica*	Mouth sores, inflamed gums, wounds
300	Limon	Lima	*Citrus aurantifolia*	Indigestion, hysteria, nervous vomiting, palpitations
301	Linden	Tila	*Tila mexicana*	Nerves, insomnia, muscle spasms, nervous indigestion
302	Living Rock	Estrella	*Ariocarpus retusus*	Sunstroke
303	Magnolia	Flor de Corazón	*Talauma mexicana*	Heart stimulant, mental senility
304	Magnolia Vine	Chizandra	*Schisandra chinensis*	Asthmatic cough, dry mouth, night sweats
305	Maidenhair Fern	Culantrillo	*Adiantum pedattum*	Menstrual cramps, bronchial congestion, sore throats
306	Maidenhair Tree	Ginkgo	*Ginkgo biloba*	Nerves, blood cells, circulation
307	Malabar	Malabar	*Solamum verbascifolium*	Digestive
308	Male Fern	Aspidio	*Dryopteris filix-mas*	Parasites
309	Mallow	Malva	*Malva rotundifolia*	Sore throat, urinary tract
310	Manna Ash	Manna	*Fraxinus ornus*	Constipation

311	Mastic	Mastiche	*Pistacia lentiscus*	Stomachache
312	Marigold	Caléndula	*Tagetes lemmoni*	Gastric irritations, gas pains, scrapes
313	Mariola	Mariola	*Parthenium incanum*	Morning sickness, liver, stomach
314	Marsh Fleabane	Cachanilla	*Pluchea sericea*	Wounds, fevers
315	Marsh Mallow Root	Malvavisco	*Althea officinalis*	Cough, sore throat, intestinal ulcers
316	Meadow Pink	Flor de la Santa Cruz	*Sabatia campestris*	Irregular menstruation
317	Meadow Sweet	Reina de los Prados	*Filipendula ulmaria*	Joints, rheumatism, digestive
318	Mescal Buttons	Mezcal	*Anhalonium lewinii*	Hysteria, asthma, gout, neuralgia, rheumatism
319	Mesquite	Mezquite	*Prosopis juliflora*	Stomach inflammations, laryngitis, eye wash
320	Mexican Day Flower	Yerba del Pollo	*Comelina coelestis*	Nose bleeds, wounds, bleeding
321	Mexican Hawthorn	Tejocote	*Crataegus pubescens,*	Cough, colds, kidney
322	Mexican Heather	Cancerina	*Cupea aequipetala*	Indigestion, dysentery, wounds, bruises, muscle pain
323	Mexican Honeysuckle	Muicle	*Jacaobinia incana*	Headache feverish conditions
324	Mexican Mock Orange	Jazmín	*Philadelphus mexicamus*	Sedative, digestive
325	Mexican Morning Glory	Jalapa	*Ipomoea purga*	Intestinal parasites
326	Mexican Oregano	Orégano	*Lippia berlandieri*	Indigestion, colic, swellings, menstrual cramp, cough
327	Mexican Papaya	Papaya	*Carica papaya*	Indigestion, intestinal parasites
328	Mexican Tarragon	Pericón	*Tagetes lucida*	Colic, common cold, fever

329	Mexican Thistle	Cardo Santo	*Cirsium undulatum*	Stomach inflammation, urinary tract inflammation, anemia
330	Milk Thistle	Cardo Lechoso	*Silybum marianum*	Liver
331	Milkweed	Lechona	*Asciepias cornut*	Asthma, cough, constipation, rheumatic
332	Mimosa	Gatuno	*Mimosa dysocarpa*	Scrapes, cuts, abrasions, burns, mouth sores
333	Mint Leaf Bee Balm	Orégano del Campo	*Monarda menthafolia*	Stomachache, fever, respiratory ailments
334	Moonpod	Raíz del Indio	*Selinocarpus*	Colic
335	Moneywort	Gorritos	*Hydrocotyle bonariense*	Thrush
336	Montezuma Cypress	Ahuehuete	*Taxodium mucronatum*	Hemorrhoids, varicose veins, congestion
337	Mormon Tea, Desert Tea	Popotillo, Retamo Real	*Ephedra torreyana*	Kidney, bladder problems, stomach disorders
338	Morning Glory	Tumba Vaqueros	*Ipomoea stans*	Kidney problems, menstrual cramps, diarrhea
339	Motherwort	Agripalma	*Leonurus cardiaca*	Cramping, stomach gas, insomnia, menopause
340	Mountain Laurel	Kalmia	*Kalmia latifolia*	Circulation, rheumatism, gastro-irritation
341	Mugwort	Estafiate	*Artemisia mexicana*	Stomach inflammations, diarrhea, cough, laryngitis
342	Mulberry	Mora	*Morus microphylla*	Sore throat
343	Muskmelon	Melón de Castilla	*Cucumis melo L*	Dyspepsia, excessive menstrual bleeding, eczema
344	Myrrh	Mirra	*Commiphora erythraea*	Bronchitis, cholesterol

345	Myrtle	Mirto	*Myrtus communis* L	Asthma, bronchitis, hemorrhoids
346	Naked-Seed Weed	Tatalencho	*Gymnosperma glatinosa*	Rheumatism, fractures
347	Nance	Nanche	*Byrsonima crassifolia*	Diarrhea, poor lactation, skin
348	Navajo Tea	Cota	*Thelesperma gracile*	Diuretic, kidney, digestive
349	Neem	Neem	*Azadirachta indica*	Skin disease, acne, boils
350	Nettles	Ortigilla	*Urtica dioica*	Stops bleeding, blood thinner
351	Night Blooming Cereus	Reina de la Noche	*Selenicereus grandiflorus*	Tachycardia, arrhythmia, palpitations
352	Night Blooming Jessamine	Huele de Noche	*Cestrum nocturnum*	Epilepsy
353	Nutmeg	Nuez Moscada	*Myristica fragans*	Stomachache, intestinal gas, overworked muscles
354	Oak	Encino	*Quercus gambelii*	Diarrhea, dandruff, mouthwash, skin abrasions
355	Olive	Olivo	*Olea europaea*	Burns sores, cuts earache, intestinal obstruction
356	Onion	Cebolla	*Allium cepa*	Appetite stimulant, diuretic, acne
357	Orange Blossom	Azahares	*Citrus aurantium*	Sedative, diuretic, astringent
358	Orange Sneezeweed	Variedad de Helenio	*Helenium hoopesii*	Headaches, hay fever, vomiting
359	Oregon Grape Root	Berberis	*Mahonia*	Psoriasis, athlete's foot, eczema, acne
360	Orris Root	Iris	*Iris florentina*	Expectorant, diuretic, remedy for chronic diarrhea
361	Ox Eye Daisy	Margarita Mayor	*Leucanthemum vulgare*	Cough, asthma, nervous excitability

362	Parsley	Perejil	*Petroselinum staivum*	Dropsy, asthma, coughs, menstruation
363	Pasque Flower	Pulsatilla	*Anemone pulsatilla*	Emotional stress, sinus pain, headaches
364	Passion Flower	Passiflora	*Passiflora edulis*	Nervousness, insomnia, stomach cramps
365	Peach	Durazno	*Prumus persica*	Intestinal parasites, asthma, menstrual difficulties, fever
366	Peanut	Cacahuate	*Arachis hypogaea*	Helps produce breast milk
367	Pecan	Nogal Pacanero	*Carya illinoensis*	Loss of appetite
368	Pencil Catus	Sacasil	*Wilcoxia poselgeri*	Fractures
369	Pennyroyal	Poleo de Monte	*Cunila lythrifolia*	Bronchitis, cough, runny nose, headaches
370	Penstemon	Lengua Azteca	*Penstemon spp.*	Rashes, bites, stings, wounds, cuts
371	Peppergrass	Berro de Huerta	*Lepidium thurberi*	Indigestion with bloating, amenorrhea, arthritis
372	Pepper Tree	Pirúl	*Schinus molle*	Bronchitis, backache, tooth and gum problems
373	Peppermint	Menta Peperita	*Mentha piperita*	Indigestion, nausea, menstrual cramps
374	Periwinkle	Teresita	*Vinca major*	Migraines, nosebleeds, urinary tract
375	Persimmon	Nispero	*Diospyros virginiana*	Chronic dysentery, sedative, diarrhea, depression
376	Peruvian Bark	Quina Roja	*Cinchona succirubra*	Chills, fever, sore throat, pimples, indigestion
377	Peyote	Peyote	*Lophophora williamsii*	Pain, toothache, child birth, rheumatism

378	Pheasant Eye	Angelico	*Adonis vernalis*	Heart, low blood pressure, regulate contractions
379	Pink Windmills	Hierba de la Hormiga	*Allionia incarnata*	Diarrhea, kidney ailments
380	Pine	Ocote	*Pinus teocote*	Rheumatism, congestion, excess mucus
381	Pineapple	Piña	*Ananas comosus*	Bronchitis, diarrhea
382	Pipsissewa	Chimaphila	*Chimaphila umbellata*	Cystitis, arthritis, kidney stones, gout
383	Plantain Seed	Plantaginis Semen	*Plantago psyllium*	Coughs, bronchitis, rashes, minor sores, boils
384	Plateau Rocktrumpet	Flor de San Juan	*Macrosiphonia lanuginosa*	Sight
385	Plumbago	Alacrán Tlachichinola	*Plumbago pulchella*	Toothache, wounds, poisonous insect bites
386	Poinsettia	Nochebuena	*Euphorbia pulcherrima*	Skin inflammation
387	Pokeweed	Fitolaca	*Phytolacca americana*	Cathartic, laxative, anti-inflammatory
388	Pomegranate	Granada	*Punica granatum*	Diarrhea, sore throat, intestinal parasites
389	Poppy Plant	Opio Amapola	*Papaver somniferum L*	Toothache, nosebleeds, insomnia
390	Poplar Buds	Populi Gemma	*Populus candicans*	Acute cold, sore throat, laryngitis
391	Porter's Loveage	Oshá	*Ligusticum porteri*	Colds, sore throat, stomachache, cuts, wounds
392	Potato	Papa	*Solanum tuberosum*	Stomachache, diarrhea, insect bite, headaches
393	Potency Wood Tree	Muira Puama	*Ptychopetalum olacoides*	Sexual dysfunction in women and men

394	Prairie Dock	Planta Magnética	*Silphium terebinthinaceim*	Coughs, lung ailments, asthma, water retention
395	Prickle Poppy	Chicalote	*Argemone mexicana*	Sedative, antispasmodic, analgesic, constipation
396	Prickle Nut	Guázima	*Guazuma tomentosa*	Gastrointestinal infirmities, bronchial problems
397	Prickly Ash Bark	Xanthoxylum	*Zanthoxylum americanum*	Diarrhea, fatigue, fever, worms, rheumatism
398	Prickly Pear Cactus	Nopal	*Opuntia spp.*	Canker sores, adult-onset diabetes, abscesses
399	Pumpkin	Calabaza	*Cucurbita mixta pang.*	Parasites
400	Puncture Vine	Abrojo Rojo	*Tribulus cistoides*	Kidney and liver problems
401	Purple Coneflower	Echinacea	*Echinacea angustifolia*	Toothache, coughs, colds, dyspepsia, snakebites
402	Purple Gromwell	Hierba de las Perlas	*Lithospermum multiflorum*	Wounds, cuts, scrapes, psoriasis, eczema
403	Purple Sage	Cenizo	*Leucophyllum laevigatum*	Colds, fever, colic
404	Queens Root	Stillingia	*Stillingia sylvatica*	Psoriasis, eczema, constipation, hemorrhoids
405	Quince	Membrillo	*Cydonia oblonga*	Diarrhea, indigestion, cough
406	Quinine	Quinina	*Cinchona officinalis*	Stimulates digestion, fevers, regulates heartbeat
407	Radish	Rábano	*Raphanus sativas*	Stomach pains, bowel movement
408	Rancher's Tea	Tabaquillo	*Hedeoma piperita*	Nausea, abscesses
409	Raspberry	Frambuesa	*Rubus idaeus L.*	Strengthen and restore womb

410	Rattlesnake Beans	Cedrón	*Simba cedron*	Spasms, convulsions, nervous problems, fever
411	Rattlesnake Weed	Orejuela de Ratón	*Euphorbia albomarginata*	Stomach ache, relieves bile
412	Ray Weed	Mariola	*Parthenium incanum*	Indigestion, liver sluggishness, mild constipation
413	Red Clover	Trébol Rojo	*Trifolium pratense*	Whooping cough, gastric problems, ulcers
414	Red Dock	Yerba Colorada	*Rumex hymenosepalus*	Diarrhea, sore throat, skin and gum problems
415	Red Texas Sage	Mirto	*Salvia microphylla*	Deafness, diaper rash
416	Red Yeast Rice	Arroz de Levadura Roja	*Monascus purpureus went.*	Lowers cholesterol levels
417	Reishi	Reishi	*Ganoderma lucidum*	Neurasthenia, insomnia, dizziness, hepatitis
418	Resurrection Plant	Doradilla	*Selaginella lepidophylla*	Urinary tract disorders, kidney stones
419	Rhatany	Crameria	*Krameria lanceolata*	Hemorrhoids, sore throat, sore gums
420	Rhubarb	Ruibarbo	*Rheum officinale*	Constipation, blood clots
421	Rice	Arroz	*Oryza sativa*	Burns, diarrhea, flux, paralysis, psoriasis
422	Rocky Mountain Bee Plant	Guaco	*Cleome serrulata*	Skin irritations, insect bites
423	Rosemary	Romero	*Rosamarinus offinalis*	Digestive disorders, rheumatism, menstruations
424	Rootbeer Plant	Hoja Santa	*Piper auritum*	Chest congestion, asthma, aches, pains

425	Rue	Ruda	*Ruta graveolens*	Menstrual cramps, earache, headache, nosebleed, colic
426	Sacred Herb	Yerba Santa	*Eriodictyon californicum*	Bruises, rheumatic pain, cough, colds, asthma
427	Saffron	Croco	*Crocus sativus*	Appetite, digestion, colic, heartburn, gas, reduces fever
428	Sage	Salvia	*Salvia hispanica*	Indigestion, eye irritations
429	Sagebrush	Chamizo Hediondo	*Artemisia tridentata*	Indigestion, fever, fungal infections, wounds
430	Sandalwood	Sándalo	*Santalum album*	Bronchitis, chapped skin, depression, oily skin
431	Sandbur	Calderona	*Krameria ramosissima*	Bruises
432	Sand Paper Tree	Anacua	*Ebretia anacua*	Ringworm
433	Sarsaparilla Root	Zarzaparrilla	*Similax medica*	Diarrhea, adult-onset diabetes, menstrual cramps
434	Sassafras	Sasafrás	*Sassafras albidum*	Fever, lice Rheumatism, Urinary tract infection
435	Savory	Té de Monte	*Satureja marcrostema*	Hangover, menstrual problems, stomach gas, fever
436	Saw Greenbriar	Cortamecate	*Simlaax bona-nox*	Dropsy, urinary complaints, rheumatism, stomach problems
437	Saw Palmetto	Serenoa	*Serenoa repens*	Stimulant, diuretic, sedative, common cold, prostate
438	Sensitive Briar	Ten Verguenza	*Mimosa latidens*	Sores
439	Senna	Hojasen	*Senna spp.*	Constipation, increases flow of gastric juices
440	Sesame	Ajonjoli	*Sesamum indicum L.*	Demulcent, digestive, excretory

#	Common Name	Spanish Name	Scientific Name	Uses
441	Seven Barks	Hydrangea	*Hydrangea arborescens*	Kidney, bladder stones, enlarged prostate
442	Siberian Ginseng	Eleuterococo	*Eleutherococcus senticosus*	Bronchitis, hypertension, impotence, low blood oxygen
443	Skunk Cabbage	Dragonzio	*Symplocarpus foetidius*	Asthma, chronic rheumatism, hysteria, epilepsy
444	Slippery Elm	Olmo	*Ulmus fulva*	Sore throats, coughs, bronchial aliments, constipation
445	Snakeroot	Echinacea	*Echinacea angustifolia*	Cold symptoms, wounds
446	Snake Broom	Escoba de Víbora	*Gutierrezia sarothae*	Arthritis, menstruation, vaginal
447	Snakeweed	Yerba de la Víbora	*Zornia diphylla*	Reduce joint soreness, rheumatoid arthritis
448	Soapberry	Jaboncillo	*Sapindus saponaria*	Arthritis, constipation, poor intestinal health
449	Solomon's Seal	Sello de Salomón	*Pollygonatum multiflorum*	Stomach inflammations, chronic dysentery, pulmonary problems
450	Sorrell	Acedera	*Rumex acetosa*	Laxative, boils
451	Spearmint	Yerba Buena	*Menth spicata*	Colic, flatulence, headache, indigestion
452	Speedwell	Veronica	*Veronica officinalis*	Asthma, bronchitis, constipation, cold
453	Spiny Hackberry	Granjéno	*Celtis pallida*	Headaches, indigestion, skin disease
454	Spurge	Golondrina	*Euphorbia prostrata*	Scorpion bite, snakebite, sores, wounds

455	Squaw Vine	Michella	*Mitchella repens*	Diarrhea, irregular menstruation, vaginal infections
456	Squill	Scilla	*Urginea maritma*	Cough, phlegm, bronchitis
457	Star Anise	Anís de Estrella	*Illicium verum*	Upset stomach
458	Stringing Nettle	Ortiga	*Urtica dioica*	Rheumatism, kidney problems, water retention
459	Stonecrop	Doradilla	*Sedum dendroideum*	Backache, earache, inflamed gums
460	Storax	Estoraque	*Liquidambar styraciflua*	Cough, cold, bronchitis, sores
461	St. Johns Wort	Hierba de San Juan	*Hypericum perforatum L*	Sores, diuretic, relieves depression
462	Sugarcane	Caña de Azucar	*Saccharum officinalis*	Hemorrhaging due to abortion, parturition, menopause, menstrual flow
463	Sumac	Zumaque	*Rhus microphylla*	Burns, cuts, scrapes, sore throats, bleeding gums
464	Sunbonnet Babies	Telenpacate	*Chaptalia*	Sores
465	Sunflower	Girasol	*Helianthus annus*	Arthritis, sore muscles, fever
466	Swamp Root	Yerba Mansa	*Anemopsis californica*	Urinary tract infections, wounds, bruises, arthritis
467	Sweet Acacia	Huizache	*Acacia farnesiana*	Sore throat, wounds, skin and gum problems
468	Sweet Clover	Trevode Cheiro	*Melilotus officinales*	Varicose veins, hemorrhoids
469	Sweet Flag	Calmus	*Acorus calmus*	Asthma, toothache, headache, hangover
470	Sweet Marjoram	Mejorana, Yerba Maté	*Mejorana hortensis*	Stomachaches and menstrual cramps

471	Sweet Orange	Naranja Dulce	Citrus sinensis	Colds, skin care, mouth ulcers, circulation
472	Sweet Sumac	Zumaque	Rhus aromatica	Bed wetting, diabetes, urethral irritations
473	Swiss Chard	Acelga	Beta vulgaris	Obesity, gastritis, constipation, anemic
474	Syrian Rue	Ruda	Peganum harmala	Mild depression, fever, infection, bacterial, fungal
475	Tag Alder	Araclán	Alnus serrulata	Impetigo, herpes, scorbutic, hay fever
476	Tamarind	Tamarindo	Tamarindus indica	Digestive, laxative, diuretic, parasitic
477	Tamarisk	Tamarisco	Tamarix aphylla	Scrapes, abrasions, burns, mouth sores, sore throat
478	Tansy	Tanceto	Chrysanthemum vulgares syn.	Delayed menstruation, fever
479	Tarbush	Ojasé	Flourensia cernua	Indigestion, wounds, fungal
480	Tasajo Cactus	Tasajillo	Opuntia leptocaulis	Relieves cough
481	Texas Croton	Barbasco	Croton texensis	Rheumatism, swollen joints, headache, earache
482	Tree Spinach	La Chaya	Cnidoscolus chayamansa	Laxative, diuretic, diabetes
483	Toadflax	Linaria	Linaria vulgares	Constipation, water retention, hemorrhoids, ulcers, jaundice
484	Tobacco	Tabaco Loco	Nicotiana glauca	Injury, hemorrhoids, insect bites, stings
485	Tolu Balsam	Bálsamo	Myroxylon balsamum	Wounds, constipation

486	Tomato	Tomate	*Lycopersicum esculentum*	Asthma, bronchitis, rashes
487	Tragacanth	Tragacanto	*Astragalus gummifer labill*	Burns, cough, diarrhea
488	Tread Softly	Mala Mujer	*Croton ciliato-glandulosus*	Warts
489	Tree Gloxina	Tlanchichinole	*Kohleria deppeana*	Kidney problems, digestive disorders, diarrhea
490	Tree of Heaven	Ailanto	*Ailanthus altissma*	Diarrhea and dysentery, amebic, nervous system
491	Tree Morning Glory	Palo del Muerto	*Ipomoea arborescens*	Purgative
492	Trixis, Threefold	Tresdoble	*Trixis californica*	Wounds, ulcers
493	Trumpet Creeper	Jazmin Trompeta	*Camsis grandiflora*	Menstrual disorder, rheumatoid pains, traumatic injures
494	Turkey Corn	Corydalis	*Dicentra canadensis*	Alleviate pain, menstrual pain, abdominal pain
495	Turmeric	Azafrán	*Curcuma longa L.*	Bronchitis, diuretic, dyspepsia, expectorant
496	Turnip	Nabo	*Brassica rapa*	Bile stones, colds, bronchitis
497	Uva Ursi	Pingüica	*Arctostaphylos uva ursi*	Kidney ailments, bladder problems, bronchitis
498	Vanilla Tree	Vanilla	*Vanilla planifolia jacks*	Flavoring
499	Various Chiles	Chile	*Capsicum*	Irritant, induce perspiration
500	Vegetable Pear	Chayote	*Sechium edule*	Kidney disorders, high blood pressure
501	Velvet-Leaf	Francia	*Hibiscus cardiophyllus*	Heart pain
502	Vervain	Verbena	*Verbena canadensis*	Colds, flu, stomach problems, bile

#	Common Name	Spanish Name	Scientific Name	Uses
503	Violet	Violeta	*Viola sp*	Headache, sedative, cough, cold
504	Virginia Skullcap	Scutellaria	*Scutellaria lateriflora*	Epilepsy, insomnia, hysteria, neuralgia, headaches
505	Walnut Tree	Nogal	*Juglans regia*	Constipation, dysentery
506	Warty Hedgehog	Alicoche	*Echinacea enneacantbus*	Mumps
507	Watercress	Berro	*Nasturtium officinale syn.*	Kidney problems, gum problems
508	Water Horehound	Marrubio	*Lycopus amerianus*	Coughs, excessive menstruation, hyper thyroids
509	Watermelon Plant	Sandia	*Citrullas lanatus*	Cystitis, dyspepsia, fever, prostate disorder
510	Wax Plant	Canelilla	*Euphorbia antisyphilitica*	Vaginal discharge, venereal disease
511	Weeping Willow	Sauce Llorón	*Salix babylonica*	Sunstroke
512	Western Coltsfoot	Tusilago	*Petasites palmatus*	Cough, sore throat, bronchial congestion
513	Western Mugwort	Estafiate	*Artemisa ludoviciana*	Dyspepsia, gastritis, intestinal inflammation, stomachaches
514	Western Peony	Peonía	*Paeonia brownii*	Uterine cramps, spasmodic cough, muscular twitching
515	Wheat Plant	Trigo	*Triticum aestivum*	Heart disease, high in fiber
516	Whistle Tree	Colorín	*Erythrina Americana*	Fever
517	White Colicroot	Aletris	*Aletris farinosa*	Diuretic tonic and sedative, colic, rheumatism
518	White Sapote	Zapote Blanco	*Casimiroa edulis*	Insomnia, nervous disorders, high blood pressure

519	Witch Hazel Leaves	Agua de Hamamelis	*Hamamelis virginiana*	Hemorrhoids, bruise pain, laryngitis, blister, burns
520	Willow	Sauz	*Salix bonplandiana*	Anti-inflammatory, headache, colds
521	Wild Indigo	Añil Silvestre	*Baptisia baracteata*	Colic, typhoid, scarlet fever, wounds, stimulate immune
522	Wild Cherry	Capulín	*Prunus serotina*	Cough, diarrhea, fever, dysentery
523	Wild Lettuce	Lechuga Silvestre	*Lactuca serriola*	Insomnia ,spasmodic coughs
524	Wild Oats	Avena	*Avena fatua*	Emotional-nervous system, stomach infections, stimulant
525	Wild Olive, Little Trumpet	Anacahuita	*Cordia boissieri*	Laryngitis, bronchitis, cough, kidney problems, headaches
526	Wild Quinine	Quinina	*Parthenium integrifolium*	Burns, fevers, inflammation of urinary passages
527	Wild Yam Root	Dioscorea	*Dioscorea villosa*	Menstrual cramps, rheumatoid arthritis
528	Willow Groundsel	Jarilla	*Senecio salignus syn.*	Arthritis, rheumatism, postpartum distress
529	Wintergreen	Gaulteria	*Gaultheria procumbens*	Digestive system, rheumatism, arthritis, sore muscles, joints
530	Wolfberry	Tomatillo	*Lycium palledum*	Rhinitis, Nausea, Intestinal spasm
531	Wood Sorrel	Raíz de la chata	*Oxalis dichondrifolia*	Venereal diseases, arthritis, kidney ailments
532	Woundwort	Vulneraria	*Stachys*	Eye wash, sties, pink eye, fever, diarrhea , mouth ,throat
533	Wormseed	Epazote del Zorrillo	*Chenopodium graveolens*	Diarrhea, vomiting, delayed menstruation

534	Wormwood	Ajenjo	*Artemisa absinthium*	Indigestion, menstrual cramps, gallbladder
535	Yam Bean	Jicama	*Pachyrhizus crosus*	Dandruff
536	Yarrow	Milenrama	*Achillea millefolium*	Circulatory system, respiratory system
537	Yellow Dock	Lengua de Vaca	*Rumex crispus*	Sore throat, wounds, abrasions, gum problems
538	Yellow Mombin	Palo de Mulato	*Spondias mombin* (L)	Diuretic, stomachache, biliousness, arthritis
539	Yellow Oleander	Ayoyote	*Thevetia thevetiodes*	Arthritis, rheumatism, hemorrhoids, pimples
540	Yellow Trumpet Bush	Esperanza	*Tecoma stans*	Diabetes, gastritis, kidney disorders, liver disorders
541	Yohimbe Tree	Arbol de Yohimbe	*Pausinystalia yohimbe*	Erectile dysfunction, female sexual disorder
542	Yucca	Palmilla	*Yucca schidigera*	Arthritis, rheumatism, constipation

Internet links referenced for medicinal plants

Note to the Reader: The following resource links are provided to the reader as additional references for material on the medicinal plant listing. You may use them to research additional information on specific plants and illnesses. At the time of publication great effort was made to ensure that all of the following Internet resource links were functioning. As you know, links come and go. Additionally, every medicinal plant listed in this book does not have a reference link. Always exercise caution with medicinal plants and always consult your doctor before taking a medicinal plant.

Acacia: http://medplant.nmsu.edu/acacia2.html

Aconite: http://earthnotes.tripod.com/aconite.htm

Aconite: http://www.herbs2000.com/herbs/herbs_aconite.htm

Adonis: http://www.lifemana.com/adonis.html

Agrimony: http://www.altnature.com/gallery/agrimony.htm

Agrimony: http://www.altnature.com/gallery/agrimony.htm

Alcelga: http://www.wanamey.org/plantas-medicinales/

Alder: http://www.henriettesherbal.com/eclectic/kings/alnus.html

Alfalfa: http://www.drugs.com/npp/alfalfa.html

Almond: http://www.botanical-online.com/medicinalsametllerangles.htm

Almond: http://www.botanical-online.com/medicinalsametllerangles.htm

Aloe Vera: http://www.gardensablaze.com/HerbAloeMed.htm

Amanita: http://www.iamshaman.com/amanita/wapaq.htm

Aspen: http://www.oakenwoods.co.uk/html/aspen.html

Aster: http://montana.plant-life.org/species/tanacet_vulgare.htm

Balsam Fir: http://www.survivaltopics.com/survival/balsam-fir-pitch/

Beetroot: http://www.herbco.com/p-949-beet-root-powder.aspx

Berenjena: http://www.ibiblio.org/pfaf/cgi-bin/arr_html?Solanum+melongena

Bergamot: http://www.ibiblio.org/pfaf/cgi-bin/arr_html?Monarda+menthifolia

Birthroot: http://www.holisticonline.com/Herbal-Med/_Herbs/h87.htm

Black Cohosh: http://www.herbalsafety.utep.edu/facts.asp?ID=27

Bloodroot: http://www.efloras.org/florataxon.aspx?flora_id=1&taxon_id=220011939

Blue Flag: http://www.herbsarespecial.com.au/free-herb-information/blue-flag.html

Blueberry: http://www.innvista.com/health/foods/fruits/blueberr.htm

Buckthorn: http://www.answers.com/topic/buckthorn?nr=1&nrls=1

Burdock: http://www.horizonherbs.com/pilot.asp?pg=burdock_seed

Burdock: http://www.pfaf.org/database/plants.php?Arctium+minus

Butternut: http://www.pfaf.org/database/plants.php?Juglans+cinerea

Buttonbush: http://museum.utep.edu/chih/gardens/plants/cephocc.htm

Cabbage: http://www.earthclinic.com/Remedies/cabbage.html#_GERD

Cacao: http://www.rain-tree.com/chocolate.htm

Calamus: http://www.drugtext.org/library/books/recreationaldrugs/calamus.htm

Calendula: http://www.planetbotanic.ca/fact_sheets/Calendula.htm

Calumba: http://www.raintreenutrition.com/calumba.htm

Caraway: http://www.ageless.co.za/herb-caraway.htm#Properties

Castor Oil: http://www.botanical.com/botanical/mgmh/c/casoil32.html

Cayenne: http://www.leaflady.org/about_cayenne.htm

Celendine: http://chestofbooks.com/health/herbs/O-Phelps-Brown/The-Complete-Herbalist/Celandine-Chelidonium-Majus.html

Celery: http://www.fairview.org/healthlibrary/content/print_ma_celery_ma.htm

Chamomile: http://medplant.nmsu.edu/Diseases/insomnia/insom_Herbs%20Link.htm#Catnip

Chaparro amargoso: http://aggie-horticulture.tamu.edu/ornamentals/nativeshrubs/castelaerecta.htm

Chaya: http://en.wikipedia.org/wiki/Chaya_(plant)

Cinquefoil: http://www.altnature.com/gallery/Cinquefoil.htm

Citrus: http://www.rain-tree.com/orange.htm

Cohosh: http://www.permaculture.info/index.php/Caulophyllum_thalictroides#Plant_Usage

Coltsfoot: http://arboretum.ucsc.edu/petasites_palmatus.html

Cosmo: http://en.wikipedia.org/wiki/User:Cosmo

Creosote: http://www.desertusa.com/mag98/april/stories/creosote.html

Culvers root: http://www.drstandley.com/herbs_culvers_root.shtml

Daphne: http://www.ibiblio.org/pfaf/cgi-bin/arr_html?Daphne+mezereum

Datura: http://www.doitnow.org/pages/525.html

Digitalis: http://www.drugs.com/npp/digitalis.html

Doggrass: http://www.herbalextractsplus.com/dog-grass.cfm

Fenogreco: http://www.hipernatural.com/en/pltfenogreco.html

Fringe Tree: http://www.herbs2000.com/herbs/herbs_fringe_tree.htm#fringe_tree_uses

Goldenseal: http://www.swedish.org/110907.cfm

Greenbrair: http://www.ibiblio.org/pfaf/cgi-bin/arr_html?Smilax+bona-nox

Guarana: http://www.medicinenet.com/guarana_paullinia_cupana-oral/article.htm

Hallucinogenic plants: http://www.erowid.org/library/books_online/golden_guide/g01-10.shtml

Herbal: http://herbal099.wordpress.com/current-entries/

Hedera: http://en.wikipedia.org/wiki/Hedera_helix

Hedera: http://www.ibiblio.org/pfaf/cgi-bin/arr_html?Hedera+helix

Henbane: http://en.wikipedia.org/wiki/Henbane#Toxicity_and_Historical_Usage

Henbane: http://www.ibiblio.org/pfaf/cgi-bin/arr_html?Hyoscyamus+niger

Herb guide http://www.azcert.org/medical-pros/herbs/hispanic-herbs.pdf

Herb uses: http://www.atihealthnet.com/pages/herbusesAB.html

Herbs Spanish: http://www.worldcrops.org/spanish.html

Herbs: http://ci-67.ciagri.usp.br/pm/

Herbs: http://food.oregonstate.edu/faq/plant/plant20a.html

Herbs: http://holisticonline.com/Herbal-Med/_Herbs/h118.htm

Herbs: http://plants.chebucto.biz/pages/Comnom.html

Herbs: http://translate.google.com/translate?hl=en&sl=es&u=http://www.bouncingbearbotanicals.com/spanish/calea-zacatechichi-hierba-sue%25C3%25B1o-p-100.html&sa=X&oi=translate&resnum=1&ct=result&prev=/search%3Fq%3Dhierba%2Bdel%2Bsueno%26hl%3Den%26rlz%3D1T4ADBF_enUS237US239

Herbs: http://www.anniesremedy.com/herb_detail97.php

Herbs: http://www.appliedhealth.com/nutri/page6.php

Herbs: http://www.casaq.com/remedy.html

Herbs: http://www.globalherbalsupplies.com/herb_information/cloves.htm

Herbs: http://www.greatdreams.com/herbal_healing.htm

Herbs: http://www.herbnet.com/Herb%20Uses_C.htm

Herbs: http://www.seedsanctuary.com/herbs/index.cfm

Hibiscus: http://www.hear.org/Pier/wra/pacific/hibiscus_insularis_htmlwra.htm

Homeopathy: http://www.elixirs.com/products.cfm?productcode=S61

Hormiga: http://www.efloras.org/florataxon.aspx?flora_id=1&taxon_id=220000445

Horseradish: http://en.wikipedia.org/wiki/Horseradish

http://desert-tropicals.com/Plants/common_names_B.html

Hydrangea: http://www.ibiblio.org/pfaf/cgi-bin/arr_html?Hydrangea+arborescens&CAN=COMIND

Hydrangea: http://www.pfaf.org/database/plants.php?Hydrangea+arborescens

Hydrastis: http://www.pfaf.org/database/plants.php?Hydrastis+canadensis

Indigo: http://www.ibiblio.org/pfaf/cgi-bin/arr_html?Baptisia+bracteata

Kolanut: http://www.angelfire.com/biz3/nutramedic/kolanut.html

Lemon Balm: http://en.wikipedia.org/wiki/Lemon_balm

Lettuce: http://www.botanical-online.com/medicinalslactucasativasangles.htm

Lime Tree: http://www.botanical.com/botanical/mgmh/l/limtre28.html

Linaria: http://en.wikipedia.org/wiki/Linaria

Liverwort: http://www.botanical.com/botanical/mgmh/l/livame36.html

Magical herbs: http://hem.passagen.se/fauna/herbs.html

Majalis: http://www.missouriplants.com/Whitealt/Convallaria_majalis_page.html

Manna: http://www.ibiblio.org/pfaf/cgi-bin/arr_html?Fraxinus+ornus&CAN=COMIND

Marshmallow: http://www.globalherbalsupplies.com/herb_information/marshmallow.htm

Meadow Sweet: http://www.isodisnatura.co.uk/filipendula_ulmaria_1_meadow_sweet.htm

Mescal: http://www.botanical.com/botanical/mgmh/m/mescal33.html#med

Milkweed: http://www.henriettesherbal.com/eclectic/kings/asclepias-syri.html

Mistletoe: http://nccam.nih.gov/health/eurmistletoe/

Motherwort: http://en.wikipedia.org/wiki/Motherwort

Mullien: http://www.botanical.com/botanical/mgmh/m/mulgre63.html

Nightshade: http://en.wikipedia.org/wiki/Deadly_nightshade

Nightshade: http://zipcodezoo.com/Plants/S/Solanum_americanum/default.asp

Nispero: http://plantarium.wordpress.com/2008/05/04/nispero-eriobotria-japonica/

Nutmeg: http://www.ageless.co.za/nutmeg.htm

Owls Claw: http://www.ibiblio.org/pfaf/cgi-bin/arr_html?Helenium+hoopesii

Pasqueflor: http://www.innvista.com/health/herbs/pasquefl.htm

Pennyroyal: http://www.mnsu.edu/emuseum/cultural/ethnoarchaeology/ethnobotany/medical1h.html

Pepperwort: http://www.plantnames.unimelb.edu.au/Sorting/Lepidium.html

Pineapple: http://en.wikipedia.org/wiki/Bromelain#Medical_uses

Pipsissewa: http://www.herbco.com/p-354-pipsissewa-herb-cs-wildcrafted.aspx

Pistacia: http://en.wikipedia.org/wiki/Mastic

Plant names: http://www.uapress.arizona.edu/onlinebks/prophet/plants.htm

Poplar: http://content.herbalgram.org/iherb/expandedcommissione/default.asp?m=79#Uses

Prairie Dock: http://www.pfaf.org/database/plants.php?Silphium+terebinthinaceum

Prikly Ash: http://www.viable-herbal.com/herbdesc3/1prickly.htm

Prunella: http://montana.plant-life.org/species/prunella_vulga.htm

Psyllium: http://www.answers.com/topic/psyllium

Quassia: http://electrocomm.tripod.com/quassia.html

Quassia: http://www.tropilab.com/quassia-ama.html

Quinine: http://www.ibiblio.org/pfaf/cgi-bin/arr_html?Parthenium+integrifolium

Radish: http://www.stuartxchange.org/Labanos.html

Rain Tree: http://www.rain-tree.com/quillaja.htm

Rain Tree: http://www.rain-tree.com/quinine.htm

Raspberry: http://www.bulkherbstore.com/articles/mamas-red-raspberry-brew

Rhubarb: http://en.wikipedia.org/wiki/Rheum_officinale

Roccella: http://www.henriettesherbal.com/eclectic/bpc1911/roccella.html

Rosa Centifolia: http://www.henriettesherbal.com/eclectic/kings/rosa-cent.html

Saffaron: http://www.herbalextractsplus.com/Fron.cfm

Sandal wood: http://www.motherherbs.com/pterocarpus-santalinus.html

Saponaria: http://www.ibiblio.org/pfaf/cgi-bin/arr_html?Quillaja+saponaria

Sassafras: http://www.mothernature.com/Library/Ency/Index.cfm/Id/3661007

Saw Palmetto: http://www.pacsoa.org.au/palms/Serenoa/repens.html

Sea Squill: http://www.maltawildplants.com/LILI/Urginea_maritima.html

Senna: http://www.theherbprof.com/hrbSenna.htm

Sesame: http://www.theepicentre.com/Spices/sesame.html

Skullcap: http://www.hort.purdue.edu/newcrop/ncnu02/v5-580.html

Skullcap: http://www.ibiblio.org/pfaf/cgi-bin/arr_html?Scutellaria+lateriflora&PRINT

Skunk Cabbage: http://www.henriettesherbal.com/eclectic/kings/dracontium.html

Slippery Elm: http://www.gardenguides.com/plants/plantguides/trees/plantguide.asp?symbol=ULRU

Snakeroot: http://www.henriettesherbal.com/eclectic/potter-comp/aristolochia.html

Snakeroot: http://www.virtualmuseum.ca/Exhibitions/Healingplants/plant_dir/seneca_snakeroot.php

Solomons Seal: http://www.ibiblio.org/pfaf/cgi-bin/arr_html?Polygonatum+multiflorum

Sorrel: http://www.viable-herbal.com/herbdesc4/1sorrel.htm

Speedwell: http://www.anniesremedy.com/herb_detail352.php

Spikenard: http://www.innvista.com/health/herbs/spikenar.htm

Squaw vine: http://www.globalherbalsupplies.com/herb_information/squaw_vine.htm#Usage

Squill: http://www.herbs2000.com/herbs/herbs_squill.htm

Stillingia: http://www.viable-herbal.com/singles/Herbs/s551.htm

Sumach: http://www.henriettesherbal.com/eclectic/kings/rhus-arom.html

Sweet Clover: http://www.delange.org/Melilotus/Melilotus.htm

Sweet Clover: http://www.medicinenet.com/sweet_clover_melilotus_officinalis-oral/index.htm

Tila: http://www.emedicinal.com/herbs/tila.php#Parts

Trumpet Creeper: http://www.pfaf.org/database/plants.php?Campsis+grandiflora

Turnip: http://electrocomm.turnipod.com/nabo_turnip.html

USDA plants: http://plants.usda.gov/index.html

Valeriana: http://zipcodezoo.com/Plants/V/Valeriana_officinalis/

Vanilla: http://unitproj1.library.ucla.edu/biomed/spice/index.cfm?displayID=27

Veronica: http://www.one-garden.org/seedbank/index.php?ID=286

Vomica: http://www.answers.com/topic/nux-vomica

Wintergreen: http://www.tryonfarm.org/share/node/394

Woundwort: http://en.wikipedia.org/wiki/Woundwort

Yellow Trumpet: http://en.wikipedia.org/wiki/Tecoma_stans

Relevant References

The following references are provided to the reader as important sources that have informed this book and that may serve to further inform the reader. They are not cited in the book.

Aikman Lonnelle. 1977, *Nature's Healing Arts*, National Geographic Association, Washington, D.C.

Alegría DE, Guerra C, Martínez G, and Meyer. 1977, *El Hospital Invisible: A Study of Curanderismo,* Archives of General Psychiatry 34: 1354-1357.

Anaya Rodolfo. 1972, *Bless Me Última*. Warner Books, NY

Anderson Allan. 2004, *An Introduction to Pentecostalism*, Cambridge University Press, Cambridge, England

Anderson Karen. 2000, *The Battle for God*. Ballantine Books, New York

Antiguo Formulario Azteca de yerbas medicinales manual imprescindible de los secretos indigenas, ND No author, Editorial Justo Sierra, México D.F.

Arenas S. 1983, *Curanderos and Mental Health Professionals: Their Perceptions of Psychopathology*, Doctoral Dissertation, Department of Psychology, Washington State University

Arzeni Charles. 1974, *Plants of Mexico*, Eastern Illinois University, Charleston, IL

Astin JA.1998, *Why patients use alternative medicine: results of a national study*. JAMA 279(19):1548-53.

Augustine Sue. 2007, *Turn Your Dreams into Realities*, Harvest House, Eugene, OR

Aun Weor, Samae. ND, *Tratado de Medicine Oculta y Magia Práctica Obra Completa*, Nous Editores, Cuernavaca, Morelos, México

Badianus Manuscript: An Aztec Herbal of 1552. Trans. Emily Walcott Emmart. 1940, Johns Hopkins Press, Baltimore, MD

Barrera M. 1978, *Mexican American Mental Health Service Utilization, Community*, Mental Health Journal 14: 35-45

Barnes, LL, S. S. Sered, eds. 2005, *Religion and Healing in America*. Oxford University Press, New York

Barnes PM, Bloom B, Hahin RL. 2008, *Complementary and alternative medicine use among adults and children: United States 2007*. National Health Statistics Reports, number 12, pp1-24, December 10 (http://www/cdc.gov/nchs/data/nhsr/hsr012.pdf, accessed 5 may 2009).

Bartholomew Robert. 2000, *Exotic Deviance: Medicalizing Cultural Idioms from Strangeness to Illness*, University Press of Colorado, Boulder, CO

Baytelman Bernardo. 2002, *Acerca de Plantas y de Curanderos*, Colección Divulgación, México DF

Beyerl Paul. 1984, *The Master Book of Herbalism*, Phoenix Publishing, Blaine, WA

Bierhorst John. 1990, *The Mythology of Mexico and Central America*, Quill, New York, NY

Bloom BL. 1975, *Changing Patterns of Psychiatric Care*, New York, Human Services Press

Bourguignon Ericka. 1973, *Religion, Altered States of Consciousness and Social Change*, The Ohio State University Press, Columbus, OH

Bourguignon Ericka. 1976, Possession Chandler and Sharp, San Francisco, CA

Brother Aloysius. 1998, *A Healer's Herbal: Recipies for Medicinal Herbs and Weeds*, Samuel Weiser Press, York Beach, ME

Brown Peter. 1981, *The Cult of Saints*, University of Chicago Press, Chicago, IL

Buckland Ray. 2003, *Advanced Candle Magick*. Llewellyn Publications, St. Paul, MN

Burruel G and N Chavez.1974, *Mental Health Outpatients Centers Relevant or Irrelevant to Mexican Americans: Beyond Clinic Walls*, University of Alabama Press, Tuscaloosa, AL

Carrasco D. 2007, *Cuando Dios y Usted Quiere: Latino Studies between Religious Powers and Social Thought*. In Blackwell Reader on Latino Studies. Edited by Juan Flores and Renato Rosaldo. Blackwell Publishers Oxford.

Caravalho Margarida de. 1995, *A Healing Journey in Brazil: a Case Study in Spiritual Surgery*, Journal of the Sociaty for Psychical Research 60:161-167

Castillo Ana. 1993, So Far From God, Norton, New York, NY

Chong Nilda. 2002, *The Latino Patient: A Cultural Guide for Health Care Providers*, Intercultural Press, Yarmouth, ME

Coe M and G Whittaker. 1986, *Aztec Sorcerers in Seventeenth Century Mexico: The Treatise on Superstitions by Hernando Ruiz de Alarcon*, Institute for Mesoamerican Studies, State University of New York, Albany, NY, publication number 7

Cohen Emma. 2007, *The Mind Possessed: The Cognition of Spirit Possession in an Afro-Brazilian Religious Tradition*, Oxford University Press, Oxford, England

Cowan Ford Karen. 1975, *Las Yerbas de la Gente: A Study of Hispano-American Medicial Plants*, Museuo of Anthropology No. 60, University of Michigan, Ann Arbor, MI

Craughwell Thomas J. 2007, *This Saint's For You*, Quirk Books, Philadelphia, PA

Cuéllar I and SB Schnee. 1987, *An Examination of Utilization Characteristics of Clients of Mexican Origin Served by the Texas Department of Mental Health and Mental Retardation, in Mental Health Issues of the Mexican Origin Population In Texas*. Hogg Foundation for Mental Health, The University of Texas, Austin, TX

Cuéllar I, R Martinez and R Gonzalez. 1983, *Clinical Psychiatric Case Presentation: Culturally Responsive Diagnostic Formulation and Treatment in an Hispanic Female*, Hispanic Journal of Behavioral Sciences 5: 93-103

Cuellar Israel and Freddy A. Paniagua. 2000, *Handbook of Multicultural Mental Health*, Academic Press, New York, NY

Current Medical Diagnosis and Treatment, Edited by Lawrence M. Tierney, Jr, et. al. 2002, Lange, New York, NY

Davidow Joie. 1999, *Infusions of Healing: A Treasury of Mexican-American Herbal Remedies*, Fireside Book, New York, NY

Day JC. *Population projections of the United States by age, sex, race, and Hispanic origin: 1995-2050, U.S. Bureau of the Census, Current Population Reports, P25-1130*. Washington. U.S. Government Printing Office. 1996. http://www.census.gov/prod/1/pop/p25-1130. Accessed May 5, 2009.

De Barrios Virginia. 1997, *The Cross in Mexico*, Editorial Minutiae Mexicana, Mexico DF

De La Torre Adela and Antonio Estrada. 2001, *Mexican Americans and Health*, University of Arizona Press, Tucson, AZ

De la Torre M and Gaston Espinoza. 2006, *Rethinking Latino(a) Religion and Idenity*. Pilgrim Press, Clevland OH.

De la Voragine Santiago. 1990, *La Leyenda Dorada I & II*, Alianza Editorial, Madrid, Spain

De Luna Anita. 2002, *Faith Formation and Popular Religion: Lessons from the Tejano Experience*, Rowman Littlefield, New York, NY

Desowitz Robert. 1997, *Who Gave Pinta to the Santa Maria? Torrid Diseases in a Temperate World*, Norton Company, New York, NY

DeStefano Anthony M. 2001, *Latino Folk Medicine: Healing Herbal Remedies from Ancient Traditions*, Ballantine Books, New York, NY

Devine MV. ND, Brujeria: *A Study of Mexican American Folk Magic*, Llewellyn's Practical Magic Series, Llewellyn Press, St. Paul, MN

Diagnostic and Statistical Manual of Mental Disorders, DSM-IV-TR, 2000, American Psychiatric Association, Washington, D.C.

Donnet Beatriz. 2000, *Brujas, Ogros, Hechiceros y Otros Asustadores*, Quarzo, Mexico DF

Dow James. 1986, *Universal Aspects of Symbolic Healing: A Theoretical Synthesis*, American Anthropologist 88:56-69

Dubin Reese. 1999, *Miracle Food Cures from the Bible*, Prentice Hall, Paramus NJ

Duke James A. 1986, *Handbook of Medicinal Herbs*, CRC Press, Boca Raton, FL

Duke James A. 2000, *Herbs of the Bible: 2000 Years of Plant Medicine*, Interweave Press, Loveland, CO

Ebright Malcolm and Rick Hendrick. 2006, *The Witches of Abiquiu*, University of New Mexico Press, Albuquerque, NM

El Libro de San. Cipriano Tesoro del Hechicero. Biblioteca Ciencias Ocultas, México DF

Erichsen-Brown Charlotte. 1979, *Medicinal and other uses of North American Plants,* Dover Publications, NY

Eisenberg DM, Davis RB, Ettner SL, Appel S, Wilkey S, Van Rompay M, et. al. *Trends in alternative medicine use in the United States, 1990-97: results of a follow-up national survey.* JAMA 280(18):1569-75. 1998

Escandón María Amparo. 1998, *Santitos,* Plaza and Janes Editores, México DF

Espinoza Gastón. 2005, *God Made a Miracle in My Life: Latino Pentescostal Healing in the Borderlands. In Religion and Healing in America.* Edited by Linda L. Barnes and Susan S. Sered. Oxford University Press, New York.

Espinoza Gastón and Mario T. García editors. 2008, *Mexican American Religion: Spirituality, activism, and culture,* Duke University Press, Durham, NC

Farmacopea Nacional. 1930, Mexico DF

Fernández James, ed. 1991, *Beyond Metaphor: The Theory of Tropes in anthropology,* University of Stanford Press, Stanford, CA

Fields Sherry. 2008, *Pestilence and Headcolds: Encountering Illness in Colonial Mexico,* Columbia University Press, New York, NY

Flaskerud JH. 1986, *The Effects of Culture-Compatible Intervention on The Utilization of Mental Health Services by Minority Clients,* Community Mental Health Journal 22: 2

Frazer James. 1922, *The Golden Bough*: A Study in Magic and Religion 3rd. Edition Macmillan, London

Galvan Macías Nélida. 1996, *Leyendas Mexicanas,* Selector Editorial, México DF

Garrett Clarke. 1987, *Spirit Possession and Popular Religion,* The John Hopkins Press, Baltimore, MD

Gonzalez-Lee Teresa and Harold Simon. 1990, *Medical Spanish: Interviewing the Latino Patient A Cross-Cultural Perspective,* Prentice Hall, New Jersey

Gonzalez-Wippler Migene. 1987, *Santería: African Magic in Latin America*, Original Products, Bronx, NY

Gonzalez-Wippler Migene. 1993, *Peregrinaje,* Editorial Llewellyn, St. Paul, MN

Goodman Felicitas D. 1988, *Ectasy, Ritual and Alternate Reality: Religion in a Pluralistic World,* Indiana University Press, Bloomington, IN

Greenfield Sidney M. 2008, *Spirits with Scalpels: The Cultural Biology of Religious Healing in Brazil,* Left Coast Press, Walnut Creek, CA

Griego y Maestas and Rudolfo Anaya. 1980, *Cuentos: Tales from the Hispanic Southwest,* The Museum of New Mexico Press, Santa Fe, NM

Harris Martin. 1998, *Curanderismo and the DSM-IV: Diagnostic and treatment implications for the Mexican American client, Julian Samora Research Institute Occasional paper #45,* Michigan State University, East Lansing, MI

Hechicerías e Idolatrías del México Antiguo, 2008, No Editor Listed, Cien de Mexico Dirección General de Publicaciones del Consejo Nacional para la Cultura y las Artes

Heiman EM and MW Kahn. 1977, *Mexican American and European Psychopathology and Hospital Course,* Archives of General Psychiatry, 34: 167-170

Heiman EM, G Burruel and N Chávez. 1975, *Factors Determining Effective Psychiatric Outpatient Treatment for Mexican Americans,* Hospital and Community Psychiatry 26: 515-17.

Herbolaría Mexicana, Guías Prácticas, México Desconocido, México DF

Hernandez-Avila I. 2005, *La Mesa del Santo Niño de Atocha and the Conchero Dance Tradition of Mexico-Tenochtitlán: Religious Healing in Urban Mexico and the United States.* In Religion and Healing in America. Edited by Linda Barnes and Susan Sered. Oxford University Press, NY

Hoffmann David. 2003, *Medical Herbalism: The Science and Practice of Herbal Medicine,* Healing Arts Press, Rochester, VT

Homenaje a Nuestras Curanderas Honoring our Healers, 1996, Edited by Luz Alvarez Martinez, Latina Press, Oakland, CA

Hoppe S and P Heller. 1975, *Alienation, Familism, and the Utilization of Services by Mexican Americans,* Journal of Health and Social Behavior 16: 304-314

Jaco EG. 1959, *Mental health of the Spanish American in Texas, in Culture and Mental Health: Cross Culture Studies,* New York: Macmillan

Johns Cupp Melanie. 2000, *Toxicology and Clinical Pharmacology of Herbal Products,* Humana Press, Totowa, NJ

Kane Charles. 2006, *Herbal Medicine of the American Southwest,* Lincoln Town Press

Kardec Allan. 1975, *The Medium's Book* A. Blackwell translator, Lake-Livraria Alan Kardec Editora Ltd.

Kardec Allan. 1987, *The Gospel According to Spiritism* J. Duncan, translator, Headquarters Publishing Co., London England

Kardec Allan, n.d., *The Spirit's Book,* A. Blackwell, translator, Lake-Livraria Alan Kardec Editora Ltd.

Kay Artschwager Margarita. 1996, *Healing with Plants: In the American and Mexican West,* The University of Arizona Press, Tucson, AZ

Keefe SE. 1978, *Why Mexican Americans Underutilize Mental Health Care Clinics: Facts and Fallacy, Family And Mental Health in the Mexican American Comm*unity, edited by J.M. Casas and S.E. Keefe. Los Angeles: Spanish-Speaking Mental Health Research Center, University of California

Keefe SE, AM Padilla and MLCarlos. 1979, *The Mexican American Extended Family as an Emotional Support System,* Human Organization 38: 144-152

Keefe SE and JM Casas. 1980, *Mexican Americans and Mental Health: A Selected Review and Recommendations for Mental Health Service Delivery*, Journal of Community Psychology 8: 303-326

Kelly Isabel. 1965, *Folk Practices in North Mexico: Birth Customs, Folk Medicine and Spiritualism in the Laguna Zone*, Latin American Monograph, No. 2 Institute of Latin American Studies, The University of Texas, Austin, TX

Kiev Ari. 1968, *Curanderismo*, The Free Press, New York, NY

King Salomón's Alleged Guide to Success

Koenig-Bricker Woodeene. 1995, *365 Saints*, Harper Collins, San Francisco, CA

Latorre Dolores. 1977, *Cooking and Curing with Mexican Herbs*, The Encino Press, Austin, TX

Lerma John. 2007, *Into the Light*, New Page Books, Franklin Lakes, NJ

Letcher Lyle Katie. 2004, *The Complete Guide to Edible Wild Plants, Mushrooms, Fruits and Nuts*, The Lyons Press, Guilford, CT

Lewis Walter and Memory Elvin Lewis. 1977, *Medical Botany: Plants Affecting Man's Health*, Wiley, NY

López Austin Alfredo. 1975, *Textos de Medicina Náhuatl*, Universidad Nacional Autónoma de México, México DF

López Alberto and Ernestina Carrillo. 2001, *The Latino Psychiatric Patient: Assessment and Treatment*, American Psychiatric Publishing, Washington, D.C.

Lozoya Xavier. 1999, *La Herbolaria en México*, Tercer Milenio, México DF

Macías Nilda. 2008, *Santos Protectores*, Diana, México DF

Macklin, June. 1979, *Curanderismo and Espiritismo: Complementary Approaches to Traditional Health Services*. In Chicano Experience. Edited by Stanley West and June Macklin, Westview Press, Boulder, CO.

Maestro EELIFFEE, *Azteca Secretos*

Magic and Medicine of Plants. 1986, Reader's Digest, New York, NY

Marcos LR. 1979, *Effect Of Interpreters On The Evaluation Of Psychotherapy In Non-English Speaking Patients*, American Journal of Psychiatry 136: 2, 171-174

Marcos LR, L. Urcuyo, M Kesselman and M Alpert. 1973, *The language barrier in evaluating Spanish-speaking patients,* Archives of General Psychiatry 29: 655-659

Marin G and VB Marin. 1991, *Research With Hispanic Populations.* Newbury Park, Calif.: Sage Publications

Martínez Maximino. 1979, *Catálogo de Nombres Vulgares y Científicos de Plantas Mexicans*, Fondo de cultura Económica, México DF

Matovina, Timothy and Gary Riebe-Estrella. 2002, *Horizons of the Sacred: Mexican Traditions in U.S. Catholicism.* Cornell University Press, Ithaca, NY

McKenna Dennis J, Kenneth Jones and Kerry Hughes with Sheila Humphrey. 2002, *The Haworth Herbal Press*, Binghamton, NY

McNeil, Norman. 1959, *Curanderos of South Texas:* Southern Methodist University, Dallas TX

Meade Harwell Thomas. 1997, *Studies in Texas Folklore Rio Grande Valley: Lore 1, Twelve Folkfore Studies with Introductions, Commentaries and a Bounty of Notes,* The Edwin Mellen Press, Lewiston, NY

Meadow A. 1982, *Psychopathology, Psychotherapy, and the Mexican American Patient In Minority Mental Health*, edited by E. Jones and S. Korchin New York: Praeger Publishers.

Meza Otilia. 1985, *Leyendas del Antiguo México*, Edamex, México DF

Moore Michael., 1979, *Medicinal Plants of the Mountain West*, Museum of New Mexico Press, Santa Fe, NM

Moore Michael. 1990, *Los Remedios: Traditional Herbal Remedies of the Southwest,* Red Crane Books, Santa Fe, NM

Moore Michael. 1995, *Herbal Materia Medica,* Fifth Edition, Southwest School of Botanical Medicine, Bisbee, AZ

National Center for Complementary and Alternative Medicine. Expanding horizons of health care: Strategic plan 2005-2009. Available from: http://nccam.nih.gov/about/plans/2005. Accessed on May 5, 2009.

National Center for Health Statistics. National Health Interview Survey (NHIS): 2007 data release [online]. Available from: http://www.cdc.gov/nchs/about/major/nhis/nhis_2007_data_release.htm. Accessed May 5, 2009.

National Center for Health Statistics. National Health Interview Survey (NHIS): Public-use data release. NHIS survey description [online]. 2008 Available from: ftp://ftp.cdc.gov/pub/Health_Statistics/NCHS/Dataset_Documentation/NHIS/2007/srvydesc.pdf. Accessed May 5, 2009

NCCAM educational campaign. Time to talk. National Center for Complementary and Alternative Medicine (online). Available from: http://nccam.nih.gov/timetotalk/. Accessed May 5, 2009.

Nott Waugh Julia. 1988, *The Silver Cradle: Las Posadas, Los Pastores, and other Mexican American Traditions,* University of Texas Press, Austin, TX

Padilla A. 1975, *Community Mental Health Services For The Spanish-Speaking/Surnamed Population,* American Psychologist 30: 892-905.

Paniagua Freddy A. 2005, *Assessing and Treating Culturally Diverse Clients: A Practical Guide,* Third Edition, Sage, Thousand Oaks, CA

Papa Jim's Magical Herb Book #1, Papa Jim's Botanica, San Antonio, TX

Paredes Américo. 1993, *Folklore and Culture on the Texas-Mexico Border,* The University of Texas Press, Austin, TX

Paredes Américo. 1970, *Folktales of Mexico,* University of Chicago, Chicago, IL

Parrilla Álvarez Laura. 2003, *Jardín Etnobotánica, Museo de Medicina Tradicional y Herbolaria,* Cuernavaca, Morelos, Instituto Nacional de Antropología e Historia, México DF

Pharmacopeia of the United States XIV. 1950, Mack Publishing Co. Easton, PA

Plantas Medicinales, Guía México Desconocido, 2001, México, DF

Polk, PA, Michael Owen Jones, Claudia J. Hernandez and Reyna C. Ronelli. 2005, *Miraculous Migrants to the City of Angeles: Perceptions of El Santo Niño de Atocha and San Simón as Sources of Health and Healing.* In *Religion and Healing in America.* Edited by Linda Barnes and Susan Sered. Oxford University Press, New York, NY

Prayers to the Saints, pamphlet, no author, no date

Pressar Patricia R. 2004, *From Fanatics to Folk: Brazilian Millenarianism and Popular Culture,* Duke University Press, Durham NC

Que Curan Las Plantas, Guía México Desconocido. 1997, No. 34, México DF

Ramirez-Najera Olga. 1997, *La Fiesta de los Tastoanes: Critical Encounters in Mexican Festival Performance,* University of New Mexico Press, Albuquerque, NM

Ríos, E. 2005, *The Ladies are Warriors: Latina Pentecostalism and Faith-based Activism in New York City.* In *Latino Religions and Civic Activism in the United States.* Edited by Gastón Espinosa, Virgilio Elizondo and Jesse Miranda. Oxford University Press, New York, NY

Rocha Arturo. 2006, *Virtud de México: El Valor de la Tradición,* Porrúa, México DF

Rogler LH, RG Malgady, and O Rodríguez. 1989, *Hispanics and Mental Health: A Framework for Research.* Malabar, FL: Robert E. Krieger Publishing Company

Rogler LH, RG Malgady, G Costantino, and R Blumenthal. 1987, *What Do Culturally Sensitive Mental Health Services Mean?,* American Psychologist 6: 565-569

Romano, Octavio. 1964, Don Pedrito Jaramillo: *The Emergence of a Mexican American Folk-Saint.* Ph.D. Dissertation, University of California, Berkeley, CA

Ross Ivan. 1999, *Medicinal Plants of the World*, Humana Press, Totowa, NJ

Ruíz de Alarcón Hernando. 1984, *Treatise on the Heathen Superstitions*, Translated and edited by J. Richard Andrews and Ross Hassig, The University of Oklahoma Press, Norman, OK

Ruiz Juan. 2002, *Medicina Traditional Purépecha*, El Colegio de Michoacán

Saints and Sinners: *Mexican Devotional Art.* 2006, A Schiffer Book for Collectors, Schiffer Publishing Co. Atglen, PA

Sams Jamie. 1994, *Earth Medicine: Ancestors' Ways of Harmony for many Moons,* HarperOne, New York, NY

Sánchez-Walsh, Arlene M. 2003, *Latino Pentecostal Identity: Evangelical Faith, Self, and Society.* Columbia University Press, New York, NY

Santeria: Sus Revelaciones, No Editor Editorial Epoca, México DF

Santiago Irizarry Vilma. 2001, *Medicalizing Ethnicity: The* Construction of Latino Identity in a Psychiatric Setting, Cornell University Press, Ithaca, NY

Sauvageau Juan. 1976, *Stories that must not die,* Vol. 3, The Oasis Press, Austin, TX

Schendel Gordon. 1968, *Medicine in Mexico: From Aztec Herbs to Betatrons,* The University of Texas Press, Austin, TX

Schultes Richard and Robert Raffauf. 1990, *The Healing Forest: Medicinal and Toxic Plants of the Northwest Amazonia*, Dioscorides Press, Portland, OR

Selig Godfrey. 1982, *Secrets of the Psalms*, Dorene Publishing, Arlington, TX

Sellner Albert. 1993, *Calendario Perpetuo de los Santos,* Editorial Sudamericana, Buenos Aires, Argentina

Smith MJ. 1985, *Ethnic Minorities: Life Stress, Social Support and Mental Health Issues*, The Counseling Psychologist 13: 537-577

Stone Martha. 1975, *At the Sign of Midnight: The Concheros Dance Cult of Mexico*, University of Arizona Press, Tucson, AZ

Sucesos y Leyendas de La Villa de Guadalupe. 2008, Crónicas y Leyendas Mexicanas, A.C., México DF

Tamara. 2002, *Brujería: Hechizos, Conjuros y Encantamientos*, Grupo Editorial Tomo, México DF

The Pharmaceutical Recipe Book. 1943, Published by The American Pharmaceutical Association

Toor Francis. 1985, *A Treasury of Mexican Folkways*, Bonanza Books, NY

Torres Eliseo. 1983, *Green Medicine: Traditional Mexican American Herbal Remedies*, Nieves Press, Kingsville, TX

Torres Eliseo. 1983, *The Folk Healer: The Mexican American Tradition of Curanderismo*, Nieves Press, Kingsville, TX

Torres Eliseo. 2006, *Healing with Herbs and Rituals: A Mexican Tradition*, University of New Mexico Press, Albuquerque, NM

Torrey EF. 1972, *The Mind Game: Witchdoctors and Psychiatrists*. New York, Emerson Hall, NY

Torrey EF. 1986, *Witchdoctors and Psychiatrists: The Common Roots of Psychotherapy and Its Future, A Shared Worldview:* The *Principle of Rumpelstiltskin*, New York: Harper & Row, Publishers, NY

Treviño FM, JG Bruhn and H. Bruce III. 1977, *Utilization of Community Mental Health Services in a Texas-Mexico Border City*, Social Science and Medicine 13A: 331-334

Treviño Roberto R. 2006, *The Church in the Barrio*, University of North Carolina Press, Chapel Hill, NC

Trotter Robert and Juan Chavira. 1997, *Curanderismo*, University of Georgia Press, Atlanta, GA

Vernon SW and RE Roberts. 1982, *Prevalence of Treated and Untreated Psychiatric Disorders in Three Ethnic Groups,* Social Science and Medicine 16: 1575-1582

Weckmann Luis. 1992, The Medieval Heritage of Mexico, Fordham University Press, NY

Weigle Marta. 1970, *The Penitentes of the Southwest,* Ancient City Press, Santa Fe, NM

Weisberg Barbara. 2004, Talking to the Dead: Kate and Maggie Fox and the rise of Spiritualism Harper, San Francisco, CA

Wignall CM and LL Koppin. 1967, *Mexican American Usage of State Mental Hospital Facilities,* Journal of Community Mental Health 3: 137-148

Wilkinson Tracy. 2007, *The Vatican's Exorcists: Driving Out the Devil in the 21st Century,* Warner Books, New York, NY

Winkelmann, John Paul. 1976, *Catholic Pharmacy,* Privately Published

Winter Evelyne. 1972, *Mexico's ancient and native remedies,* Editorial Fournier, Mexico DF

Wood Horation and Arthur Osol. 1943, *United States Dispensatory* 23rd Edition, J.B Lippincott Company Philadelphia, PA

Yamamoto J. 1968, *Cultural Problems in Psychiatric Therapy,* Archives of General Psychiatry 19: 44-49.

Zavaleta Antonio. 1998, *El Niño Fidencio: Un Santo Popular para el Nuevo Milenio,* SOCIOTAM, Revista Internacional de Ciencias Sociales y Humanidades, Vol. VIII, No. 2, pp. 149-208

Zellner William W and Marc Petrowsky. 1998, *Sects, Cults, and Spiritual Communities: A Sociological Analysis,* Praeger, Westport, CT

Index

A

Abedul 103, 386
Abre Camino 182, 192, 223, 237, 310
ADD 101
ADHD 101, 308, 374
Afro-Cuban 60
Aganyú 62
Agua Bendita 225
Aguacate 109, 385
Agua Florida 54, 310
Aire 92, 151, 152, 377
Ajo 67, 333, 397
Ajo macho 67, 333
Alabanza 31
Alamo 109, 114, 385, 393
Alcachofa 119, 385
Alfalfa 99, 131, 384, 417
Alfileres 305, 306
Algebrista 41
Algodoncillo 121, 394
All heal 82, 122, 384
Almendra 88, 99, 384
Almond 88, 99, 384, 417
Aloe Vera 88, 91, 93, 102, 109, 220, 309, 321, 322, 384, 417

Aloysius Gonzaga 189
Altamisa 86, 114, 125, 396
Alternative vii, xx, xxi, 7, 23, 31, 114, 116, 117, 340, 342, 352, 353, 362, 364, 368, 374, 427, 431, 436
Aluminum Triangle 207
Alum Rock 54, 61, 74, 133, 134, 149, 155, 156, 258, 263, 264, 311
Amapola 144, 396, 406
Amarillo 54
Ambrosia 91, 109, 123, 384, 389
American Pharmaceutical 322, 439
Américo Paredes 436
Ammonia 55, 218, 271, 310
Anacahuita 103, 415
Anemic 118, 131, 412
Anestésico 97
Angels Trumpet 91
Anodino 97
Anodyne 97
Ansiedad 144
Anthelminic 124
Antibacterial 122, 386
Antidysenteric 89
Antiemetic 133

Antiemético 133
Antiespasmódico 91
Antihelmíntico 124
Antihepatotoxic 181
Antiseptic 122, 392, 398
Ant weed 103
Anxiety 144, 156, 157, 223, 268, 376, 389, 392, 400
Aphrodisiac 203, 204, 385
Apples 14, 196, 304
Arbol de la Cera 83, 386
Ari Kiev 53
Arthritis 95, 97, 132, 286, 384, 385, 386, 388, 389, 390, 393, 394, 396, 399, 405, 406, 410, 411, 415, 416
Artichoke 119, 385
Ash Wednesday 49
Aspen 114, 385, 417
Aspirin xxi, 54, 115, 155
Assistants 14, 32
Association 54, 101, 145, 257, 307, 323, 361, 376, 377, 426, 430, 439
Asustado 144, 148, 149, 154, 155, 156, 266
Aurorita 48
Autism 308
Avocado 109, 113, 385
Azarcon 88
Aztec xix, 6, 7, 46, 56, 65, 67, 101, 111, 239, 278, 279, 385, 428, 438
Aztec Herbal 7, 46

B

Baby's head 161
Badianus Manuscript 6
Balthazar 71
Banana 14, 113, 385
Bandera 32
Baraja 40, 62, 63, 64, 372
Barba de Maíz 392

Barley 123, 386
Barrida 2, 75, 101, 133, 153, 159, 167, 378
Basil 23, 83, 86, 89, 125, 133, 140, 141, 144, 149, 155, 169, 197, 219, 228, 230, 231, 236, 238, 249, 292, 298, 311, 324, 326, 330, 392
Bearberry 386
Bedwetting 123, 124, 393
Bee Brush 103, 386
Berengena 118, 395
Berro 405, 414
Bicarbonate of soda 121
Bilberry 103, 386
Bile 100, 101, 111, 112, 386, 388, 399, 408, 413
Bilis 100, 101, 145
Birthwort 386
Bitter Wood 88, 386
Blackberry 121, 387
Black Cherry 131
Black Cohosh 116, 387, 418
Black Cumin 88, 387
Black Mustard Seed 225, 250, 310
Black Pepper 387
Bladder 98, 99, 124, 386, 391, 396, 410, 413
Bleeding 43, 55, 115, 264, 392, 402, 411
Blessed Kateri, Tekakwitha 25
Blessed Thistle 82, 88, 387
Blood 4, 91, 92, 100, 101, 102, 103, 111, 112, 114, 116, 118, 119, 120, 121, 131, 167, 168, 174, 176, 177, 238, 264, 290, 292, 322, 364, 384, 387, 388, 394, 395, 398, 401, 406, 408, 410, 413, 414
Blood Root 116, 121
Blue Ribbon 194
Blue Wax 247
Boils 388, 391, 406, 410

442

Boldo 83, 107, 387
Bonesetter 1, 38, 41, 91
Borage 82, 83, 106, 111, 122, 387
Borraja 82, 99, 106, 111, 122, 387
Botanica 369, 436
Botica 45, 46, 371
Bougainvillea 387
BPHC 363
Bracero 18, 19
Bricklebush 119, 388
Bronchitis 385, 386, 387, 389, 391, 392, 393, 395, 398, 399, 400, 405, 406, 409, 410, 411, 413, 415
Brook Mint 388
Broth 54
Bruise 385, 386, 387, 388, 389, 390, 391, 392, 395, 396, 402, 409, 411, 415
Bruja 41, 173, 204, 221, 263, 264, 272, 275, 283, 294, 313, 430
Brujo 2, 26, 41, 59, 136, 137, 165, 173, 174, 221, 264, 295, 310, 311
Buckeye Seed 169
Buddha 67, 219
Buñuelos 71
Burro Bush 91
Button Snakeroot 389

C

Cachana 397
Cactus 12, 96, 120, 192, 193, 320, 321, 407, 412
Caída de la Mollera 84, 85, 373
Cajita 22
Cajón 22
Calamus 89, 418
Calendula 82, 92, 114, 395, 418
California Pepper Tree 227
CAM 352, 353, 354
Camillus de Lellis 105

Camphor 54, 83, 91, 93, 109, 389
Caña fistula 82
Cancer 76, 114, 115, 116, 130, 145, 375, 385, 387, 390, 395
Candelaria 49, 62
Candle 24, 29, 53, 64, 65, 77, 92, 94, 98, 103, 108, 116, 125, 126, 131, 135, 138, 150, 151, 152, 155, 156, 157, 159, 162, 164, 165, 166, 172, 175, 176, 178, 184, 187, 190, 196, 197, 200, 201, 208, 209, 217, 218, 221, 225, 229, 230, 231, 232, 234, 243, 246, 247, 250, 255, 256, 257, 265, 275, 276, 281, 284, 285, 290, 298, 302, 324, 372, 428
Candlewood 118, 389
Candy 61, 71
Canela 88, 122, 391
Cardo Santo 82, 88, 99, 118, 403
Cargo Cult 33
Caridad del Cobre 62
Carlos Gómez ix, 176, 267
Carminative 105
Carminativo 105
Carnation 390
Cartomancy 40
Cáscara Sagrada 249, 250, 386
Castor bean 82
Castor Bean 390
Castor oil 54, 419
Cataplasma 54, 371
Catártico 105
Catemaco, Veracruz 41
Cathartic 105, 406
Catholic Church 28, 42, 47, 48, 52, 54, 59, 74, 102, 116, 145, 252, 289, 292, 294, 306, 319, 340, 370
Catholicism 23, 42, 49, 52, 78, 162, 289, 340, 435

Catholic Priest 26, 27, 28, 46, 47,
    49, 73, 102, 111, 179, 201,
    252, 268, 270, 289, 379
Cayenne 390, 419
Cebada 123, 386
Cebolla 404
Cedar 25, 121, 390
Cedro 121, 393
Celandine 121, 390, 419
Celedonia 390
Celo 134
Cenizo 49, 55, 115, 163, 407
Century Plant 83, 320, 390
Certified Nurse Midwife 81, 85
CNM 81, 85, 86
Chakras 4
Chamizo Hediondo 386, 409
Chamomile 82, 86, 88, 89, 100,
    161, 390, 397, 419
Champurrado 71
Changó 62, 231
Chaparral 238, 390
Chaya 119, 120, 412, 419
Cherokee xix
Cherry Juice 96
Chicken Soup 54, 83, 111
Chiflado 266
Chipil 100, 105
Christ Child 78, 324
Chuparosa 220
Cilantro 92, 144, 392
Cinnamon 23, 88, 122, 178, 190,
    191, 196, 220, 271, 297, 391
Citrus Tea 101
Clairvoyant 148
CLAS 344, 347, 348, 349, 350,
    351, 352
Clavel 390
Clavo 391
Clinic 121, 428
Cloth Doll 281
Clove 82, 95, 169, 333, 334, 391,
    421

Coagulant 55
Coagulante 55
Coconut water 130
Cod liver oil 54
Coffee grounds 23
Cofradia 147
Cola de Caballo 103, 123, 399
Cold 81, 82, 83, 92, 100, 104, 110,
    111, 113, 114, 123, 124, 151,
    152, 156, 161, 184, 203, 321,
    322, 377, 384, 385, 386, 387,
    389, 390, 391, 392, 393, 395,
    396, 398, 399, 400, 402, 406,
    407, 409, 410, 411, 412, 413,
    414, 415
Cold food 110, 113, 114, 152
Coldness 123, 124
Colibri 220
Cólico 87, 88
Cologne 141
Colombia 341
Come to me 2, 104, 108, 171, 201
Comino Negro 88, 387
Complementary Care 117
Compuesto 38, 82, 271
Confraternity 33, 147
Congestion 83, 322, 384, 386, 393,
    395, 397, 399, 401, 406, 408,
    414
Constantino vi, 12, 132, 204, 324,
    325
Constipation 385, 387, 388, 389,
    390, 393, 395, 397, 398, 401,
    403, 407, 408, 409, 410, 412,
    414, 416
Copal 134, 143, 225, 239, 271, 278,
    287, 326, 392, 395
Copper Coin 102, 169
Coraje 100, 101
Coral Beans 100
Coriander 92, 102, 144, 169, 392
Corn 61, 86, 99, 102, 110, 115,
    119, 120, 125, 333, 392, 413

444

Corn Silk 86, 99, 115, 125
Cosme 42, 94, 116
Cottonwood 109, 393
Cough 82, 83, 123, 384, 385, 386, 387, 389, 390, 391, 392, 393, 394, 395, 396, 397, 398, 399, 401, 402, 403, 404, 405, 407, 408, 409, 410, 411, 412, 413, 414, 415
Cow Lard 14
Cramp 384, 385, 389, 391, 392, 395, 396, 397, 398, 400, 401, 402, 405, 409, 411, 414, 415, 416
Cranberry 103, 393
Crazy 62, 112, 147, 190, 250, 251, 286, 295, 299, 307, 308
Credo 133, 153, 155
Croton 131, 412, 413
Cuachalate 400
Cucurbita 407
Cucurucho 91
Cudweed 83, 393
Cult 33, 41, 47, 52, 61, 78, 189, 300, 313, 314, 315, 369, 428, 439, 440
Culto 47, 61
Cultural Bound Syndrome 144
Cultural Broker Programs 94, 358, 360
Cultural Competency Resources 43, 84, 343, 344, 345, 349, 350, 351, 352, 355, 356, 358, 361, 363
Cumin 88, 387
Cupping 152
Curandera 1, 2, 37, 38, 42, 54, 55, 56, 57, 58, 59, 63, 171, 241, 251, 263, 368
Curanderismo ix, xx, 2, 3, 4, 5, 6, 7, 8, 11, 19, 21, 22, 26, 31, 35, 37, 38, 39, 40, 41, 42, 43, 48, 49, 53, 55, 57, 58, 61, 62, 66, 81, 109, 111, 152, 154, 158, 162, 165, 168, 169, 192, 231, 238, 243, 249, 257, 270, 273, 279, 281, 283, 287, 290, 292, 296, 304, 305, 324, 337, 339, 340, 341, 342, 355, 368, 381, 426, 432, 434, 439
Curanderismo Research 3, 4, 37, 42, 337, 339, 368
Curandero v, vi, vii, xix, xx, xxi, 1, 2, 7, 8, 11, 15, 17, 18, 19, 20, 22, 23, 25, 27, 29, 30, 31, 34, 35, 36, 37, 38, 40, 41, 42, 43, 44, 45, 46, 48, 49, 52, 53, 54, 55, 56, 57, 58, 59, 60, 63, 65, 66, 69, 70, 72, 74, 76, 81, 82, 83, 84, 85, 88, 90, 92, 94, 95, 97, 98, 99, 100, 101, 102, 103, 104, 106, 107, 108, 109, 110, 113, 114, 115, 116, 118, 119, 120, 121, 122, 123, 124, 125, 126, 129, 130, 131, 132, 133, 134, 135, 136, 137, 138, 139, 140, 141, 142, 143, 145, 146, 147, 149, 150, 151, 153, 155, 157, 158, 159, 160, 161, 162, 163, 165, 166, 167, 168, 169, 172, 173, 175, 177, 178, 179, 180, 181, 182, 183, 184, 185, 187, 189, 190, 191, 192, 193, 194, 195, 196, 197, 198, 199, 200, 201, 202, 203, 204, 206, 207, 208, 209, 211, 212, 213, 214, 218, 219, 221, 222, 223, 224, 225, 227, 228, 229, 230, 231, 232, 233, 234, 235, 236, 237, 238, 239, 243, 244, 246, 247, 248, 249, 250, 251, 252, 253, 254, 255, 256, 257, 258, 260, 261, 263, 264, 265, 266, 267, 268, 269, 270, 271, 272, 273, 274, 275, 276, 278, 279, 280, 281, 282, 284, 285,

286, 287, 288, 290, 291, 292,
293, 294, 296, 297, 298, 299,
300, 301, 302, 304, 305, 306,
307, 309, 310, 311, 314, 315,
319, 320, 322, 323, 325, 326,
327, 328, 329, 331, 332, 334,
336, 337, 338, 339, 340, 341
Curar 1, 56
Cure xix, xx, 2, 12, 13, 15, 18, 25,
27, 30, 60, 76, 89, 90, 92, 98,
106, 112, 117, 119, 124, 125,
132, 133, 148, 149, 152, 153,
154, 155, 285, 306, 328, 329,
361, 362, 374, 430
Curse 130, 164, 174, 186, 282, 283,
284, 327
Cystitis 391, 392, 406, 414

D

Dada 62
Damiana 86, 104, 203, 204
Dandelion 103, 123
Darkness 74, 136, 190
Day of the Dead 51, 266
Deer's Eye 150, 154
Depression 139, 140, 141, 156, 205,
255, 268, 405, 409, 411, 412
Desarrollo Espiritual 299
Descruce 218
Desert Anemone 394
Desert Broom 394
Despojo 162
Devil v, 40, 41, 67, 68, 69, 71, 101,
173, 174, 195, 263, 266, 267,
286, 292, 298, 304, 313, 379,
394, 440
Diabetes 93, 97, 119, 120, 130,
185, 376, 385, 388, 391, 392,
396, 397, 399, 407, 409, 412
Diabetic Neuropathy 30
Día de los Muertos 51, 266
Diuretic 385, 388, 395, 397, 401,
404, 409, 411, 412, 413

Divina Providencia 64, 221, 230
Divination 40, 63, 279
Divine Spirit of Light 108
Don v, ix, 14, 15, 50, 56, 58, 66, 78,
88, 121, 129, 165, 169, 185,
189, 195, 212, 221, 285, 291,
308, 354, 438
Don Pedrito Jaramillo v, 50, 58, 78,
438
Don Perfecto ix, 129, 169
Dragon Blood Powder 394
Dry 395

E

Earache 91
Edema 106, 391, 400
Egg 2, 74, 75, 84, 96, 100, 133,
143, 153, 174, 175, 258, 305,
306, 311, 323
Eggplant 395
Egg White 96, 133, 323
Elder Flower 395
Elegguá 62
Elephant 395
El Niño Fidencio v, vi, vii, xxii, 3, 4,
9, 11, 12, 15, 17, 18, 19, 20,
22, 23, 24, 25, 28, 37, 42, 47,
58, 61, 78, 99, 115, 116, 130,
132, 139, 150, 157, 163, 175,
179, 185, 191, 193, 202, 204,
207, 208, 212, 213, 214, 222,
223, 227, 237, 255, 296, 315,
323, 324, 327, 332, 337, 339,
340, 368, 440
Embrujada 297
Emenagogo 106
Emetic 89
Emmenagogue 106
Emollient 393
Emotional Stress 122
Empacho 87, 88, 89, 101, 373, 374
Encino 121, 434
Enebro 83, 103

Enema 89
Enrique López de la Fuente 12
Envidia 134, 135, 139, 229, 332
Envy 134, 135, 139, 140, 142, 229, 300, 301, 324, 334
Epazote de Zorrillo 82
Epilepsy 98, 389, 393, 399, 410
Epsom salts 89
Escapulario 146
Espanto 150
Espinazo, Nuevo León 12, 14, 28, 31, 78, 134, 150, 151, 337
Espiritista 39
Espuelas de Dama 400
Estampa 141, 218, 220, 309
Estandarte 32
Estramonio 400
Estrella de Anís 411
Estropajo 54
Eucalipto 395
Eucalyptus 395
Eupatorium 91
Euphorbia Herb 107
Evangelical 2, 28, 56, 289, 292, 365, 371
Evening Dew 161
Evil 2, 25, 34, 35, 40, 41, 45, 53, 57, 60, 70, 74, 84, 95, 96, 97, 98, 100, 124, 127, 134, 135, 137, 139, 140, 141, 143, 146, 153, 154, 158, 162, 163, 167, 168, 173, 174, 175, 178, 191, 194, 196, 197, 219, 221, 225, 229, 235, 236, 248, 250, 251, 252, 256, 257, 258, 263, 264, 265, 267, 268, 269, 270, 271, 272, 273, 274, 275, 276, 277, 278, 279, 281, 282, 286, 287, 288, 289, 291, 294, 296, 298, 299, 300, 301, 302, 304, 305, 306, 307, 308, 309, 312, 314, 315, 324, 325, 327, 362, 365, 377

Evil Eye 2, 84, 143, 153, 154, 258, 306, 307, 308, 362, 377
Exhaustion 394
Expectorant 404
Extreme Unction 102
Ex-Voto v, 73, 336
Eyes 68, 69, 99, 153, 174, 180, 190, 191, 229, 236, 250, 288, 297, 300, 384, 392, 397

F

Faith v, ix, xxi, 20, 21, 22, 23, 24, 27, 28, 30, 31, 32, 34, 42, 47, 48, 53, 56, 57, 60, 63, 67, 70, 75, 76, 77, 79, 90, 108, 117, 119, 122, 130, 132, 135, 142, 143, 145, 146, 147, 157, 163, 165, 175, 179, 196, 207, 212, 214, 230, 232, 234, 235, 236, 237, 241, 243, 244, 251, 253, 259, 283, 298, 299, 302, 314, 315, 318, 319, 320, 324, 325, 326, 328, 329, 330, 332, 365, 371, 372, 376, 430, 437, 438
Fall Equinox 51
Fantasma 265
Fava Bean 395
Feast of the Assumption 50
Feast of the Epiphany 49
Federally Qualified Health 86, 121
Feet 32, 34, 69, 85, 107, 123, 124, 155, 224, 290, 291, 309, 331, 384, 398
Fennel 395
Fenogreco 396, 397, 420
Fenugreek 118, 119
Fetish 281
Fever 82, 87, 111, 112, 113, 123, 124, 133, 134, 154, 322, 384, 387, 388, 389, 390, 391, 392, 394, 395, 396, 397, 402, 404, 405, 407, 408, 409, 411, 412, 414, 415

Feverfew 396
Fidencistas 27, 28, 29, 33, 340
Fiestas 27, 29, 31, 48
Fig 392
Flax 89, 96, 121
Flor de Corazón 401
Flor de Jamaica 114
Flor de Manita 398
Flor de San Juan 406
Flor de Saúco 395
Florifundo 91
Flowers 29, 75, 77, 309, 333, 334
Folk Catholicism 52, 78, 340
Folk Healer 439
Folk Illness 5, 85, 373, 376
Folk Massage 38, 90
Folk Medicine 14, 368, 371, 374, 430, 434
Folk Psychiatry 53
Folk Remedies 104, 338, 341, 374
Folk Saints v, 28, 47, 48, 78, 271, 319, 324, 369, 370
Fontanel 84, 85, 373
Forest Elves 19, 48
Four O'clock 103
FQHC 86, 121
Frankincense 396
Fresh Honey 54
Fresno 395
Frialdad 123
Frialdad de la matriz 123
Fright Sickness 132
Fruit 14, 61, 75, 110, 119, 193, 320, 418, 434
Funnel 91

G

Gabriel the Archangel 86, 196, 201, 234, 327
Gallbladder 389, 396, 416
Garlic 29, 67, 74, 75, 82, 91, 95, 102, 114, 168, 169, 177, 178, 191, 219, 222, 232, 258, 286, 304, 309, 322, 333, 334
Garlic Bath 177, 191
Gas 87, 89, 105, 234, 387, 390, 392, 395, 397, 402, 409
Gaspar 71
Gay Feather 397
Gentian 397
Geranio 397
Giant Hyssop 88, 115, 144
Gift ix, 1, 2, 3, 8, 16, 17, 22, 37, 38, 56, 57, 63, 129, 132, 136, 148, 168, 194, 251, 255, 301, 330, 338
Ginger 397
Girasol 411
Glaucoma 389
Goat's Milk 130, 293, 294
Gobernadora 99, 103, 118, 141, 196, 301
God 3, 11, 14, 15, 16, 20, 21, 22, 23, 24, 27, 28, 29, 30, 32, 34, 40, 46, 53, 54, 56, 57, 58, 62, 63, 69, 73, 75, 76, 90, 94, 102, 107, 115, 117, 122, 129, 130, 132, 136, 140, 141, 146, 148, 151, 153, 157, 158, 165, 168, 169, 173, 179, 180, 184, 189, 191, 201, 202, 205, 206, 207, 208, 212, 224, 229, 230, 234, 236, 237, 239, 241, 243, 248, 251, 252, 253, 255, 256, 258, 259, 260, 261, 263, 264, 283, 291, 292, 293, 296, 298, 299, 302, 304, 305, 314, 315, 320, 323, 326, 328, 329, 330, 331, 332, 364, 398, 426, 428, 431
Goldenrod 397
Gordolobo 393
Gout 385
Granada 406
Green Alcohol 97

Green Cloth 135
Green Pouch 249
Greta 88
Guardian Angel 21, 138, 301
Guardias 14, 17
Guava 398
Gum Tree 134

H

Habas de San Ignacio 89, 181
Hackberry Bark 115
Hair 76, 77, 266, 282, 294, 321
Handflower 398
Hangover 409
Headache xxi, 217, 385, 386, 390, 394, 397, 409, 410, 411, 412, 415
Head of Garlic 74, 258, 286, 333
Healer xx, 1, 3, 8, 12, 15, 18, 30, 39, 41, 42, 56, 62, 104, 108, 124, 168, 293, 308, 328, 339, 361, 376
Healing Missions 213
Healing Practices xx, 6, 17
Healing Rituals 25, 28, 75, 124, 168, 251, 338
Healing Traditions xix, 3, 4, 28, 55, 57, 58
Healthcare 380
Heart 2, 3, 6, 20, 22, 24, 30, 49, 56, 58, 66, 97, 99, 107, 115, 131, 146, 165, 171, 179, 183, 190, 191, 195, 201, 205, 207, 221, 241, 243, 246, 255, 283, 317, 319, 320, 325, 326, 384, 387, 390, 391, 401, 406, 413, 414
Heated 104, 123
Hechicera 293
Heliotrope 396
Helpers 14, 17, 33, 48, 87, 319
Hemorrhoids 385, 387, 389, 397, 399, 407, 411, 412, 416

Hens Eggs 258
Hepatica 114, 400
Herb 15, 23, 30, 45, 82, 83, 107, 109, 115, 125, 133, 144, 149, 197, 202, 221, 250, 266, 281, 324, 327, 338, 369, 375, 376, 381, 390, 398, 409, 418, 419, 420, 421, 422, 423, 425, 436
Herbalist xx, 1, 15, 38, 45, 164, 340
Herbal Laxatives 89
Herbal Mixtures 38, 82
Herbal Remedies 44, 109, 115, 429, 430, 436, 439
Herbs 2, 25, 30, 34, 38, 44, 45, 54, 104, 106, 109, 125, 129, 131, 140, 141, 144, 159, 180, 230, 231, 238, 288, 298, 311, 326, 333, 368, 371, 417, 418, 419, 420, 421, 422, 423, 425, 428, 430, 434, 438, 439
Herb Shops 149
Hibiscus 114, 239, 398, 413, 421
Hierba Amarga 91, 109, 123, 384
Hierba del Burro 91
Hierba del Golpe 103
Hierbanís 88, 97
Hierbería 23, 30, 38, 43, 44, 45, 46, 47, 65, 66, 72, 82, 88, 96, 109, 120, 130, 131, 133, 135, 149, 154, 155, 164, 169, 181, 191, 193, 197, 200, 201, 213, 219, 220, 243, 250, 266, 275, 281, 299, 309, 312, 324, 383
Higuera 392
Higuerilla 82, 390
Hinojo 86, 395
Hispanic xix, 26, 136, 343, 344, 345, 347, 363, 371, 372, 380, 420, 429, 432, 435, 437
Hoja Santa 408
Holy Bark 250
Holy Bible 46, 56, 57, 125, 168, 237, 259

Holy Card 141
Holy Cross 27, 50
Holy Death 47, 312, 313, 314
Holy Infant of Prague 231
Holy Innocents 121, 160
Holy Rosary 66, 132, 157, 232, 288, 296
Holy Spirit 22, 32, 47, 49, 56, 57, 96, 100, 136, 191, 232, 234, 236, 243, 244, 248, 255, 261, 314, 325, 329, 330
Holy Trinity 65, 126, 221, 229, 230, 231, 232, 234, 264, 326
Holy Water 100, 130, 131, 133, 143, 145, 157, 159, 164, 165, 225, 250, 252, 271, 278, 287, 290, 291, 292, 294, 302, 306, 310
Holy Week 50
Honey 54, 61, 82, 121, 122, 140, 178, 196, 230, 231
Honeysuckle 82, 114, 402
Hookworms 124
Horehound 88, 109, 144, 169, 398, 414
Horsetail 103, 123, 399
Hot 18, 54, 71, 104, 110, 111, 113, 114, 124, 133, 134, 151, 152, 156, 161, 169, 230, 238, 333, 334
Hot Coals 124, 133, 134
Hot food 110, 111
Hot water bottle 54
HRSA 344, 345, 346, 355, 363
Huele de Noche 97
Huesero 38, 41, 91, 368
Huichol 40
Hummingbird 220, 272, 273, 399
Humoral Theory 113, 151
Hypochondriac 293

I

Immaculate Conception 51, 138
Immune System 118

Incense 25, 55, 59, 74, 75, 125, 134, 143, 163, 164, 165, 215, 225, 239, 270, 271, 278, 287, 302, 326
Incontinence 392
Incubus 286, 287
Indian Plantain 91, 119, 399
Indigestion 89, 114, 384, 386, 387, 389, 390, 391, 392, 393, 394, 395, 396, 397, 398, 399, 400, 401, 402, 405, 407, 408, 409, 410, 412, 416
Indio 4, 25, 47, 399
Induce Vomiting 89, 181
Infection 55, 83, 91, 92, 93, 101, 121, 125, 375, 380, 386, 388, 392, 393, 394, 395, 398, 399, 409, 411, 412, 415
Inflammation 91, 385, 386, 388, 391, 398, 402, 403, 406, 410, 414, 415
Injerto 97, 395
Inmortal 385
Insect 384, 385, 386, 390, 392, 393, 394, 406, 408, 412
Insomnia 144, 386, 388, 389, 390, 396, 397, 400, 401, 405, 406, 408, 414, 415, 419
Internet v, vii, 7, 24, 26, 30, 31, 33, 37, 42, 43, 44, 45, 46, 59, 95, 114, 117, 121, 135, 163, 210, 219, 268, 304, 329, 337, 338, 341, 343, 344, 367, 417
Intestinal 85, 88, 89, 101, 124, 384, 388, 390, 391, 392, 395, 399, 400, 402, 404, 405, 406, 410, 414, 415
Iodine 54
Ipecac 54, 399

J

Jabón de la Paloma 54
Jalisco 40

Jamie Sams ix, xix, 17, 114, 335, 375
Jealousy 25, 134, 135, 221, 300, 301, 332, 334
Jicama 416
Jimson Weed 197, 400
Job 35, 41, 52, 65, 126, 139, 146, 172, 180, 184, 194, 199, 205, 207, 210, 218, 220, 223, 224, 226, 227, 228, 229, 230, 231, 232, 233, 234, 235, 236, 237, 238, 239, 249, 256, 257, 275, 291, 292, 297, 302, 303, 326, 332, 334
John the Conqueror 102, 184, 197, 298
José Fidencio Sintora vi, 12
Juan Soldado 41, 47, 50
Juliana 108, 118, 400
Juniper Berry 169
Just Judge 164, 165, 200, 201, 225, 247
Justo Juez 164, 165, 201, 225, 247

K

Kerosene 54
Kidney 99, 101, 102, 103, 375, 376, 384, 386, 387, 388, 389, 390, 392, 393, 396, 397, 398, 399, 400, 402, 406, 407, 408, 410, 411, 413, 414, 415, 416
Kidneywood 91, 103
Kidneywort 114, 400
King Salomón 434
Kleinman 87, 355

L

La Coste 139
Lactation 394
La Gavia 13
Lágrimas de San Pedro 250
La Llorona 48
Larkspur 400
Larry Dossey 102, 367, 375
La Santísima Muerte 380
Latido 87, 89
Latino xx, 1, 4, 5, 6, 7, 8, 22, 23, 25, 26, 38, 40, 41, 42, 43, 44, 46, 53, 55, 56, 57, 61, 66, 70, 72, 77, 78, 81, 85, 87, 91, 97, 108, 109, 113, 120, 132, 136, 137, 138, 143, 144, 145, 147, 148, 152, 156, 158, 159, 161, 162, 167, 173, 177, 180, 183, 187, 189, 191, 199, 218, 239, 243, 247, 263, 265, 266, 269, 270, 275, 277, 279, 281, 282, 283, 308, 315, 319, 320, 337, 338, 339, 340, 341, 342, 363, 364, 365, 366, 371, 428, 430, 431, 434, 437, 438
Latinos xx, 5, 6, 7, 8, 23, 26, 31, 42, 46, 54, 58, 63, 66, 67, 69, 89, 96, 123, 138, 152, 160, 161, 208, 213, 217, 239, 247, 249, 263, 278, 279, 287, 292, 301, 304, 308, 310, 311, 319, 339, 340, 341, 342, 363, 364, 365, 366, 372, 377
Laurel 82, 83, 88, 92, 386
Lavender 62, 83, 116, 122, 180, 333, 400
Laxative 54, 89, 386, 389, 392, 395, 396, 406, 410, 412
Lead oxide 88
Lechona 109, 403
Lechuga 401, 415
Lechuza 137, 175, 272, 273, 286
Lemon Balm 144, 400, 422
Lemon Grass 30, 90, 91, 96, 97, 116, 122, 163, 400
Lemons 14, 54, 185, 227, 258
Lettuce 401, 415, 422
Lice 385, 400, 409
Licorice Root 83

Lily of the Valley 401
Limón 30, 88, 91, 96, 103, 133,
    163, 400
Limpia 36, 44, 70, 153, 167, 219,
    228, 229, 258, 274, 287, 301,
    304, 305, 306
Linaza 96, 121, 396
Linden 141, 144, 401
Liniment 91
Linimento 54, 91
Linimento Blanco 54
Liquid Amber 134
Liquid Retention 106
Lirio de los Valles 401
Liver 54, 181, 385, 387, 389, 393,
    400, 402, 403, 407, 408, 416
Loción Siete Machos 169, 250
Lodestone 102, 219, 220
Lord's Prayer 75, 178, 191, 306
Loteria 374
Luck 34, 61, 67, 106, 121, 125,
    130, 134, 139, 140, 156, 157,
    158, 168, 169, 178, 191, 218,
    219, 220, 237, 239, 263, 282,
    283, 298, 299, 301, 304, 309,
    323, 324
Lunar Eclipse 160
Lupus 117, 118

M

Magic 2, 20, 55, 65, 67, 102, 166,
    169, 193, 201, 208, 231, 257,
    260, 277, 284, 307, 321, 368,
    372, 379, 430, 431, 432, 435
Magnolia 401
Maguey 83, 320, 321, 390
Malabar 109, 401, 437
Mal Aire 152
Mala Mujer 413
Malaria 390, 401
Maldad 150
Mal de Ojo 2, 84, 101, 143, 145,
    153, 154, 258

Maldición 164, 282
Mallow 82, 391, 399, 401, 402
Mal Puesto 90
Malva 82, 391, 401
Malverde, Jesus 50
Manda 76, 166, 265, 318
Manteca de Coyote 55, 122
Manteca de Puerco 55
Margarita 86, 404, 433
Marigold 82, 92, 114, 385, 388,
    395, 402
Marijuana 97, 181, 248, 260, 389
Marjoram 411
Marrubio 88, 109, 144, 398, 414
Matarique 30, 91, 119, 120, 399
materia 22, 28, 29, 31, 32, 38, 219,
    318
Materia 1, 3, 22, 75, 319, 436
Maximón 47
Mayan xix
Mayans 239
Mayordomo 33, 78
Medicina de Patente 38
medicinal plant 3, 83, 106, 417
Medicinal Plant 2, 3, 6, 21, 38, 46,
    55, 65, 66, 83, 89, 90, 92,
    103, 106, 109, 111, 112, 115,
    121, 125, 164, 181, 338, 381,
    382, 383, 417, 435, 438
Melchor 71
Memory 91, 182, 249, 323, 434
Menopause 411
Menstruation 387, 388, 389, 402,
    405, 408, 410, 411, 412, 414,
    415
Menta 385, 405
Mentalista 39
Mercado Sonora 3, 36, 80, 127,
    170, 215, 262
Mercurochrome 54
Mesquite 322, 402
Mexican Day Flower 402
Mexican Oregano 86, 402

Mexican Thistle 118, 403
Mexico v, vi, ix, xix, 3, 6, 9, 11, 12,
    13, 18, 19, 26, 28, 29, 30, 36,
    38, 41, 42, 43, 46, 48, 52, 54,
    55, 59, 72, 73, 77, 78, 80, 85,
    86, 87, 97, 103, 104, 112,
    114, 115, 116, 127, 137, 151,
    170, 177, 181, 208, 213, 215,
    251, 295, 308, 312, 315, 318,
    325, 330, 331, 336, 337, 340,
    377, 381, 427, 428, 429, 430,
    431, 432, 434, 435, 436, 437,
    438, 439, 440
Midwife 15, 38, 81, 82, 85, 86, 106,
    159
Miguelito 47
Milagritos 72
Milenrama 91, 106, 416
Milkweed 109, 403, 422
Mineral Oil 54
Mint 83, 88, 89, 112, 114, 122,
    197, 219, 298, 385, 388
Mint Bee Balm 114
Miracle 19, 27, 30, 32, 33, 48, 51,
    59, 72, 73, 76, 77, 78, 102,
    116, 117, 143, 147, 157, 189,
    207, 213, 224, 237, 238, 254,
    259, 260, 290, 317, 318, 319,
    320, 326, 330, 331, 372, 380,
    430, 431
Mirto 92, 123, 408
Misa de Gallo 71
Misión de Sanación 30
Mistletoe 97, 395, 422
Moist 111, 334
Mojo Bag 67
Money 13, 14, 23, 29, 34, 59, 60,
    62, 67, 72, 77, 125, 129, 130,
    134, 135, 146, 166, 168, 169,
    173, 174, 175, 177, 189, 191,
    213, 226, 234, 237, 244, 245,
    249, 250, 283, 299, 301, 302
Moon 160, 183, 219

Moons 438
Mora 82, 387
Mormon Tea 88
Morning Glory 97, 413
Mother Earth xxi, 8
Muicle 82, 111, 114, 402
Muina 100
Mulberry 82, 387
Mustard Seed 83, 102, 166, 169,
    190, 225, 250, 310, 322, 324
Myrrh 134, 197, 225, 278, 298, 398
Myrtle 123

N

Nagual 137
Naranja 83, 121, 386, 412
Narciso Negro 134, 271
Nasturtium 118, 396, 414
National Geographic 282, 378, 426
Native American xix, 7, 25, 26, 39,
    48, 374
Naturalist 38, 39
Natural Pharmacy xxi
Naturista 38
Naturopathic xx
Nausea 89, 133, 181, 384, 388, 390,
    391, 392, 397, 405, 407, 415
NCCAM 352, 353, 422, 436
Needles 305, 306, 321, 323
Nettle 118, 399, 411
New Age 7, 243, 379
Night Blooming Jasmine 97
Nightmares 156
Niño Perdido 48, 138, 139, 141,
    142
Noche Buena 51, 71
Nogal 405, 414
Nopal 96, 119, 192, 193, 407
Novena 147, 162, 238, 380
Nuestra Señora de la Merced 51
Nuez 91, 389
Nuez Moscada 91

Nutmeg 91, 423

O

Oak 121, 436
Obbatala 62
Occam's Razor 296
Ochosi 62
Ochún 62
Ocultista 39
Ofrenda 75, 76
Oggún 62
Oils 3, 39, 44, 59, 65, 105, 193, 247, 310, 311
Old Testament 67, 146, 169
Olivo 13, 404
Olmo 82, 410
Olodumare 62
Omen 273, 303
OMH 347, 348, 363
Orishia 62
Ortigilla 118
Ouija Board 278, 279, 379
Our Father 24, 75, 139, 155, 230, 231, 232, 239, 258, 286, 325, 326
Our Lady of Good Counsel 214
Our Lady of Lourdes 16
Our Lady of Miracle 51
Our Lady of Pharmacy 46
Our Mother of Mercy 51
Owl 175, 273, 286
Oyá 62

P

Padre Nuestro 75, 155, 178, 230
Palma Bendita 309
Palm Sunday 309
Palo Blanco 115
Palo De Brasil 131
Pancho Villa 41, 47, 50, 220, 247, 296
Papa 368, 406, 436

Papaya 402
Parasite 124, 388, 402, 405, 406
Parasites 375, 401, 407
Parche Guadalupano 54, 90
Parchment paper 65, 157, 192, 235, 313
Parsley 86, 118, 122, 123, 301, 322, 393, 405
Partera 1, 38, 39, 85, 86, 87, 159, 241, 373
Partero 15
Pasmo 86, 111, 123, 394
Passiflora 405
Passion Flower 405
Pastorela 51, 70, 71, 372
Pecan 405
Pencas de Nopal 192
Pennyroyal 82, 83, 86, 395, 405, 423
Peonía 288, 414
Peppermint 23, 405
Pepper Tree 227, 238, 405
Peregrinación 76, 317
Perejil 86, 116, 118, 123, 288, 393, 405
Perfume 44, 96, 125, 129, 135, 157, 184, 193, 201, 205, 218
Pericón 402
Persimmon 141, 144, 405
Peruvian Bark 405
Pesar 145
Phantom 265
Pharmacology 3, 342, 433
Piedra Alumbre 74, 133, 149, 155, 258
Piedra Imán 102, 191, 192, 219
Pilgrimage 52, 66, 72, 73, 76, 77, 78, 207, 317, 318, 319, 329, 330, 331
Piloncillo 54
Pine Oil 55
Pink Ribbon 194
Pink Windmill 99, 115

Pinworm 124
Pirul 101, 141, 227
Plateau Rocktrumpet 406
Plutarco Elías Calles 13
Poleo 83, 86, 88, 388, 395, 405
Poleo Chino 395
Pomada 14, 99
Pomada del Niño Fidencio 99
Pomegranate 82, 406
Poppy 144, 385, 389, 396, 406, 407
Popular Saints 47, 370
Pork 113
Posada 51, 70, 71, 372, 436
Possession 3, 159, 252, 263, 268, 269, 270, 289, 290, 300, 307, 308, 315, 379, 428, 429, 431
Post Traumatic Stress Disorder (PTSD) 144
Potato 406
Potions 44, 193
Powder 44, 88, 116, 167, 168, 176, 177, 178, 190, 191, 193, 247, 261, 280, 297, 305, 310, 311, 394, 418
Prenda 76
Prescription 32, 44, 46, 52, 99, 103, 109, 112, 115, 229, 230, 354, 369
Prickly Pear 193, 407
Prodigiosa 119, 131, 388
Project 3, 4, 37, 42, 337, 339, 358, 368
Promesa 33, 71, 72, 76
Promise 16, 24, 33, 71, 72, 76, 77, 140, 143, 150, 151, 162, 183, 203, 223, 260, 293, 313, 314, 318, 330, 365
Propitiate 24
Prostate 409, 410, 414
Protection 2, 17, 24, 34, 53, 60, 61, 66, 67, 77, 106, 110, 111, 134, 138, 141, 151, 159, 160, 200, 217, 218, 219, 221, 225, 231, 236, 250, 255, 259, 271, 272, 287, 289, 309, 310, 317, 327, 334, 345, 386
Protestant 168, 287
Psalm 5 250
Psalm 7 222
Psalm 8 229
Psalm 10 274
Psalm 13 132
Psalm 14 197
Psalm 16 162
Psalm 17 278
Psalm 19 246
Psalm 22 137
Psalm 23 273, 328
Psalm 26 254
Psalm 28 142, 143
Psalm 33 103
Psalm 37 181
Psalm 56 195
Psalm 60 138
Psalm 61 163
Psalm 62 136, 163, 376, 387
Psalm 71 261
Psalm 119 213, 237
Psalm 126 189
Psalm 132 211, 224
Psalm 134 227
Psalm 135 34
Psalm 138 193
Psychic 98, 173, 174, 175, 266, 276
Psychologist xx, 270, 436, 437, 439
Pumpkin 124, 407
Purga 89, 402
Purgante 89
Purgative 54, 89, 105, 386, 393, 413
Purple Sage 115, 407

Q

Quinine 407, 415, 424

R

Rage 204, 206, 288
Real de Catorce 40, 78
Receta 32, 45, 99
Red Dock 408
Remedio casero 54
Resources 343, 344, 345, 358, 363
Respiratory 83, 384, 385, 386, 392, 395, 400, 401, 416
Restorative 55, 132
Resurrection Plant 408
Retiro 257
Rheumatism 95, 97, 384, 386, 387, 388, 389, 391, 392, 394, 396, 397, 399, 402, 405, 406, 407, 408, 409, 410, 411, 412, 414, 415, 416
Rice 19, 61, 102, 119, 166, 225, 284, 287, 310, 324, 371, 373, 374, 376, 408
Ritual 2, 5, 44, 61, 64, 66, 75, 79, 96, 100, 118, 126, 133, 134, 151, 153, 155, 159, 162, 172, 173, 174, 175, 178, 180, 181, 193, 219, 225, 228, 235, 245, 258, 266, 270, 271, 273, 274, 278, 284, 288, 294, 297, 301, 305, 306, 311, 326, 364, 378, 432, 439
Romero 83, 141, 230, 231, 236, 326, 330, 408
Rootbeer Plant 408
Rosemary 23, 55, 83, 134, 140, 141, 149, 190, 191, 197, 209, 228, 230, 231, 236, 238, 239, 261, 271, 292, 298, 326, 330, 408
Ruda 92, 121, 141, 230, 231, 236, 326, 330, 409, 412
Rue 92, 121, 140, 141, 149, 228, 230, 231, 236, 238, 292, 326, 330, 409, 412

S

Sábila 384
Sabino macho 390
Sacamuelas 41
Sacasil 12, 405
Sacred Heart 66, 131, 190, 221, 255
Sacred Heart of Jesus 190, 255
Saffron 409
Sage 25, 55, 92, 96, 105, 115, 121, 122, 145, 163, 164, 392, 407, 408, 409, 435, 436
Sagebrush 386, 409
Sagrado Corazón 131, 190, 221, 255
Sahagún 46
Sahumerio 96, 270, 271, 287, 378
Saint Adelaide 197
Saint Agapitus 88
Saint Andrew 114, 193
Saint Ann 179, 184
Saint Anthony 49, 50, 54, 162
Saint Anthony Abad 49
Saint Anthony of Padua 50
Saint Bartholomew 144
Saint Benedict Labre 237
Saint Bernadette 23
Saint Bernard of Clairvaux 126
Saint Blaise 82
Saint Brigid 227
Saint Catherine of Sweden 86
Saint Cecilia 86
Saint Chad 137
Saint Columba 176
Saint Cornelius 92
Saint Cyriacus 54, 69
Saint Daniel 182
Saint Denis 271
Saint Domitian 124
Saint Dorothy 193, 196
Saint Dymphna 54, 144
Saint Eduviges 243
Saint Edwin 237

Saint Elizabeth 135
Saint Erasmus 88
Saint Eugene de Mazenod 143
Saint Faustina Kowalska 244
Saint Felicitas 98
Saint Flora 211
Saint Francis Xavier 219
Saint George 138
Saint Gerard 86
Saint Gregory the Great 224
Saint Gudule 206
Saint Gummarus 172
Saint Helen 185, 199
Saint Homobonus 271
Saint Isadore 50
Saint Ivo 250
Saint James 50, 96, 138, 319
Saint James the Greater 96
Saint Joachim 177
Saint Joan of Arc 138, 247
Saint John of the Cross 130
Saint John Salle 224, 227
Saint John the Baptist 50
Saint John the Evangelist 256
Saint Joseph 50, 62, 107, 145, 166, 167, 378
Saint Joseph the Worker 50, 107
Saint Jude 51, 140, 142, 143, 247
Saint Justice 50
Saint Lawrence 90
Saint Lazarus 61, 122
Saint Leopold 213
Saint Louis 92
Saint Lucy 154
Saint Marculf 122
Saint Margaret 176, 272
Saint Margaret Clitherow 272
Saint Maria Goretti 159
Saint Marina 86
Saint Mark 50
Saint Martha 213
Saint Martin of Porres 51
Saint Matilda 141
Saint Matthais 180
Saint Maximilian Kolbe 244, 248
Saint Odilo 252
Saint Patient 51
Saint Patron v, x, 25, 26, 32, 33, 42, 45, 61, 66, 73, 75, 76, 77, 79, 82, 86, 90, 94, 98, 99, 103, 105, 107, 108, 114, 119, 122, 131, 132, 135, 138, 141, 142, 145, 146, 154, 155, 156, 157, 159, 162, 176, 179, 182, 189, 191, 193, 197, 199, 211, 213, 218, 220, 224, 225, 230, 243, 244, 247, 254, 271, 272, 286, 291, 319, 365, 370
Saint Peter 50, 123, 250
Saint Peter of Verona 250
Saint Quentin 82
Saint Scholastica 227
Saint Stanislaus 116, 118
Saint Thomas Aquinas 227
Saint Thomas More 137
Saint Timothy 88
Saint Valentine 49, 98
Saint Vincent de Paul 265
Saint Willibrord 98
Sal 167
Salaciones 304
Salada 121, 218, 220, 255
Salt 54, 88, 157, 168, 219, 230, 231, 300, 312, 396
Salted 121, 299
Salve 14, 39, 123
Salvia 30, 34, 90, 96, 103, 116, 118, 121, 133, 163, 164, 389, 392, 408, 409
SAMHSA 363, 378
San Alberto Mago 51
San Alejo 94, 118, 164, 172, 190, 197, 200, 235, 256, 257, 275, 276, 290, 292, 370
San Antonio Abad 49
San Antonio de Padua 50

San Bartolomé 98
San Basilio 100
San Benito 180
San Buenaventura 50
San Camilo 50
San Casimiro 191
San Cayetano 211
San Cipriano 65, 135, 172, 176, 180, 193, 200, 278, 281, 290, 300
San Cristóbal 62, 140, 163, 278, 286
Sanctuaries 33
Sándalo 167, 409
Sandalwood 168, 409
San Eduardo 172, 191, 194
San Elías 50
San Francisco de Asís 78
San Gabriel Arcángel 196, 201, 234, 327
San Gil 122
Sangradora 41
Sanguinaria 116, 121, 387
San Humberto 62
San Ignacio de Loyola 50, 94, 148, 157, 164, 172, 180, 190, 197, 200, 275, 276, 292, 309
San Isidro Labrador 50, 198, 218, 231
San José 50
San José Obrero 50
San Juan Bautista 50
San Judas Tadeo 370
San Justo 50
San Lázaro 60, 61, 62
San Marcos 50, 103, 121, 155
San Martín Caballero 220, 222
San Mauricio 92, 278, 291
San Miguel Arcángel 251, 290
San Nicolás of Flue 143
San Norberto 62
San Onofre 166
San Pablo 50, 62

San Paciente 51
San Pantaleón 119
San Pascual Bailón 142
San Pedro 50, 62, 151, 250
San Rafael Arcángel 116
San Ramón 62, 86, 105
San Ramón Nonato 86, 105
San Roque 51
San Santiago 50, 319, 369, 430, 438
Santa Agueda 116, 159, 243
Santa Bibiana 180
Santa Catalina de Siena 114
Santa Cecilia 105
Santa Clara 50, 146
Santa Inés 177, 246
Santa Isabel 146
Santa Juliana 108, 118
Santa Lourdes 133
Santa María Magdalena 50
Santa Martha 213
Santa Teresa 47, 369
Santa Teresa de Avila 47
Santería Orisha 61
Santero 60, 61, 300, 312
Santísima Trinidad 230
Santo Daniel 246
Santo José María Escrivá 131
San Tomás 90
Santo Niño de Atocha 32, 47, 62, 78, 246, 260, 373, 432, 437
Santoral 48, 49, 52
Santos Populares 47, 370
Santuario 33
Satan 236, 267, 290, 314
Satanic Cult 41, 313, 314, 315
Saúco 395
Sauz 82, 83, 114, 115, 415
Scapular 146, 147, 377
Scared 59, 93, 94, 107, 133, 150, 153, 155, 156, 162, 174, 185, 210, 233, 242, 244, 248, 253, 255, 265, 266, 272, 273, 274, 280, 288, 302, 305, 306, 310, 312, 313

Schizophrenia 52, 60, 156, 157, 297, 299, 300, 379
Sedante 144
Sedative 398, 400, 401, 402, 404, 405, 407, 409, 414
Semana Santa 50
Semilla de Calabaza 124
Semillas de Mostaza Negra 250
Señora de la Medalla Milagrosa 51
Serenar 161
Sereno 161
Seven Archangel 196
Seven Day Candle 116, 172, 197, 200, 232
Seven Male Billy Goat's Lotion 169
Shamanism vii, 2, 7, 25, 39, 337, 379
Shape Shift 273
Sherry Fields 43
Siete Machos 169, 249, 250, 271
Sinusitis 391
Smoke 25, 126, 134, 150, 155, 227, 285, 378
Smoking-House Cleansing 270
Soap 14, 54, 83, 193
Sobadora 1, 38, 39, 90, 91, 368
Socorro Constantino 12
Sopa 111
Soplador 41
Soplar 98
Soporific 144
Soporífico 144
Sores 122, 322, 384, 386, 390, 391, 392, 394, 396, 397, 398, 399, 400, 401, 403, 404, 406, 407, 409, 410, 411, 412
Sorrell 410
Sortilegios 194
Soul Loss 5, 8, 70, 134, 308
Souls 34, 37, 155, 162, 182, 252, 370
Sour Orange Tree 83
Spanish Tarot 16, 17, 40, 63, 64

Spearmint 112, 133, 149, 410
Spell 59, 61, 65, 66, 67, 69, 123, 127, 136, 137, 140, 145, 158, 165, 168, 169, 170, 172, 173, 174, 175, 177, 178, 184, 191, 194, 195, 221, 225, 232, 238, 250, 262, 263, 264, 274, 275, 276, 277, 280, 282, 284, 294, 297, 298, 300, 301, 304, 308, 310, 311, 312, 327, 380
Spider Web 54
Spirit Box 22
Spirit Channeling 3, 49
Spiritism 35, 370, 433
Spirit Mediums 1, 23
Spiritual Bath 141, 227, 230, 294, 327
Spiritual Cleansing 70, 141, 143, 167, 175, 178, 191, 219, 228, 230, 232, 250, 258, 272, 274, 278, 305, 324, 338
Spiritual Debt 265
Spiritual Development 214, 299
Spiritual Healing Baths 159, 169
Spiritual Helpers 15, 17
Spiritual Lotions 44
Spoiled 68, 89, 266, 267
Spring Equinox 50
Star Anise 102, 197, 298, 411
Stimulant 132, 389, 391, 397, 401, 404, 409, 415
Storax 134, 239, 271, 411
Straight Pins 305, 306
Strep Infection 121
Styptic 55
Succubus 287, 379
Suerte 139, 158, 238, 323, 378
Sugar 23, 54, 119, 120, 134, 178, 190, 239, 271, 388
Sulfur 54, 122
Sumac 82, 411, 412
Summer Solstice 50
Sunflower 385, 411

Supernatural illness 124, 264
Susto 5, 8, 84, 90, 132, 133, 134, 141, 144, 145, 148, 149, 156, 258, 274, 285, 307, 376, 377
Susto Pasado 90, 134
Sweet Flag 89, 411
Sympathetic magic 193, 257, 307
Syncretism 42, 48

T

Taboo 58, 113, 114, 282, 378
Taboo: Mexican Witchcraft 282
Talisman 3, 44, 65, 66, 67, 105, 140, 150, 218, 220, 284, 299, 368, 372
Tamales 71
Tamaulipas 29, 318
Tarbush 121, 412
Tarot 16, 17, 40, 63, 64, 372, 379
Tarragon 402
Taumaturgo 48
Tejano 142, 430
Tenedoras 87
Teodoro von Wernich 12
Thaumaturge 48
Three Kings 49, 64, 71, 225
Three Kings Incense 225
Thrush 121
Thyme 396
Tinieblas 74, 286
Tlanchalagua 390
Tlanchichinole 413
Tobacco 25, 55, 134, 155, 271, 399, 412
Toltec xix
Tomasito 48
Tomates marinos 271
Tomatillo 415
Tomatoes 14, 122
Tomato juice 96, 122
Tomillo 118, 396
Tonic 43, 55, 118, 132, 386, 391, 414

Tonsillitis 384, 397
Toothache 83, 387, 388, 391, 392, 393, 394, 396, 397, 400, 405, 406, 407, 411
Toronjil 397
Torreón, Coahuila 13
Trabajo 2, 61, 145, 165, 173, 220, 275, 298
Traditional cures xx
Trance medium 3, 22, 28, 32, 39, 47, 214, 300, 318
Tranquilizer 144
Trastornado 299
Tree Spinach 119, 412
Trigo 116, 414
Tumba Vaquero 34, 97, 288
Tuna 193
Turibius 26
Turnera Diffusa 104, 393

U

Ulcers 114, 238, 384, 387, 390, 391, 394, 397, 399, 400, 401, 402, 408, 412, 413
Uña de Gato 390
Uncrossing 218
Unguent 92, 123
Unguento 92
Untie Knot 185, 206
Urinary tract infection 125, 393, 398, 409
Uterus 123, 124, 387

V

Valle de las Cuevas 12
Vanilla 413, 426
Vapor Rub 54
Varicose Veins 389, 411
Vatican 6, 379, 440
Ven a mi 201
Ventosa 152
Verbena 209, 219, 221, 330, 401, 413

Vervain 219, 221, 330, 413
Vinegar 54, 113
Violet 54, 61, 144, 414
Violeta 144, 414
Virgen de Dolores 51
Virgen de Guadalupe 9, 32, 48, 51, 77, 145, 157, 166, 167, 203, 220, 253, 317, 318, 319, 330, 331, 336
Virgen de la Candelaria 62
Virgen de la Regla 62
Virgen del Carmen 50, 62
Virgen del Chorrito 78
Virgen de los Remedios 51
Virgen de Salud 51
Virgen de San Juan de Los Lagos 78
Virgen de San Juan del Valle 76
Virgin of Pain 51
Virgin of Remedies 51
Vitamin 115, 118
Volcanic 54
Volcánico 91
Votive Candle 3, 9, 29, 217, 218, 275

W

Walnut 414, 432
Warts 387, 390, 393, 413
Watercress 414
Water retention 393, 397, 407, 411, 412
Weight loss 388, 390
Western Mugwort 414
Wheat seed 166, 287, 324
Willow xxi, 82, 83, 115, 394, 414, 415
Witch v, 136, 172, 173, 175, 204, 272, 275, 276, 280, 283, 294, 295, 304, 312, 415

Witchcraft 2, 4, 14, 26, 34, 41, 65, 90, 98, 123, 127, 130, 136, 140, 147, 153, 165, 172, 173, 176, 177, 178, 191, 200, 201, 202, 204, 205, 218, 219, 232, 251, 255, 262, 263, 264, 265, 270, 275, 276, 277, 280, 281, 282, 283, 284, 287, 289, 290, 292, 294, 295, 299, 306, 307, 308, 309, 311, 312, 315, 334, 379, 380
Wormseed 384, 415
Wormwood 416

Y

Yam bean 416
Yarrow 89, 91, 105, 106, 416
Yellow Wax Candle 209
Yerba Buena 219, 410
Yerba del Golpe 395
Yerba del pasmo 123, 394
Yerba del Pollo 402
Yerba del Sapo 389
Yerba Mansa 394, 411
Yerba Maté 411

Z

Zacate de Limón 91, 96, 103, 133, 163, 400
zarzamora 121
Zarzamora 387
Zarzaparrilla 409

Made in the USA
Lexington, KY
27 March 2015